Basic Epidemiological Methods and Biostatistics

The Jones and Bartlett Series in Health Science and Physical Education

AIDS Smartbook, Kopec

Anatomy and Physiology: An Easy Learner, Sloane

Aquatic Exercise, Sova

Aquatics: The Complete Reference Guide for Aquatic Fitness Professionals, Sova

Aquatics Activities Handbook, Sova

An Athlete's Guide to Agents, Ruxin

Basic Epidemiological Methods and Biostatistics, Page, et al.

Basic Law for the Allied Health Professions, Second Edition, Cowdrey/Drew

The Biology of AIDS, Third Edition, Fan, et al.

Bloodborne Pathogens, National Safety Council

A Challenge for Living: Dying, Death, and Bereavement, Corless, et al.

CPR Manual, National Safety Council

Dawn Brown's Complete Guide to Step Aerobics, Brown

Drugs and Society, Fourth Edition, Hanson/Venturelli

Drug Use in America, Venturelli

Dying, Death, and Bereavement: Theoretical Perspectives and Other Ways of Knowing, Corless, et al.

Emergency Encounters: EMTs and Their Work, Mannon

Essential Medical Terminology, Stanfield

Ethics Consultation: A Practical Guide, La Puma/Schiedermayer

First Aid, National Safety Council

First Aid and CPR, Second Edition, National Safety Council

First Aid and CPR, Infants and Children, National Safety Counicl

Fitness and Health: Life-Style Strategies, Thygerson

Fostering Emotional Well-Being in the Classroom, Page/Page

Golf: Your Turn for Success, Fisher/Geertsen

Grant Application Writer's Handbook, Reif-Lehrer

Health and Wellness, Fourth Edition, Edlin/Golanty

Health Eucation: Creating Strategies for School and Community Health, Gilbert/Sawyer

Healthy Children 2000, U.S. Department of Health and Human Services

Healthy People 2000, U.S. Department of Health and Human Services

Healthy People 2000–Summary Report, U.S. Department of Health and Human Services

Human Aging and Chronic Disease, Kart, et al.

Human Anatomy and Physiology Coloring Workbook and Study Guide, Anderson

An Introduction to Epidemiology, Timmreck

Introduction to Human Disease, Third Edition, Crowley

Introduction to the Health Professions, Second Edition, Stanfield/Hui

Managing Stress: Principles and Strategies for Health and Wellbeing, Seaward

Medical Terminology, Second Edition, Stanfield/Hui

Medical Terminology with Vikki Wetle, RN, MA, Video Series, Wetle

National Pool and Waterpark Lifeguard/CPR Training, Ellis & Associates

The Nation's Health, Fourth Edition, Lee/Estes

Omaha Orange: A Popular History of EMS in America, Post

Oxygen Administration, National Safety Council

Planning, Program Development, and Evaluation: A Handbook for Health Promotion, Aging, and Health Services, Timmreck

Perspectives on Death and Dying, Fulton/Metress

Primeros Auxilios y RCP, National Safety Council

Safety, Second Edition, Thygerson

Skill-Building Activities for Alcohol and Drug Education, Bates/Wigtil

Sports Equipment Management, Walker/Seidler

Sports Injury Care, Abdenour/Thygerson

Statistics: An Interactive Text for the Health and Life Sciences, Krishnamurty et al.

Stress Management, National Safety Council

Teaching Elementary Health Science, Third Edition, Bender/Sorochan

Weight Training for Strength and Fitness, Silvester

Basic Epidemiological Methods and Biostatistics

A Practical Guidebook

Randy M. Page

University of Idaho
Moscow, Idaho

Galen E. Cole

Centers for Disease Control and Prevention
Atlanta, Georgia

Thomas C. Timmreck

California State University
San Bernardino, California

JONES AND BARTLETT PUBLISHERS

Sudbury, Massachusetts

BOSTON TORONTO LONDON SINGAPORE

World Headquarters
Jones and Bartlett Publishers
40 Tall Pine Drive
Sudbury, MA 01776
978-443-5000
info@jbpub.com
www.jbpub.com

Jones and Bartlett Publishers Canada
2406 Nikanna Road
Mississauga, ON L5C 2W6
CANADA

Jones and Bartlett Publishers International
Barb House, Barb Mews
London W6 7PA
UK

Portions of this book first appeared in *Basic Epidemiology Methods and Biostatistics: A Workbook* by Cecil Slome, et al., © 1986 by Jones and Bartlett Publishers.

Library of Congress Cataloging-in-Publication Data

Page, Randy M.
Basic epidemiological methods and biostatistics : a practical guidebook / Randy M. Page, Galen E. Cole, Thomas C. Timmreck.
p. cm.
Includes bibliographical references and index.
ISBN 0-86720-869-4
1. Epidemiology—Statistical methods. 2. Epidemiology—Research. 3. Biometry. 4. Epidemiology—Problems, exercises, etc. I. Cole, Galen E. II. Timmreck, Thomas C. III. Title.
[DNLM: 1. Epidemiologic Methods—programmed instruction. 2. Biometry—programmed instruction. 3. Research Design—programmed instruction. WA 18 P133b 1995]
RA652.2.M3P34 1995
614.4′072--dc20
DNLM/DLC
for Library of Congress 94-22670
CIP

Acquisitions Editor: Joseph E. Burns
Production Editor: Judy Songdahl
Manufacturing Buyer: Dana L. Cerrito
Design: Katherine Harvey
Editorial Production Service: Ocean Publication Services
Typesetting: Camden Type 'n Graphics
Cover Design: Marshall Henrichs
Printing and Binding: D. B. Hess
Cover Printing: New England Book Components

Printed in the United States of America

02 01 10 9 8 7 6 5 4

Contents

Preface

In our analysis of introductory epidemiology courses, we have learned that there is no such thing as a "typical" epidemiology course, epidemiology instructor, or student of epidemiology. Instructors of introductory epidemiology courses differ widely in educational and professional background, in their approaches to teaching epidemiology concepts, and even in the subject matter that they present. Students in epidemiology courses come from a wide range of health science program areas—schools of public health, school and community health education programs, and schools of pharmacy, medicine, nursing, dentistry, and allied medicine. Epidemiology courses are also offered in graduate and professional schools, universities, four-year colleges, and community colleges. Keeping all of these variables in mind, we prepared an easy-to-understand, application-oriented guidebook for learning the basic principles of epidemiologic investigation that is suitable for the diverse groups of students who take epidemiology courses.

This book will guide you in learning the basic concepts and principles of epidemiology and biostatistics. Special emphasis has been placed upon application of the epidemiologic concepts that are presented. Throughout the text, you are given numerous opportunities to apply and test your learning through problems and application exercises. Answers to problems are provided to check for learning and mastery. The last chapter of the book—Chapter 10—is devoted entirely to evaluating understanding. Even students with a limited background in mathematics or statistics can master the problems that we present—only a basic calculator is necessary.

To enhance your learning, we placed key terms in bold-faced print and listed them in the order in which they appear in the text at the end of each chapter. Key terms are defined in the glossary for ease of reference, and chapter objectives, summaries, and review questions are included to guide your learning. Appendix B contains a listing of epidemiology and biostatistics resource books for student reference and further reading. We include several examples of current epidemiologic studies to give you a fresh sense of how epidemiologic methods are used in addressing current health problems.

We have enhanced this text by including material from the Centers for Disease Control and Prevention's *Principles of Epidemiology: An Introduction to Applied Epidemiology and Biostatistics, Self-Study Course Manual.* The chapters on organizing epidemiologic data and investigating an outbreak are from this manual. We have also used some material from this manual in our discussion of basic epidemiologic concepts, historical overview, and rates. Some of the problems at the end of chapters were adapted from this manual.

Some additional key features of this book include:

- numerous problems for student practice and application
- examples of key principles
- historical overview of epidemiology
- description of the uses of epidemiology in community and public health practice
- an emphasis on the role of behavioral epidemiology in disease prevention and health promotion
- use of current epidemiologic studies as illustrations of epidemiologic principles
- an entire section on the Behavioral Risk Factor Surveillance System
- discussion of computer resources for analysis of epidemiologic data
- entire chapters devoted to:

  epidemiologic rates and rate adjustment
  thinking through a study
  organizing epidemiologic data
  investigating outbreaks
  avoiding pitfalls in conducting epidemiologic research

Acknowledgments

This book is an outgrowth of an earlier work by Cecil Slome, Donna Brogan, Sandra Eyres, and Wayne Lednar, entitled *Basic Epidemiological Methods and Biostatistics: A Workbook*. We appreciate their ability to take complex concepts and make them highly understandable and relevant for the beginning epidemiologist. Following their example, our goal in this new work is to make the sometimes difficult-to-master concepts of epidemiologic study highly palatable, interesting, and understandable.

We are especially grateful for the efforts of Joseph Burns, our senior editor, who encouraged and guided us through the lengthy process of preparing this manuscript. We appreciate his devotion to quality and to this book.

This book is also a product of quality reviews provided by Steve Dorman, University of Florida; Gail Frank, California State University Long Beach; John Morgan, Loma Linda University; William Oleckno, Northern Illinois University; Paul Sarvela, Southern Illinois University at Carbondale; Alex Taylor, Department of Health, San Bernardino; and Elena Yu, San Diego State University. We appreciate their service; their comments were especially important in crafting this work.

This book would not have been possible without the support of our families and children. For their patience and assistance we are grateful.

Lastly, we acknowledge those to whom this book was written—the readers. As students of epidemiology we hope that the pages that lie before you will help you develop an appreciation for epidemiology and the basic skills that will serve you in your health science career.

1 Introduction to Epidemiology

OBJECTIVES

On completion of this chapter, you will be able to:

- Define epidemiology
- Explain why epidemiology is the basic science of community and public health and its uses
- Define behavioral epidemiology
- Describe significant historical events in the field of epidemiology
- Describe the uses of epidemiology in community health and individual decision-making
- Describe how host, agent, and environmental factors interact in causing various diseases and health conditions and how an understanding of these factors can lead to effective prevention and control measures
- Describe the various stages of the natural history of disease and elements comprising the chain of infection
- Describe common source, propagated, and mixed epidemic patterns of disease
- Identify the functions of epidemiology in promoting public health
- Explain the importance of descriptive epidemiology

What is epidemiology?

Epidemiology is the study of the distribution and determinants of health events in human populations. Epidemiology also includes the application of this study to the control of health problems (Last, 1988). For this reason, epidemiology is often referred to as the basic science of public health. Epidemiology uses biostatistical tools and methods to quantify the distribution and determinants of health events in groups of people rather than individuals.

Epidemiologic tools or methods are used to describe many types of health events. Originally, epidemiology was concerned with epidemics of communicable diseases. More recently, epidemiologic methods have been applied to chronic diseases (Brownson, Remington, and Davis, 1993), injuries, violence, birth defects, maternal–child health, occupational health, and environmental health (Green, 1990).

What is behavioral epidemiology?

Increasingly, behaviors related to health and well-being (amount of exercise, seat-belt use, etc.) are recognized as valid subjects for applying epidemiologic methods (Centers for Disease Control and Prevention, 1992). This application of epidemiology is known as **behavioral epidemiology.** Thus, health-related events include such occurrences as deaths, diseases, birth, utilization of health services, and behaviors that are related to health status (e.g., patterns of exercise, cigarette smoking).

Why is epidemiology known as the "basic science of public health"?

Epidemiology is known as the basic science of public and community health because it provides data for directing public health action. Epidemiologists use scientific methods in analyzing the health of communities. Such analyses can then be applied to planning the control and prevention of disease in communities. Epidemiology is the fundamental science underlying all aspects of public health—infectious disease, chronic disease, unintentional and intentional injuries, maternal and child health, family planning, mental health, nutrition, health education and promotion, health planning, health services administration, and medical care delivery.

Mausner and Kramer (1985, p. 1) discuss how the science of epidemiology serves as the foundation for public health prevention and control programs:

> . . . epidemiology is concerned with the *frequencies* and types of illnesses and injuries in *groups* of people and with the *factors* that influence their distribution. This implies that disease is not randomly distributed throughout a population, but rather that subgroups differ in the frequency of different diseases. Further, knowledge of this uneven distribution can be used to investigate causal factors and thus to lay the groundwork for programs of prevention and control.

What do epidemiologists do?

The range of activities that epidemiologists are involved with is very broad. The following list outlines these activities:

1. Collecting and analyzing vital records (i.e., births and deaths)
2. Collecting and analyzing morbidity data from hospitals, health agencies, clinics, physicians, and industry
3. Monitoring diseases or other community health problems
4. Investigating outbreaks leading to control or prevention of epidemics and other community health problems
5. Designing and implementing research studies and health surveys
6. Designing and implementing health registries for problems of interest such as birth defects, cancer incidence, or drug and medication use
7. Screening for disease
8. Evaluating the effectiveness of existing or newly proposed treatment methods
9. Describing the clinical course as well as the natural history of disease
10. Identifying individuals or subgroups of the general population at increased risk of developing certain diseases
11. Identifying links in the etiology of disease
12. Identifying public health problems and measuring the extent of their distribution, frequency, or effect on the public's health
13. Evaluating health programs
14. Providing data necessary for health planning or decision making by health agency administrators or health policy makers

HISTORICAL OVERVIEW

The First Epidemiologists

Hippocrates

Hippocrates, who lived from 460 B.C. to 377 B.C., is often credited with being the "first epidemiologist" because he attempted to explain disease occurrence on a rational basis instead of from a supernatural viewpoint. His observations and explanations of disease occurrence are included in three of his books: *Epidemic I, Epidemic II,* and *On Airs, Waters, and Places*. Lacking sophisticated epidemiological methodology, Hippocrates recognized the association of various diseases with such factors as place (geography), water conditions, climate, eating habits, and housing (Fox, Hall, and Elveback, 1970). The following excerpt from

On Airs, Waters, and Places, demonstrates his intuitive understanding of the possible relationship between these factors and disease frequency:

> Whoever wishes to investigate medicine properly should proceed thus: in the first place to consider the seasons of the year, and what effects each of them produces. Then the winds, the hot and the cold, especially such as are common to all countries, and then such as are peculiar to each locality. In the same manner, when one comes into a city to which he is a stranger, he should consider most attentively the waters which the inhabitants use, whether they be marshy and soft, or hard and running from elevated and rocky situations, and then if saltish and unfit for cooking; and the ground, whether it be naked and deficient in water, or wooded and well watered, and whether it lies in a hollow, confined situation, or is elevated and cold; and the mode in which the inhabitants live, and what are their pursuits, whether they are fond of drinking and eating to excess, and given to indolence, or are fond of exercise and labor.[1]

Hippocrates introduced the terms "epidemic" and "endemic," terms still used in modern epidemiologic practice. Furthermore, his theory about the causes of disease dominated medical opinion for more than 2,000 years. Hippocrates' theory evolved from his personal observations and was heavily influenced by Greek thinking. Postulating that the body was composed of four humors (phlegm, blood, yellow bile, black bile), Hippocrates believed that disease was the result of imbalances in humors in the body. Treatment of disease was based upon means believed to restore humoral balance—this explains the use of blood-letting as a medical treatment of "blood diseases" or the use of enemas to treat "black bile diseases."

A major tenet of his theory of disease causation was that "constitution" had a major influence on the balance of humors in the body. "Constitution" referred to the geography, climate, foods of a particular area, and the movements of the stars and planets, especially meteors and comets.

Galen

Galen (129-199 A.D.), a surgeon in the Roman army and often regarded as the "father of experimental physiology," elaborated on Hippocrates' theory. In addition to the "constitution," Galen asserted that "procatartic factors" and "temperament" influenced health and disease. Galen defined "procatartic factors" as the way of life a person led. "Temperament" was believed to be the innate qualities of the body—tendencies to have more or less of one or more humors. Various temperaments were not only associated with a particular disease vulnerability but also with a particular

---

[1]*On Airs, Waters, and Places* was translated and republished in 1938 in *Medical Classics* 3:19-42.

personality type (Duncan, 1988). Thus was borne the notion that lifestyle factors and personality can influence health and disease (Fox, Hall, and Elveback, 1970).

Galen was instrumental in shifting Hippocrates' emphasis on "constitution" away from profound environmental influences such as geography and climate to "miasmas." **Miasma** is a general term for particles in the air. In fact, the term for the disease malaria literally means "bad air." Bad miasmas or vapors emanating from sources such as waste, stagnant water, or decaying animals were thought to cause disease. Miasma theory persisted for centuries. An example of miasma theory can be taken from the great plague epidemics in Europe. A commonly used preventive action was the mass killing of dogs and cats because it was believed that their bad breath was responsible for the plague. Unfortunately, this action compounded the problem since these animals were helpful in controlling the population of rats that carried plague-infested fleas. On the other hand, good smells were believed to drive plague away. Thus, perfumes and flowers were used for this purpose. The popular children's rhyme shows that the miasma theory of plague was dominant: "Ring around the rosies, Pocket full of posies, Ashes, Ashes, They all fall down." The good smell from a pocket full of posies was believed to keep away plague. Yet it was common for those who fell down and died with plague to have had a pocket full of posies—but to no avail.

Thomas Sydenham

Some consider Thomas Sydenham (1624-1689) to be the "English Hippocrates" because he revived the

> Hippocratic idea of epidemic constitutions and industriously studied variations in epidemics of different diseases with respect to season, year, and age of sufferer. In particular, he was insistent that observation should have precedence over theory in the study of the natural history of disease (Fox et al., 1970, p. 21).

For this reason Sydenham is often referred to as the "father of epidemiology," despite the fact that his conclusions contributed little to true understanding of disease causes. Fox et al. (1970, p. 21) commented that "Apparently he [Sydenham] considered that undefined atmospheric changes resulted in 'epidemic constitutions' which, by grafting themselves onto any existing illness, gave to all concurrent illness a common character determined by the particular 'constitution'."

Noah Webster

Noah Webster (1758-1843), the compiler of the first American dictionary, was a very important American epidemiologist. After studying influenza, yellow fever, and scarlet fever epidemics, he noted that epidemics were related to certain environmental factors that combined to affect large numbers of people within the same time period. He published his results and conclusions in a book entitled *Epidemic and Pestilential Diseases.*

The Concept of Contagion and Germ Theory of Disease

Hieronymous Fracastorius

The notion that disease could be caused by germs was largely popularized by an Italian poet and physician, Hieronymous Fracastorius (1478-1553). His belief that disease was transmitted from one person to another by particles too small to be seen was put forth in his book *Des Res Contagiosa.* Calling this transmission process "contagion," he hypothesized that minute particles could be spread by close personal contact and conveyed person-to-person by "fomes" or inanimate objects (Duncan, 1988). Fracastorius is best known for his epic poem about two lovers, entitled *Syphilidis, sive Morbi Gallici,* which translates as Syphilis, the "French Disease."

Fox et al. (1970, p. 21) comment on the historical impact of Fracastorius' concept of contagion:

> Although this concept was respected enough in his time that he prevailed upon Pope Paul III to transfer the Council of Trent to Bologna because of the prevalence of a contagious disease in Trent, this work and its vitally important concept were virtually forgotten for the next two hundred years. While Fracastorius must be credited with the first formal expression of contagion, the idea had long been implicit in the attitudes towards sufferers from at least one dread disease, leprosy. Ramses II and Moses were among the early lepraphobes and, by 1200 A.D., the Christian church was sanctioning such practices as the conduct of antemortem funeral services for the leper who was then provided with his bell and cup and prohibited from further contact with his fellow man or who, in more extreme circumstances, might actually be burned alive or burned at the stake.

Igmatz Semmelweis

A Hungarian obstetrician, Igmatz Semmelweis (1818-1865) was instrumental in demonstrating that puerperal fever, commonly referred to as "child-bed fever," could be reduced when physicians washed their hands before delivering a baby. Duncan (1988, pp. 21-22) explains how Semmelweis' contribution was regarded:

> This great contribution resulted in Semmelweis being suspended from his position for 6 months and subsequently being subjected to a variety of harassments. He left Vienna abruptly and returned to his home in Budapest, where he became head of the maternity hospital and wrote a book on his findings on puerperal fever. His theory was regarded by many of his colleagues as evidence of insanity. Eventually, he was sent back to Vienna as a mental patient. When examined at the mental hospital, it was discovered that he had a cut on his finger that had

> probably resulted during one of his last operations. He died of the fever he had first recognized as being the same thing as puerperal fever. Unlike Fracastorius, Semmelweis' ideas did live on after him, although acceptance was slow.

Edward Jenner

The discovery of the microscope several years after the death of Fracastorius made it possible for scientists to view the microorganisms that Fracastorius had theorized to exist. Several other significant events led to greater acceptance for a "germ theory of disease." Edward Jenner experimented with inoculating healthy people with a formulation of material taken from cowpox lesions (a related but less serious infection than smallpox). His work led to the discovery of an effective smallpox vaccination in the late 1700s (Winklestein, 1992).

Louis Pasteur

A major event that advanced the emergence of the germ theory of disease occurred when Louis Pasteur demonstrated effective immunization to prevent rabies in 1885. The demonstration was made despite Pasteur's being unable to isolate the rabies virus. This event did much to dispel miasma theory.

Birth of Vital Statistics

John Graunt

An important early contributor to epidemiology was John Graunt, a London haberdasher who published a landmark analysis of mortality data in 1662. He was the first to quantify patterns of birth, death, and disease occurrence, noting male-female disparities, high infant mortality, urban–rural differences, and seasonal variations (CDC, 1992).

William Farr

No one built upon Graunt's work until the mid-1800s, when William Farr began to systematically collect and analyze Britain's mortality statistics. Farr, considered the father of modern vital statistics and surveillance, developed many basic practices used today in vital statistics and disease classifications. He extended the epidemiologic analysis of morbidity and mortality data, looking at the effects of marital status, occupation, and altitude. He also developed many epidemiologic concepts and techniques still in use today (CDC, 1992).

Early Classic Epidemiologic Studies

James Lind

James Lind conducted an experimental epidemiologic study of the etiology and treatment of scurvy. Here is his description of this experiment (1753) in his own words, as cited in Lilienfeld and Lilienfeld (1980, pp. 30-31):

> On the 20th of May, 1747, I took twelve patients in the scurvy, on board the SALISBURY at sea. Their cases were as similar as I could have them. They all in general had putrid gums, the spots and lassitudes, with weakness of their knees. They lay together in one place, being a proper apartment for the sick in the fore-hold; and had one diet common to all, viz., water-gruel sweetened with sugar in the morning; fresh mutton broth often times for dinner; at other times puddings, boiled biscuit with sugar, etc; and for supper, barley and raisins, rice and currents, sago and wine, or the like. Two of these were ordered each a quart of cyder a day, upon an empty stomach; using a gargle strongly acidulated with it for their mouths. Two others took two spoonsful of vinegar three times a day, upon an empty stomach; having their gruels and their other food well acidulated with it, as also the gargle for their mouth. Two of the worst patients, with the tendons in the ham rigid (a symptom none of the rest had), were put under a course of sea water. Of this, they drank a half a pint every day, and sometimes more or less as it operated by way of a gentle physic. Two others had each two oranges and one lemon given them every day. These they eat with greediness, at different times, upon an empty stomach. They continued but six days under this course, having consumed the quantity that could be spared. The two remaining patients took the bigness of a nutmeg tree three times a day, of an electuary recommended by a hospital-surgeon, made of garlic, mustard seed, rad raphan, balsam of Peru, and gum myrrh; using for common drink, barley-water well acidulated with tamarinds; by a decoction of which, with the addition of cremor tartar, they were gently purged three or four times during the course.
>
> The consequence was, that the most sudden and visible good effects were perceived from the use of the oranges and lemons; one of those who had taken them being at the end of six days fit for duty. The spots were not indeed at that time quite off his body, nor his gums sound; but without any other medicine, than a gargarism of elixir vitriol, he became quite healthy before we came into Plymouth, which was on the 16th of June. The other was the best recovered of any in his condition; and being now deemed pretty well, was appointed nurse to the rest of the sick.

Lind was able to conclude from the results of this experiment that eating citrus fruits successfully treated scurvy and that consuming these fruits would also prevent the occurrence of scurvy. Lind's epidemiologic work led the British navy to require that limes or lime juice be included in the diet of seamen since 1795, resulting in the nicknaming of British seamen as "limeys" (Lilienfeld and Lilienfeld, 1980).

P. L. Panum

P. L. Panum is acknowledged for his classic epidemiologic study of measles on the Faroe Islands. Lilienfeld and Lilienfeld (1980, pp. 39-40) relate the following account of the study:

> A cabinetmaker from Copenhagen landed in the Faroe Islands on March 28, 1846, and developed symptoms of measles early in April. The population of the Faroes at the time numbered 7864; 6100 came down

with measles between the end of April and October and 170 deaths occurred. The islanders had experienced measles in the past, but there had been no cases between 1781 and 1846.

The Danish government sent a twenty-six-year-old physician, P. L. Panum, to deal with the epidemic situation; to his observations, we owe much of our knowledge of measles. Panum personally visited fifty-two villages and made observations on several thousand cases of measles of which he personally treated 1000. He obtained information on "the circumstances and dates of their exposure to infection, the dates on which the exanthem [rash] appeared on them and the time that elapsed thereafter before other residents broke out with the exanthem." From these observations, he concluded that the period from exposure to development of the rash (the incubation period) is usually thirteen to fourteen days and that the patient is infectious at the time that the rash is breaking out, or had just broken out, and possibly for a few days prior to the eruption, although he was not certain about this. He did not find the disease to be transmissible during the period of desquamation (when the rash disappears with the shedding of the skin), which was the prevalent view of the time. From these observations on personal contacts, he concluded that measles can be transmitted only by direct contact between infected and susceptible individuals. It is not conveyed by miasma nor does it arise spontaneously, at least not in the Faroe Islands. He also suggested that one attack of measles conferred lifelong immunity, since none of the ninety-eight inhabitants who had had measles before 1781 developed the disease in 1846. His hypothesis was validated when the Faroes had another measles epidemic in 1875 and only persons under thirty years of age became ill.

John Snow

John Snow (1813-1858),[2] an anesthesiologist, conducted a series of investigations in London that later earned him the title "the father of field epidemiology." Twenty years before the discovery of the microscope, Snow conducted studies of cholera outbreaks to discover the cause of the disease and to prevent its recurrence. His work classically illustrates the sequence from descriptive epidemiology to hypothesis generation to hypothesis testing to public health application.

Snow conducted his study in 1854 when an epidemic of cholera developed in the Golden Square of London. He began his investigation by determining where in this area persons with cholera lived and worked. He then used this information to map the distribution of cases on what epidemiologists call a spot map. His map is shown in Figure 1.1.

Because Snow believed that water was a source of infection for cholera, he marked the location of water pumps on his spot map, and then looked for a relationship between the distribution of cholera case households and the location of pumps. He noticed that more case households

---

[2]Much of the remainder of this chapter is adapted from Centers for Disease Control and Prevention, *Principles of epidemiology: An introduction to applied epidemiology and biostatistics, 2d ed*. Atlanta, GA: Centers for Disease Control and Prevention, 1992.

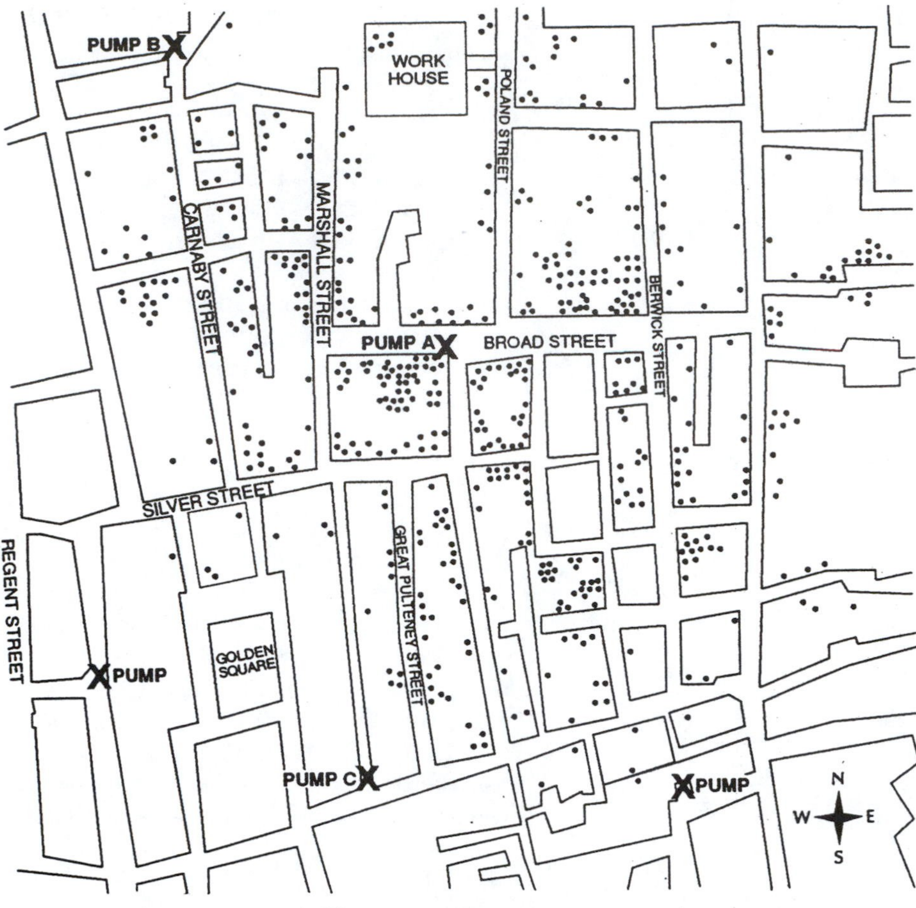

FIGURE 1.1 *Distribution of cholera cases in the Golden Square area of London, August–September 1854*

clustered around the Broad Street pump (Pump A) than around Pumps B or C, and he concluded that the Broad Street pump was the most likely source of infection. Questioning residents who lived near the other pumps, he found that they avoided Pump B because it was grossly contaminated, and that Pump C was located too inconveniently for most residents of the Golden Square area. From this information, it appeared to Snow that the Broad Street pump was probably the primary source of water for most persons with cholera in the Golden Square area. He realized, however, that it was too soon to draw that conclusion because the map showed no cholera cases in a two-block area to the east of the Broad Street pump. Perhaps no one lived in that area. Or perhaps the residents were somehow protected.

Upon investigating, Snow found that a brewery was located there and that it had a deep well on the premises where brewery workers, who also lived in the area, got their water. In addition, the brewery allotted workers a daily quota of malt liquor. Access to these uncontaminated rations could explain why none of the brewery's employees contracted cholera.

To confirm that the Broad Street pump was the source of the epidemic, Snow gathered information on where persons with cholera had obtained their water. Consumption of water from the Broad Street pump was the one common factor among cholera patients (Figure 1.2). According to legend, Snow removed the handle of that pump and aborted the outbreak.

Snow's second major contribution involved another investigation of the same outbreak of cholera that occurred in London in 1854. In a London epidemic in 1849, Snow had noted that districts with the highest mortalities had water supplied by two companies: the Lambeth Company and the Southwark and Vauxhall Company. At that time, both companies obtained water from the Thames River at intake points that were below London. In 1852, the Lambeth Company moved their water works to above London, thus obtaining water that was free of London sewage. When cholera returned to London in 1853, Snow realized the Lambeth Company's relocation of its intake point would allow him to compare districts that were supplied with water from above London with districts that received water from below London. Table 1.1 shows what Snow found when he made comparisons for cholera mortality over a 7-week period during the summer of 1854.

The data in Table 1.1 show that the risk of death from cholera was more than 5 times higher in districts served only by the Southwark and Vauxhall Company. Interestingly, the mortality rate in districts supplied by both companies falls between the rates for districts served exclusively by either company. These data were consistent with the hypothesis that water obtained from the Thames below London was a source of cholera. Alternatively, the populations supplied by the two companies may have differed in a number of other factors which affected their risk of cholera.

To test his water supply hypothesis, Snow focused on the districts served by both companies because the households within a district were generally comparable except for their water supply company. In these districts, Snow identified the water supply company for every house in which a death from cholera had occurred during the 7-week period. Table 1.2 shows his findings.

This additional study added support to Snow's hypothesis, and demonstrates the sequence of steps used today to investigate outbreaks of disease. Snow developed a testable hypothesis based on a characterization of the cases and population at risk by time, place, and person. He then tested this hypothesis with a more rigorously designed study, ensuring that the groups to be compared were comparable. After this study, efforts to control the epidemic were directed at changing the location of the water intake of the Southwark and Vauxhall Company to avoid sources of contamination. Thus, with no knowledge of the existence of microorganisms, Snow demonstrated through epidemiologic studies that water could serve as a vehicle for transmitting cholera and that epidemiologic information could be used to direct prompt and appropriate public health action.

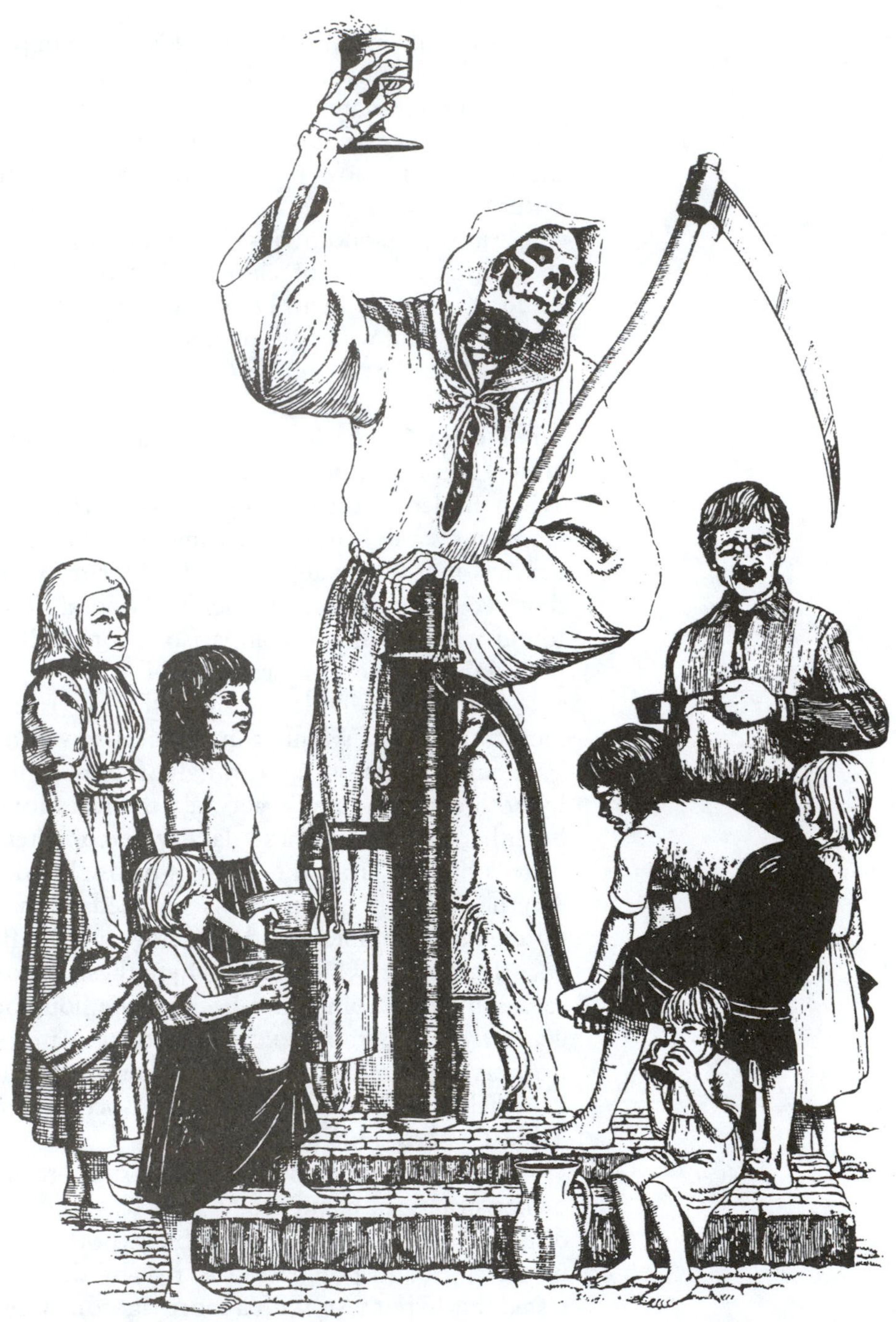

FIGURE 1.2 *Water contaminated with deadly cholera flowed from the Broad Street pump*

TABLE 1.1 Mortality from cholera in the districts of London supplied by the Southwark and Vauxhall Company and the Lambeth Company, July 9-August 26, 1854

Districts with water Supplied by	*Population (1851 Census)*	*Deaths from Cholera*	*Cholera Death Rate per 1,000 Population*
Southwark and Vauxhall Co. only	167,654	844	5.0
Lambeth Co. only	19,133	18	0.9
Both companies	300,149	652	2.2

SOURCE: Snow, 1936 as cited in CDC, 1992.

TABLE 1.2 Mortality from cholera in London related to the water supply of individual houses in districts served by both the Southwark and Vauxhall Company and the Lambeth Company, July 9-August 26, 1854

Water Supply of Individual House	*Population (1851 Census)*	*Deaths from Cholera*	*Death Rate per 1,000 Population*
Southwark and Vauxhall Co.	98,862	419	4.2
Lambeth Co.	154,615	80	0.5

SOURCE: Snow, 1936 as cited in CDC, 1992.

Joseph Goldberger

Joseph Goldberger and his associates (1923) conducted a classic epidemiologic investigation that led to a clear demonstration that pellagra is not an infectious disease, as was widely believed at the time. Goldberger's observation that nurses and attendants who had close contact with inmates in asylums did not develop pellagra led him to hypothesize that pellagra was related to diet rather than to infectious agents (MacMahon and Pugh, 1970). He experimentally proved in two orphanages and two wards of a state mental institution that by changes in diet pellagra could be induced as well as relieved. Pellagra was later determined to be the result of a dietary deficiency of nicotinic acid, a B-complex vitamin. You can read the account of this fascinating study in Goldberger's own words in *Public Health Reports,* 1923, Volume 38, pp. 2361-2368.

Modern Epidemiology

In the mid- and late-1800s, many others in Europe and the United States began to apply epidemiologic methods to investigate disease occurrence. At that time, most investigators focused on acute infectious diseases. In the 1900s, epidemiologists extended their methods to noninfectious diseases. A classic example of this is Golberger's work on pellagra—a disease generally believed in the early 1900s to be infectious. As discussed in the previous section, Goldberger and associates (1923) demonstrated through the use of both observational and experimental epidemiologic studies that pellagra resulted from a dietary deficiency of a vitamin. This vitamin was later determined to be nicotinic acid.

Since the Second World War an explosion has been seen in the development of research methods and the theoretical underpinnings of epidemiology, and the application of epidemiology to the entire range of health-related outcomes, behaviors, knowledge, and attitudes. The studies by Doll and Hill (1950) linking smoking to lung cancer and the study of cardiovascular disease among residents of Framingham, Massachusetts (Dawber, Kannel, and Lyell, 1963; Gordon, Castelli, Hjortland, Kannel, and Dawber, 1977), are two classic examples of how pioneering researchers have applied epidemiologic methods to chronic diseases since World War II. More recent examples include the Bogalusa Heart Study (Freedman, Chear, Srinivasan, Webber, and Berenson, 1985), Multiple Risk Factor Intervention Trial (Stamler, Wentworth, and Neaton, 1986), Stanford Heart Disease Prevention Trials (Farquhar, Fortmann, and Maccoby, 1985), Pawtucket Heart Health Program (Elder, McGraw, and Abrams, 1986), and North Karelia Study (McAlister, Puska, Salonen, Tuomilehto, and Koskela, 1982). During the 1960s and early 1970s health workers applied epidemiologic methods to eradicate smallpox worldwide. This was an achievement of unprecedented proportions for applied epidemiology.

Today, public health workers throughout the world accept and use epidemiology routinely. Epidemiology is often practiced or used by non-epidemiologists to characterize the health of their communities and to solve day-to-day problems. This landmark in the evolution of the discipline is less dramatic than the eradication of smallpox, but is no less important in improving the health of people everywhere.

USES OF EPIDEMIOLOGY

Epidemiology and the information generated by epidemiologic methods have many uses.[3] These are categorized and described below.

Population or Community Health Assessment

To set policy and plan programs, public health officials must assess the health of the population or community they serve and must determine whether health services are available, accessible, effective, and efficient. To do this, they must find answers to many questions: What are the actual and potential health problems in the community? Where are these problems? Who is at risk? Which problems are declining over time? Which ones are increasing or have the potential to increase? How do these patterns relate to the level and distribution of services available? The methods of epidemiology provide ways to answer these and other questions. With

[3]Adapted from Centers for Disease Control and Prevention, *Principles of epidemiology: An introduction to applied epidemiology and biostatistics, 2d ed.* Atlanta, GA: Centers for Disease Control and Prevention, 1992.

answers provided through the application of epidemiology, public health officials can make informed decisions that will lead to improved health for the populations they serve.

Individual Decisions

People may not realize that they use epidemiologic information in making their daily decisions. When they decide to stop smoking, take the stairs instead of the elevator, order a salad instead of a cheeseburger with french fries, or choose one method of contraception instead of another, they may be influenced consciously or unconsciously by epidemiologists' assessments of risk. Since World War II, epidemiologists have provided information related to all those decisions. In the 1950s epidemiologists documented the increased risk of lung cancer among smokers; in the 1960s and 1970s, epidemiologists noted a variety of benefits and risks associated with different methods of birth control; in the mid-1980s, epidemiologists identified the risk of human immunodeficiency virus (HIV) infection associated with certain sexual and drug-related behaviors; more positively, epidemiologists today continue to document the role of exercise and proper diet in reducing the risk of heart disease. These and hundreds of other epidemiologic findings are directly relevant to the choices that affect people's health over a lifetime.

Completing the Clinical Picture

When studying a disease outbreak, epidemiologists depend on clinical physicians and laboratory scientists for proper diagnosis of individual patients. But epidemiologists also contribute to physicians' understanding of the clinical picture and natural history of disease. For example, in late 1989 three patients in New Mexico were diagnosed as having myalgias (severe muscle pains in the chest or abdomen) and unexplained eosinophilia (an increase in the number of one type of white blood cell). Their physician could not identify the cause of their symptoms, or put a name to the disorder. Epidemiologists began looking for other cases with similar symptoms, and within weeks had found enough additional cases of eosinophilia–myalgia syndrome to describe the illness, its complications, and its rate of mortality. Similarly, epidemiologists have documented the course of HIV infection from the initial exposure to the development of a wide variety of clinical syndromes that include acquired immunodeficiency syndrome (AIDS). They have also documented numerous conditions associated with cigarette smoking—from pulmonary and heart disease to lung and cervical cancer.

Search for Causes

Much of epidemiologic research is devoted to a search for causes, factors which influence one's risk of disease. Sometimes this is an academic pursuit, but more often the goal is to identify a cause so that appropriate public health action can be taken. It has been said that epidemiology can never prove a causal relationship between an exposure and a disease. Nevertheless, epidemiology often provides enough information to support effective action. An example of this is the withdrawal of a specific brand of tampon that was linked by epidemiologists to toxic shock syndrome.[4] Frequently, epidemiology and laboratory science converge to provide the evidence needed to establish causation. For example, a team of epidemiologists was able to identify a variety of risk factors during an outbreak of pneumonia among persons attending the American Legion Convention in Philadelphia in 1976, but the outbreak was not "solved" until the Legionnaires' bacillus was identified in the laboratory almost 6 months later.

PROBLEM

In the early 1980s, epidemiologists recognized that AIDS occurred most frequently among men who had sex with men and among intravenous drug users. How can this information be used for population or community health assessment, individual decisions, and search for causes?

SOLUTION

Population or community health assessment. Two high-risk behaviors have been identified. If either of these behaviors is common in the community, public health officials can expect a substantial number of AIDS cases over time. Therefore, public health officials need to ask, How common are these behaviors in our community? (Another way of phrasing this question is, How large are the groups of persons in our community who engage in these behaviors?) Where are they located? What types of public health programs might be most effective in reaching these groups? Answers to these questions should help officials develop appropriate policies and programs.

Individual decisions. The individual can use this information to make choices regarding sexual behavior and the use of intravenous drugs. For example, the findings might convince someone who occasionally uses intravenous drugs to stop.

Search for causes. Research asks, What specifically about these behaviors might be associated with disease? Are people who more frequently engage in these behaviors at greater risk of the disease? What other risk factors can we identify? What common pathway might there be? Could AIDS be caused by some toxic agent (chemical) used by both groups? Could it be caused by an infectious agent transmitted by exchange of blood, like hepatitis B? Could it be caused by sheer immunologic overload? By addressing these questions and hypotheses with epidemiologic and laboratory methods, researchers identified the mode of transmission (and prevention strategies) and, eventually, the causative virus.

---

[4]Rely (brand) tampons, which consisted of polyester foam and cross-linked carboxymethylcellulose, were withdrawn from the market in 1980 by the Procter and Gamble Company. In 1985 tampons containing polyacrylate were withdrawn. Tampons currently on the market are made of cotton and/or rayon (Schuchat and Broome, 1991).

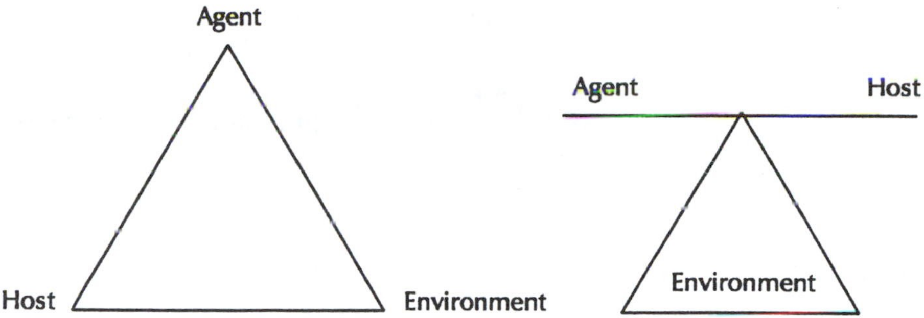

FIGURE 1.3 *Epidemiologic triangle and triad (balance beam)*

THE EPIDEMIOLOGIC TRIAD

Epidemiologic methods are used to search for causes of disease. A variety of models of disease causation have been proposed. The traditional model of infectious disease causation is the **epidemiologic triangle** or **triad.** It has three components: an external agent, a susceptible host, and an environment that brings the host and the agent together. In this model, the environment influences the agent, the host, and the route of transmission of the agent from a source to the host. Figure 1.3 shows two versions of this model in diagram form.

Agent Factors

Agent originally referred to an infectious microorganism—a bacterium, virus, parasite, or other microbe. Generally, these agents must be present for disease to occur. That is, they are necessary but not always sufficient to cause disease.

Does the concept of agent have applicability beyond infectious diseases?

As epidemiology has been applied to noninfectious conditions, the concept of agent in this model has been broadened to include chemical and physical causes of disease. These include chemical contaminants, such as the L-tryptophan contaminant responsible for eosinophilia–myalgia syndrome, and physical forces such as repetitive mechanical forces associated with carpal tunnel syndrome. For some noninfectious diseases the epidemiologic triangle does not work well because it is not always clear whether a particular factor should be classified as an agent or as an environmental factor.

Host Factors

Host factors are intrinsic factors that influence an individual's exposure, susceptibility, or response to a causative agent. Age, race, sex, socioeconomic status, and behaviors (smoking, drug abuse, lifestyle, sexual practices and contraception, and eating habits) are some of the many host factors that affect a person's likelihood of exposure. Age, genetic composition, nutritional and immunologic status, anatomic structure, presence of disease or medications, and psychological makeup are some of the host factors that affect a person's susceptibility and response to an agent.

Environmental Factors

Environmental factors are extrinsic factors that affect the agent and the opportunity for exposure. Generally, environmental factors include physical factors such as geology, climate, and physical surroundings (e.g., a nursing home, hospital); biologic factors such as insects that transmit the agent; and socioeconomic factors such as crowding, sanitation, and the availability of health services.

Agent, host, and environmental factors interrelate in a variety of complex ways to produce disease in humans. Their balance and interactions are different for different diseases. When we search for causal relationships, we must look at all three components and analyze their interactions to find practical and effective prevention and control measures.

KEY CONCEPTS IN EPIDEMIOLOGY

Although epidemiologic methods can be applied to all types of disease, injury, and health conditions, the chain of infection for infectious diseases is better understood. In addition, infectious diseases remain an important focus of state and local public health department activities. Therefore, a description of some of the key concepts of infectious disease epidemiology are presented below. These concepts are rooted in infectious disease, but are also relevant to noninfectious diseases.

Natural History and Spectrum of Disease

Natural history of disease refers to the progress of a disease process in an individual over time, without intervention. The process begins with exposure to or accumulation of factors capable of causing disease. Without medical intervention, the process ends with recovery, disability, or death. The stages in the natural history of disease are shown in Figure 1.4. Most diseases have a characteristic natural history (poorly understood for many diseases) although the time frame and specific manifestation of disease may vary from person to person. With a particular individual, the usual course of a disease may be halted at any point in the progression by preventive and therapeutic measures, host factors, and other influences.

As shown in Figure 1.4, the natural history begins with the appropriate exposure to or accumulation of factors sufficient to begin the disease process in a susceptible host. For infectious disease, the exposure usually

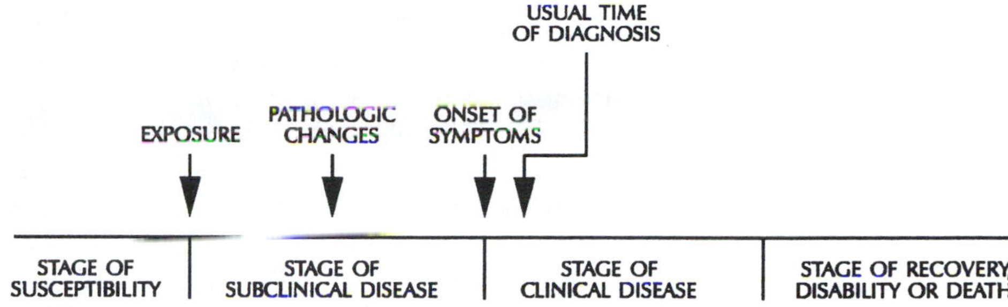

FIGURE 1.4 *Natural history of disease*

is a microorganism. For cancers, the critical factors may require both cancer initiators, such as asbestos fibers or components in tobacco smoke (for lung cancer), and cancer promoters, such as estrogens (for endometrial cancer).

Usually a period of subclinical or inapparent pathologic changes follows exposure, ending with the onset of symptoms. For infectious diseases, this period is usually called the **incubation period;** for chronic diseases, this period is usually called the **latency period.** This period may be as brief as seconds for hypersensitivity and toxic reactions or as long as decades for certain chronic diseases. Even for a single disease, the characteristic incubation period has a range. For example, for hepatitis A, the range is about 2 to 6 weeks. For leukemia associated with exposure to the atomic bomb blast in Hiroshima the range was 2 to 12 years, with a peak at 6 to 7 years. Although disease is inapparent during the incubation period, some pathologic changes may be detectable with laboratory, radiographic, or other screening methods. Most screening programs attempt to identify the disease process during this phase of its natural history, since early intervention may be more effective than treatment at a later stage of disease progression.

The onset of symptoms marks the transition from subclinical to clinical disease. Most diagnoses are made during the stage of clinical disease. In some people, however, the disease process may never progress to clinically apparent illness. In others, the disease process may result in a wide spectrum of clinical illness, ranging from mild to severe or fatal.

Three terms are used to describe an infectious disease according to the various outcomes that may occur after exposure to its causative agent.

- **Infectivity**—the proportion of exposed persons who become infected
- **Pathogenicity**—the proportion of infected persons who develop clinical disease
- **Virulence**—the proportion of persons with clinical disease who become severely ill or die

For example, hepatitis A virus in children has low pathogenicity and low virulence since many infected children remain asymptomatic and few develop severe illness. In persons with good nutrition and health, measles virus has high pathogenicity but low virulence since almost all infected persons develop the characteristic rash illness but few develop the life-threatening presentations of measles—pneumonia or encephalitis. In persons with poorer nutrition and health, measles is a more virulent disease, with mortality as high as 5 to 10%. Finally, rabies virus is both highly pathogenic and virulent, since virtually 100% of all infected persons who do not receive treatment progress to clinical disease and death.

What challenges do the natural history and spectrum of disease present to public health workers and clinicians?

Because of the clinical spectrum, cases of illness diagnosed by clinicians in the community often represent only the "tip of the iceberg." Many additional cases may be too early to diagnose or may remain asymptomatic. For the public health worker, the challenge is that persons with inapparent or undiagnosed infections may nonetheless be able to transmit them to others. Such persons who are infectious but have subclinical disease are called **carriers.** Frequently, carriers are persons with incubating disease or inapparent infection. Persons with measles, hepatitis A, and several other diseases become infectious a few days before the onset of symptoms. On the other hand, carriers may also be persons who appear to have recovered from their clinical illness, such as chronic carriers of hepatitis B virus.

Chain of Infection

As described earlier, the traditional model of disease causation (epidemiologic triangle) illustrates that infectious diseases result from the interaction of agent, host, and environment. More specifically, transmission occurs when the agent leaves its **reservoir** or host through a **portal of exit,** and is conveyed by some **mode of transmission,** and enters through an appropriate **portal of entry** to infect a susceptible **host.** This is sometimes called the **chain of infection** and is illustrated in Figure 1.5.

Reservoir

The **reservoir** of an agent is the habitat in which an infectious agent usually lives, grows, and multiplies. Reservoirs include humans, animals, and the environment. The reservoir may or may not be the source from which an agent is transferred to a host. For example, the reservoir of *Clostridium botulinum* is soil, but the source of most botulism infections is improperly canned food containing *C. botulinum* spores.

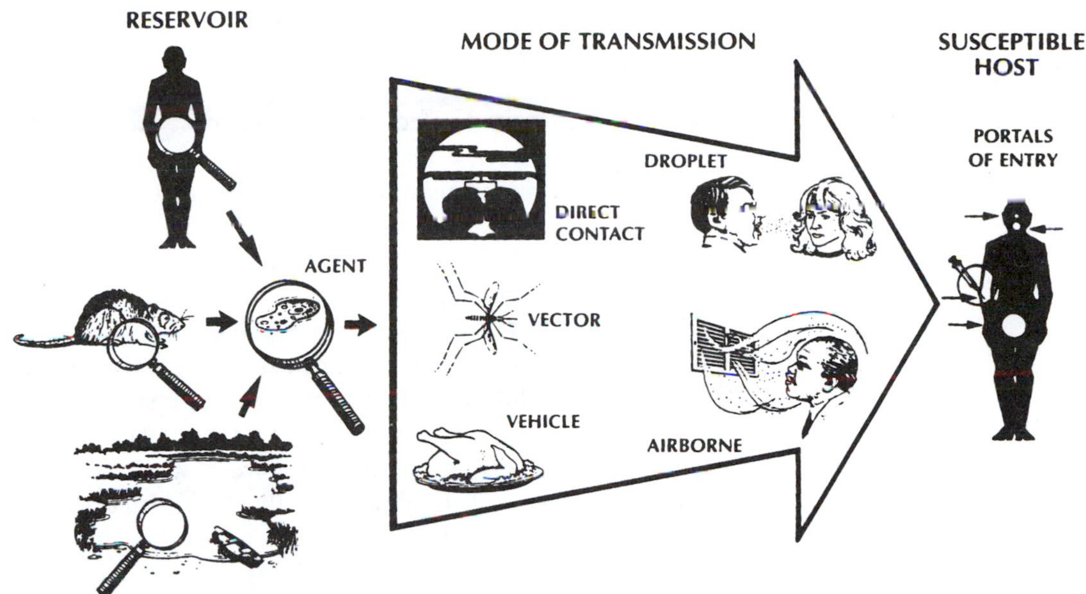

FIGURE 1.5 *Chain of infection*

Human Reservoirs. Many of the common infectious diseases have human reservoirs. Diseases which are transmitted from person to person without intermediaries include sexually transmitted diseases, measles, mumps, streptococcal infection, most respiratory pathogens, and many others. Smallpox was eradicated after the last human case was identified and isolated because humans were the only reservoir for the smallpox virus. Two types of human reservoirs exist:

- persons with asymptomatic disease
- carriers

What is a carrier and what are the different types of carriers?

A **carrier** is a person without apparent disease who is nonetheless capable of transmitting the agent to others. Carriers may be **asymptomatic carriers,** who never show symptoms during the time they are infected, or may be **incubatory** or **convalescent carriers,** who are capable of transmission before or after they are clinically ill. A **chronic carrier** is one who continues to harbor an agent (such as hepatitis B virus or *Salmonella typhi*—the agent of typhoid fever) for an extended time (months or years) following the initial infection. Carriers commonly transmit disease because they do not recognize they are infected and consequently take no special precautions to prevent transmission. Symptomatic persons, on the other hand, are usually less likely to transmit infection widely because their symptoms increase their likelihood of being diagnosed and treated, thereby reducing their opportunity for contact with others.

Animal Reservoirs. Infectious diseases that are transmissible under normal conditions from animals to humans are called **zoonoses.** In general, these diseases are transmitted from animal to animal, with humans as incidental hosts. Such diseases include brucellosis (cows and pigs), anthrax (sheep), plague (rodents), trichinosis (swine), and rabies (bats, raccoons, dogs, and other mammals).

Another group of diseases with animal reservoirs is that caused by viruses transmitted by insects and caused by parasites that have complex life cycles, with different reservoirs at different stages of development. Such diseases include St. Louis encephalitis and malaria (both requiring mosquitoes) and schistosomiasis (requiring fresh water snails). Lyme disease is a zoonotic disease of deer incidentally transmitted to humans by the deer tick.

Environmental Reservoirs. Plants, soil, and water in the environment are also reservoirs for some infectious agents. Many fungal agents, such as those causing histoplasmosis, live and multiply in the soil. The primary reservoir of Legionnaires' bacillus appears to be pools of water, including those produced by cooling towers and evaporative condensers.

Portal of Exit

Portal of exit is the path by which an agent leaves the source host. The portal of exit usually corresponds to the site at which the agent is localized. Thus, tubercule bacilli and influenza viruses exit the respiratory tract, schistosomes through urine, cholera vibroes in feces, *Sarcoptes scabiei* in scabies skin lesions, and enterovirus 70, an agent of hemorrhagic conjunctivitis, in conjunctival secretions. Some bloodborne agents can exit by crossing the placenta (rubella, syphilis, toxoplasmosis), and others exit by way of the skin (percutaneously) through cuts or needles (hepatitis B) or blood-sucking arthropods (malaria).

Modes of Transmission

After an agent exits its natural reservoir, it may be transmitted to a susceptible host in many ways. These modes of transmission are classified as:

- Direct
  - –Direct contact
  - –Droplet spread
- Indirect
  - –Airborne
  - –Vehicleborne
  - –Vectorborne
    - * Mechanical
    - * Biologic

In **direct transmission,** there is essentially immediate transfer of the agent from a reservoir to a susceptible host by direct contact or droplet spread. **Direct contact** occurs through kissing, skin-to-skin contact, and sexual intercourse. Direct contact refers also to contact with soil or vegetation harboring infectious organisms. Thus, infectious mononucleosis ("kissing disease") and gonorrhea are spread person-to-person by direct contact. Hookworm is spread by direct contact with contaminated soil. **Droplet spread** refers to spray with relatively large, short-range aerosols produced by sneezing, coughing, or talking. Droplet spread is classified as direct because transmission is by direct spray over a few feet, before the droplets fall to the ground.

In **indirect transmission**, an agent is carried from a reservoir to a susceptible host by suspended air particles or by animate (**vector**) intermediaries. Most vectors are arthropods such as mosquitoes, fleas, and ticks. These may carry the agent by purely mechanical means. For example, flies carry *Shigella* on their appendages; fleas carry *Yersinia pestis* (the agent that causes plague) in the gut and deposit the agent on the skin of a new host. In mechanical transmission, the agent does not multiply or undergo physiologic changes in the vector. This is in contrast to instances in which an agent undergoes part of its life cycle inside a vector before being transmitted to a new host. When the agent undergoes changes within the vector, the vector is serving as both an intermediate host and as a mode of transmission. This type of transmission is **biologic transmission.**

Guinea worm disease and many other vectorborne diseases have complex life cycles which require an intermediate host until the agent has completed that part of its life cycle. Follow the life cycle of *Dracunculus medinensis* (Guinea worm) illustrated in Figure 1.6.

Dracunculiasis Eradication in Ghana

The reported incidence of dracunculiasis (guinea worm disease) in Ghana declined substantially during 1992—the third consecutive year in which reports of known cases declined. During 1992, more than 33,000 cases of dracunculiasis were prevented as a result of control interventions instituted in 1991. Trained village-based health workers used visual aids (flip charts and posters) to provide health education in all villages where the disease is endemic. Schoolteachers in areas where the disease is endemic were provided 10,000 teacher's manuals; in addition, they were provided one million pamphlets about prevention of dracunculiasis for distribution to schoolchildren. Sixty-six percent of households in villages where the disease is endemic received cloth filters and instruction for filtering unsafe drinking water. Unsafe water sources in 266 villages were treated with temephos. Because of the rapid reduction in dracunculiasis, Ghana has declined from second to the third most highly endemic country for this problem (Centers for Disease Control and Prevention, 1993).

Start
Infected individual approaches water source containing noninfected copepods ("water fleas" or "cyclops").
Infected individual enters water. When blister (caused by adult female worm) comes into contact with water, it rapidly becomes an ulcer through which the adult female worm releases first-stage larvae. The larvae are ingested by copepods.
Within 10 to 14 days larvae ingested by copepods develop into infective third-stage larvae.
Susceptible individual consumes water containing infected copepods.
Infected individuals are symptom free for 10 to 14 months then ingested third-stage larvae mature into adult worms.
The adult female worm provokes the formation of a painful blister in the skin of the infected individual.

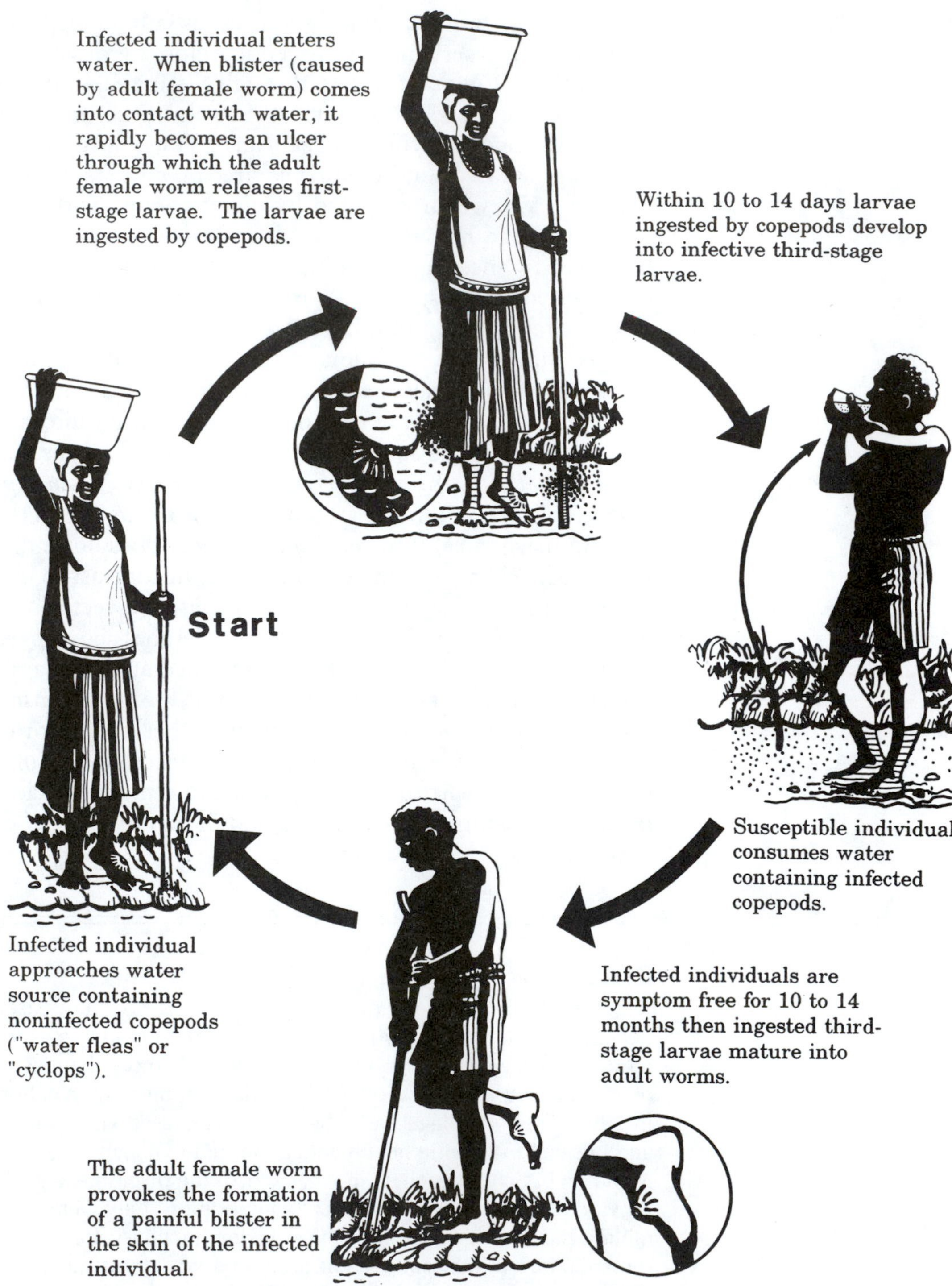

The agent, *Dracunculus*, develops in the intermediate host (fresh water copepod). Man acquires the infection by ingesting infected copepods in drinking water.

FIGURE 1.6 *The complex life cycle of* Dracunculus medinensis *(Guinea worm)*

Because the agent undergoes part of its life cycle in the intermediate host, the agent cannot be transmitted by the intermediate host until the agent has completed that part of its life cycle. Therefore, this is an indirect, vectorborne, biologic transformation.

Vehicles that may indirectly transmit an agent include food, water, biologic products (blood), and fomites (inanimate objects such as handkerchiefs, bedding, or surgical scalpels). As with vectors, vehicles may passively carry an agent—as food or water may carry hepatitis A virus—or may provide an environment in which the agent grows, multiplies, or produces toxin—as improperly canned foods may provide an environment in which *C. botulinum* produces toxin.

Airborne transmission is by particles that are suspended in air. There are two types of these particles: **dust** and **droplet nuclei**. Airborne **dust** includes infectious particles blown from the soil by the wind as well as material that has settled on surfaces and become resuspended by air currents. **Droplet nuclei** are the residue of dried droplets. The nuclei are less than 5 microns in size and may remain suspended in the air for long periods, may be blown over great distances, and are easily inhaled into the lungs and exhaled. This makes them an important means of transmission for some diseases. Tuberculosis, for example, is believed to be transmitted more often indirectly through droplet nuclei, than directly through droplet spread. Legionnaires' disease and histoplasmosis are also spread by airborne transmission.

Portal of Entry

An agent enters a susceptible host through a **portal of entry**. The portal of entry must provide access to tissues in which the agent can multiply or a toxin can act. Often to enter a new host organisms use the same portal that they use to exit a source host. For example, influenza virus must exit the respiratory tract of the source host and enter the respiratory tract of the new host. The route of transmission of many enteric (intestinal) pathogenic agents is described as "fecal–oral" because the organisms are shed in feces, carried on inadequately washed hands, and then transferred through a vehicle (such as food, water, or cooking utensil) to the mouth of a new host. Other portals of entry include the skin (hookworm), mucous membranes (syphilis, trachoma), and blood (hepatitis B).

Host

The final link in the chain of infection is a susceptible **host**. Susceptibility of a host depends on genetic factors, specified acquired immunity, and other general factors which alter a person's ability to resist infection or to limit pathogenicity. An individual's genetic makeup may either increase or decrease susceptibility. General factors which defend against infection include the skin, mucous membranes, gastric acidity, cilia in the respiratory tract, the cough reflex, and nonspecific immune response. General factors that may increase susceptibility are malnutrition, alcoholism, and disease or therapy that impairs the nonspecific immune response. Specific acquired immunity refers to protective antibodies that are directed against a specific agent. Individuals gain protective antibodies in two ways: 1) They develop antibodies in response to infection, vaccine, or toxoid—this is called **active immunity**; or 2) They acquire their mothers' antibodies before birth through the placenta or receive injections of antitoxins or immune globulin—this is called **passive immunity**.

What is herd immunity?

Note that the chain of infection may be interrupted when an agent does not find a susceptible host. This may occur if a high proportion of individuals in a population is resistant to an agent. These persons limit the spread of disease to the few who are susceptible by reducing the probability of contact between infected and susceptible persons. This concept is called **herd immunity**. The degree of herd immunity necessary to prevent or abort an outbreak varies by disease. In theory, herd immunity means that not everyone in a community needs to be resistant (immune) to prevent disease spread and occurrence of an outbreak. In practice, herd immunity has not prevented outbreaks of measles and rubella in populations with immunity levels as high as 85 to 90%. In highly immunized populations, the relatively few susceptible persons are often clustered in population subgroups, usually defined by socioeconomic or cultural factors. If the agent is introduced into one of these subgroups, an outbreak may occur.

What are the implications for community health in knowing how an agent exits and enters a host and what its modes of transmission are?

By knowing how an agent exits and enters a host and what its modes of transmission are, we can determine appropriate control measures. In general, we should direct control measures against the link in the infection chain that is most susceptible to interference, unless this is impractical.

For some diseases, the most appropriate intervention may be directed at controlling or eliminating the agent at its source. In the hospital, patients may be treated and/or isolated with appropriate "enteric precautions," "respiratory precautions," "universal precautions," and the like for different exit pathways. In the community, soil may be decontaminated or covered to prevent the agent's escape.

Sometimes, we direct interventions at the mode of transmission. For direct transmission, we may provide treatment to the source host or educate the source host to avoid the specific type of contact associated with transmission. In the hospital, since most infections are transmitted by direct contact, handwashing is the single most important way to prevent disease from spreading. For vehicleborne transmission, we may decontaminate or eliminate the vehicle. For fecal–oral transmission, we may also try to reduce the risk of future contamination by rearranging the environment and educating the persons involved to practice better personal hygiene. For airborne transmission, we may modify ventilation or air pressure and filter or treat the air. For vectorborne transmission, we usually attempt to control (i.e., reduce or eradicate) the vector population.

Finally, we may apply measures that protect the portals of entry of a susceptible host or reduce the susceptibility of the potential host. For example, a dentist's mask and gloves are intended to protect the dentist from a patient's blood, secretions, and droplets, as well as to protect the patient from the dentist. Prophylactic antibiotics and vaccination are strategies to improve a potential host's defenses.

Epidemic Disease Occurrence

The amount of a particular disease that is usually present in a community is the baseline level of the disease. This level is not necessarily the preferred level (which should be zero); it is the observed level. Theoretically, if no intervention occurred and if the level is low enough not to deplete the pool of susceptible persons, the occurrence of the disease should continue at the baseline level indefinitely. Thus, the baseline level is often considered the expected level of the disease. For example, over the past 4 years the number of reported cases of poliomyelitis has ranged from 5 to 9. Therefore, assuming there is no change in population, we would expect to see approximately 7 reported cases next year.

Different diseases in different communities show different patterns of expected occurrence: 1) a persistent level of occurrence with a low-to-moderate disease level is referred to as an **endemic** level; 2) a persistently high level of occurrence is called a **hyperendemic** level; 3) an irregular pattern of occurrence, with occasional cases occurring at irregular intervals, is called **sporadic**.

Occasionally, the level of disease rises above the expected level. When the occurrence of a disease within an area is clearly in excess of the expected level for a given time period, it is called an **epidemic**. Public health officials often use the term **outbreak**, which means the same thing, because it is less provocative to the public. When an epidemic spreads over several countries or continents and affects a large number of people, it is called a **pandemic**.

HIV/AIDS Pandemic

The following are conclusions from *AIDS in the World 1992* (Mann, Tarantola, and Netter) about the HIV/AIDS pandemic and were cited by Goldsmith (1992, p. 445):

- The magnitude of the pandemic has increased more than 100-fold since AIDS was discovered in 1981. In early 1992 at least 12.9 million people worldwide were estimated to be infected with HIV (7.1 million men, 4.7 million women, and 1.1 million children)—up from an estimated 10,000 total in 1981. Of these, 1 in 5 have developed AIDS and nearly 2.5 million have died.
- In the next 3 years, 3.8 million people will develop AIDS. This exceeds the total number who developed the disease up to now. Also from 1992 through 1995, an additional 5.7 million adults and 1.2 million children will become infected with HIV.
- The spread of AIDS has not been stopped in any community or country. At least 40,000 to 80,000 new HIV infections are anticipated in the United States this year. Last year, more than 75,000 new HIV infections occurred in Europe. In the past 5 years, the number in Africa tripled; it is now more than 7.5 million. The infection continues to spread unabated in the Caribbean, Central America, and South America.
- HIV is spreading to new communities and countries around the world. It was reported recently from the Pacific island nations of Fiji and Samoa. Within only a few years, it has exploded in southeast Asia, infecting more than 1 million people in Thailand, Burma, and India. China, Pakistan, the Philippines, and Indonesia are on the verge of national epidemics. By the year 2000, the largest proportion of infections—42%—will be in Asia. Sub-Saharan Africa will have 31%, Latin America 8%, and the Caribbean 6%.

Why do epidemics occur?

Epidemics occur when an agent and susceptible hosts are present in adequate numbers, and the agent can effectively be conveyed from a source to the susceptible hosts. More specifically, an epidemic may result from the following:

- A recent increase in amount or virulence of the agent
- The recent introduction of the agent into a setting where it has not been before
- An enhanced mode of transmission so that more susceptible persons are exposed
- Some change in the susceptibility of the host response to the agent
- Factors that increase host exposure or involve introduction through new portals of entry

Epidemic Patterns

We sometimes classify epidemics by how they spread through a population, as shown below:

- Common source
  - Point
  - Intermittent
  - Continuous
- Propagated
- Mixed
- Other

A **common source outbreak** is one in which a group of persons is exposed to a common noxious influence, such as an infectious agent or a toxin. If the group is exposed over a relatively brief period, so that everyone who becomes ill develops disease at the end of one incubation period, the common source outbreak is further classified as a **point source outbreak.** The epidemic of leukemia cases in Hiroshima following the atomic bomb blast and an epidemic of hepatitis A among college football players who unknowingly drank contaminated water after practice one day each had a point source of exposure. When the number of cases in a point source epidemic is plotted over time, the resulting epidemic curve classically has a steep upslope and a more gradual downslope (a "log-normal distribution"). Figure 1.7 is an example of a typical log-normal distribution of a point source outbreak.

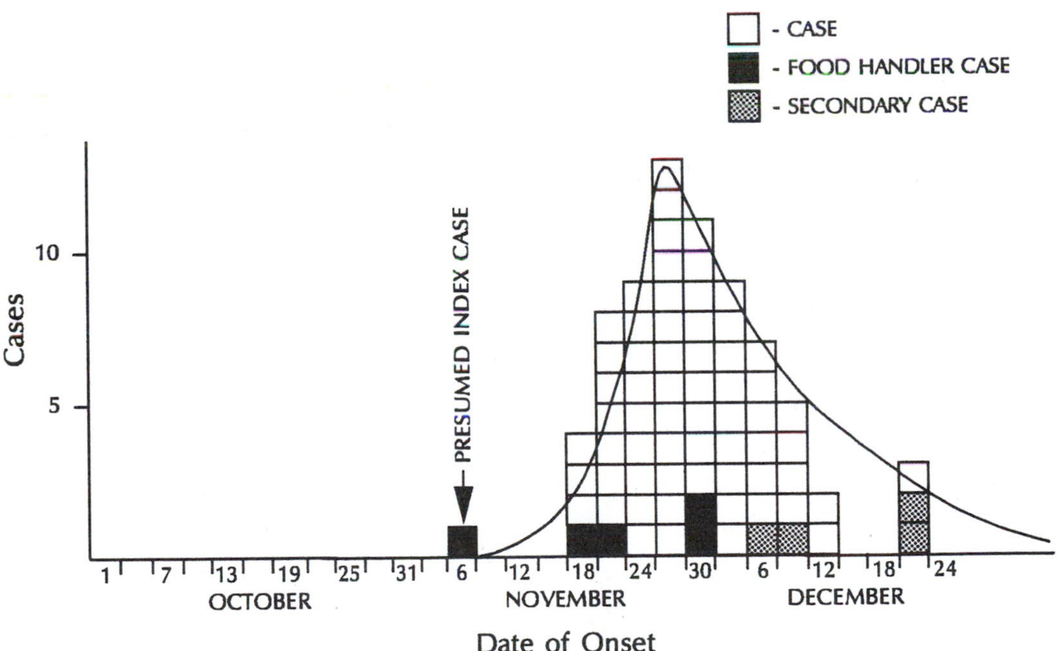

SOURCE: CDC, unpublished data, 1979

FIGURE 1.7 *Example of common source outbreak with point source exposure: Hepatitis A cases by date of onset, Fayetteville, Arkansas, November–December 1978, with log-normal curve superimposed*

In some common source outbreaks, cases may be exposed over a period of days, weeks, or longer, with the exposure being either **intermittent** or **continuous**. Figure 1.8 is an epidemic curve of a common source outbreak with continuous exposure. When we plot the cases of a continuous common source outbreak over time, the range of exposures and range of incubation periods tends to dampen and widen the peaks of the epidemic curve. Similarly, when we plot an intermittent common source outbreak, we often find an irregular pattern that reflects the intermittent nature of the exposure.

An outbreak that does not have a common source, but spreads gradually from person to person—usually growing as it spreads—is called a **propagated outbreak**. Usually transmission is by direct person-to-person contact, as with syphilis. Transmission may also be vehicleborne, as in the transmission of hepatitis B or HIV by sharing needles, or vectorborne, as in the transmission of yellow fever by mosquitoes.

In a propagated epidemic, cases occur over more than one incubation period. In theory, the epidemic curve of a propagated epidemic would have a successive series of peaks reflecting increasing numbers of cases in each generation. The epidemic usually wanes after a few generations, either because the number of susceptible persons falls below some critical level, or because intervention measures become effective. Figure 1.9 shows such an epidemic curve.

In reality, few propagated outbreaks provide as classic a pattern as that shown in Figure 1.9. For many diseases, the variability of time of

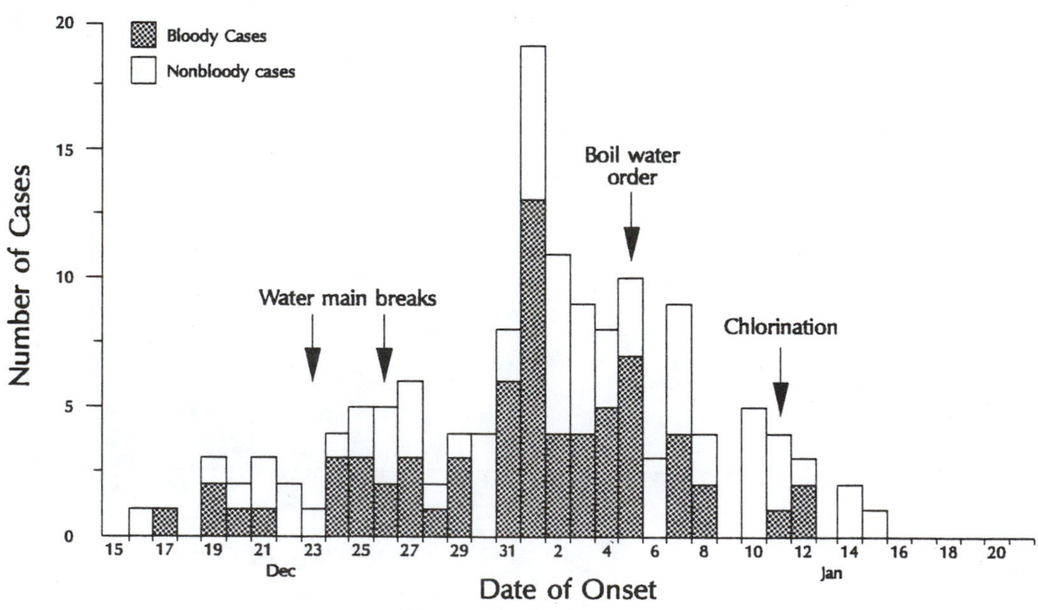

SOURCE: CDC, unpublished data, 1990

FIGURE 1.8 *Example of common source outbreak with continuous exposure: Diarrheal illness in city residents by date of onset and character of stool, Cabool, Missouri, December 1989–January 1990*

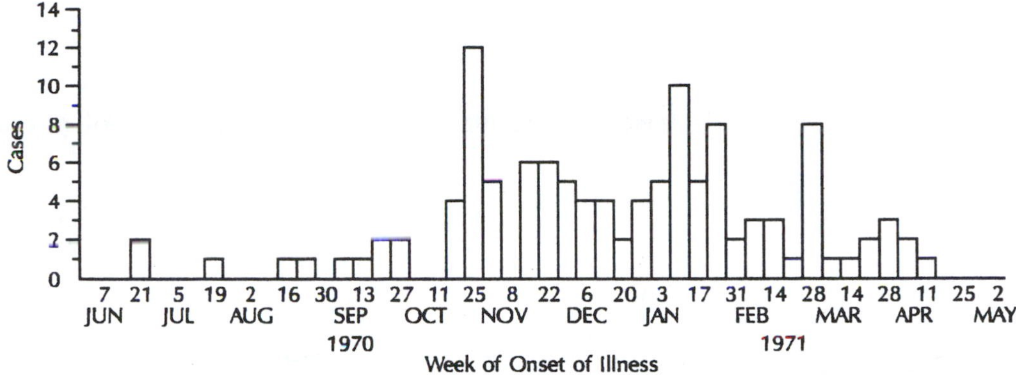

FIGURE 1.9 *Example of a propagated epidemic that does not show the classic pattern: Infectious hepatitis cases by week of onset, Barren County, Kentucky, June 1970–April 1971*

exposure and range of incubation periods tend to smooth out the peaks and valleys, as shown in Figure 1.10. For influenza, the incubation period is so short and transmission is so effective that its epidemic curve may look like that of a point source epidemic.

Some epidemics have features of both common source epidemics and propagated epidemics. The pattern of a common source outbreak followed

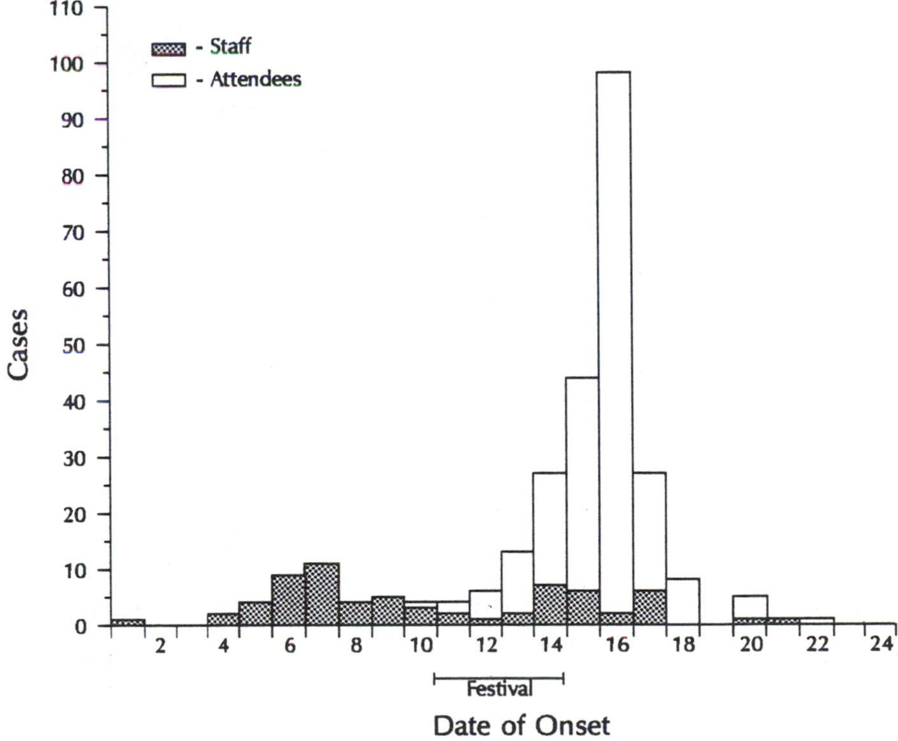

FIGURE 1.10 *Example of a mixed epidemic: Shigella cases at a music festival by day of onset, Michigan, August 1988*

by secondary person-to-person spread is not uncommon. These are called **mixed epidemics**. Finally, some epidemics are neither common source nor propagated person-to-person. Outbreaks of zoonotic or vectorborne diseases may result from sufficient prevalence of infection in host species, sufficient presence of vectors, and sufficient human–vector interaction. Examples include the epidemic of Lyme disease that affected several states in the northeastern United States in the late 1980s and the large epidemic of St. Louis encephalitis in Florida in 1990.

EPIDEMIOLOGY IN PUBLIC HEALTH PRACTICE

Epidemiology is an essential tool for carrying out four fundamental functions: public health surveillance, disease investigation, analytic studies, and program evaluation. These are the key areas through which epidemiology contributes to the promotion of the public's health.

Public Health Surveillance

Through **public health surveillance**, a health department or other health agency systematically collects, analyzes, interprets, and disseminates health data on an ongoing basis (Thacker and Berkelman, 1988). Public health surveillance, which has been called "information for action" (Orenstein and Bernier, 1990), is how a health department/agency takes the pulse of its community. By knowing the ongoing patterns of disease occurrence and disease potential, a health department/agency can effectively and efficiently investigate, prevent, and control disease in the community.

At the local level, the most common source of surveillance data is reports of disease cases received from health-care providers who are required to report patients with certain "reportable" diseases, such as cholera or measles or syphilis. In addition, surveillance data may come from laboratory reports, surveys, diseases registries, death certificates, and public health program data such as immunization coverage. Data also may come from investigations of cases or clusters of cases reported to the health department.

Most health departments use simple surveillance systems. They monitor individual morbidity and mortality case reports, record a limited amount of information on each case, and look for patterns by time, place, and person. Unfortunately, with some reportable diseases, a health department may receive reports of only 10% to 25% of the cases that actually occur. Nevertheless, health departments have found that even a simple surveillance system can be invaluable in detecting problems and guiding public health action.

Disease Investigation

As noted above, surveillance is considered information for action. When a health department receives a report of a case or cluster of cases of a disease, its first action is to investigate. The investigation may be as limited as a telephone call to the health-care provider to confirm or clarify the circumstances of the reported case, or it may be as extensive as a field investigation coordinating the efforts of dozens of people to determine the extent and cause of a large outbreak.

The objectives of such investigations vary. With a communicable disease, one objective may be to identify additional unreported or unrecognized cases in order to control the spread of the disease. For example, one of the hallmarks of investigations of sexually transmitted disease is the identification of the sexual contacts of case patients. When these contacts are interviewed and tested, they are often found to have asymptomatic infections. By providing treatment that these contacts had not realized they needed, the health department prevents them from spreading the disease further.

For other diseases, the objective of an investigation may be to identify a source or vehicle of infection which can be controlled or eliminated. For example, the investigation of a case of botulism usually focuses on identifying the vehicle contaminated with botulinum toxin, such as food that was improperly canned. Once the investigators have identified the vehicle, they can establish how many other people may have been exposed and how many continue to be at risk, and take action to prevent their exposure. In Taiwan, investigators of a cluster of botulism cases implicated consumption of canned peanuts prepared by a single manufacturer (Chou, Hwang, and Malison, 1988). Then they initiated a nationwide recall of that product from warehouses, stores, and homes to reduce the risk of exposure for others.

For some diseases, the objectives of an investigation may be simply to learn more about the disease itself—its natural history, clinical spectrum, descriptive epidemiology, and risk factors. In the nationwide outbreak of toxic shock syndrome in 1980, early investigations focused on establishing a case definition based on clinical symptoms, and on describing the populations at risk. From this, investigators were able to develop hypotheses which they could test with analytic studies. The investigators conducted a series of increasingly specific studies narrowing specific risk factors from menstruating women to tampon users to users of a specific brand of tampon. This information prompted the withdrawal of that tampon brand from the market, and started subsequent research to identify what factors in the composition and use of the tampon caused the syndrome to develop (CDC, 1990).

Field investigations of the type described above are sometimes referred to as "shoe-leather epidemiology," conjuring images of dedicated, haggard epidemiologists beating the pavement in search of additional cases to interview and clues to identify the source and mode of transmission.

Analytic Studies

Surveillance and case investigation sometimes are sufficient to identify causes, modes of transmission, and appropriate control and prevention measures. Sometimes they provide clues or hypotheses that must be assessed with appropriate analytic techniques. The focus of this book is on these analytic techniques.

Investigators initially use descriptive epidemiology (see following section) to examine clusters of cases or outbreaks of disease. They examine the incidence of the disease or health event and its distribution by time, place, and person. They calculate rates and identify parts of the population that are at higher risk than others. When they find a strong association between exposure and disease, the investigators may implement control measures immediately. More often, investigators find that descriptive studies, like case investigations, generate hypotheses which they then can test with analytic studies.

Epidemiologists must be familiar with all aspects of an analytic study, including its design, conduct, analysis, and interpretation. In addition, the epidemiologist must be able to communicate the study's findings.

Evaluation

Evaluation of control and prevention measures is another responsibility of the epidemiologist. Evaluation frequently addresses both **effectiveness** and **efficiency. Effectiveness** refers to the ability of a program to produce results in the field. Effectiveness differs from **efficacy**, which is the ability of a program to produce results under ideal conditions. Finally, **efficiency** refers to the ability of a program to produce the intended results with a minimum expenditure of time and resources. Evaluation of an immunization program, for example, might compare the stated efficacy with the field effectiveness of the program, and might assess the efficiency with which acceptable results are achieved.

THE EPIDEMIOLOGIC APPROACH

Like a newspaper reporter, an epidemiologist determines what, when, where, who, and why. However, an epidemiologist is more likely to describe these concepts in slightly different terms: case definition, time, place, person, and causes.

Case Definition

A **case definition** is a set of standard criteria for deciding whether a person has a particular disease or other health-related condition. By using a standard case definition, we ensure that every case is diagnosed in the same way, regardless of when or where it occurred, or who identified it. We can then compare the number of cases of the disease that occurred in one time or place with the number that occurred at another time or another place. For example, with a standard case definition, we can compare the number of cases of hepatitis A that occurred in New York City in 1994 with the number that occurred there in 1990. Or, we can compare the number of cases that occurred in New York in 1994 with the number that occurred in San Francisco in 1994. With a standard case definition, when we find a difference in disease occurrence, we know it is likely to be a real difference rather than the result of differences in how cases were diagnosed.

A case definition consists of clinical criteria and, sometimes, limitations on time, place, and person. The clinical criteria usually include confirmatory laboratory tests, if available, or combinations of symptoms (subjective complaints), signs (objective physical findings), and other findings.

A case definition may have several sets of criteria, depending on how certain the diagnosis is. For example, during an outbreak of measles, we might classify a person with a fever and rash as having a suspect, probable, or confirmed case of measles, depending on what additional evidence of measles is present. In other situations, we temporarily classify a case as suspect or probable until laboratory results are available. When we receive the laboratory report, we then reclassify the case as either confirmed or "not a case," depending on the laboratory culture results. In the midst of a large outbreak of a disease caused by a known agent, we may permanently classify some cases as suspect or probable because it is unnecessary and wasteful to run laboratory tests on every patient with a consistent clinical picture and a history of exposure (e.g., chickenpox). However, case definitions should not rely on laboratory culture results alone, since organisms are sometimes present without causing disease.

Case definitions may also vary according to the purpose for classifying the occurrences of a disease. For example, health officials need to know as soon as possible if someone has symptoms of plague or foodborne botulism so that they can begin planning what actions to take. For such rare but potentially severe communicable diseases, in which it is important to identify every possible case, health officials use a **sensitive**, or "loose" case definition. On the other hand, investigators of the causes of a disease outbreak want to be certain that any person included in the investigation really had the disease. The investigator will prefer a **specific**, or "strict" case definition. For instance, in an outbreak of *Salmonella agona,* the investigators would be more likely to identify the source of the infection if they included only persons who were confirmed to have been infected with that organism, rather than including everyone with acute diarrhea. The only disadvantage of a strict case definition is an underestimate of the total number of cases.

Numbers and Rates

A basic task of health departments is counting cases in order to measure and describe morbidity. When physicians diagnose a case of a reportable disease, they send a report of the case to their local health department. These reports are legally required to contain information on time (when the case occurred), place (where the patient lived), and person (the age, race, and sex of the patient). The health department combines the reports and summarizes the information by time, place, and person. From these summaries, the health department determines the extent and patterns of disease occurrence in the area, and identifies clusters or outbreaks of disease.

A simple count of cases, however, does not provide all the information a health department or particular health professional may need. To compare the occurrence of a disease at different locations or during different times, a health department converts the case counts into **rates,** which relate the number of cases to the size of the population in which they occurred. In Chapter 2 we will discuss rates further.

Rates are useful in many ways. With rates, groups in a community with an elevated risk of disease or other health events can be identified. These **high-risk groups** can be further assessed and targeted for special intervention; the groups can be studied to identify **risk factors** that are related to the occurrence of disease. Individuals can use knowledge of these risk factors to guide their decisions about behaviors that influence health.

Descriptive Epidemiology

In descriptive epidemiology, we organize and summarize data according to time, place, and person. These three characteristics are sometimes called **epidemiologic variables.**

Compiling and analyzing data by time, place, and person is desirable for several reasons. First, the investigator becomes intimately familiar with the data and with the extent of the public health problem being investigated. Second, the data analysis provides an easily communicated, detailed description of the health of a population. Third, such analysis identifies the populations that are at greatest risk of acquiring a particular disease. This information provides important clues to the causes of the disease, and these clues can be turned into testable hypotheses.

Time

Disease rates change over time. Some of these changes occur regularly and can be predicted. For example, the seasonal increase of influenza cases with the onset of cold weather is a pattern familiar to nearly everyone. By knowing when flu outbreaks will occur, health care professionals can time flu shot campaigns effectively. Other disease rates change unpredictably. By examining events that precede an increase or decrease in disease rates, we may identify causes and appropriate actions to control or prevent further occurrences of the disease.

Depending on what condition we are describing, we may be interested in a period of years or decades, or we may limit the period to days, weeks, or months when the number of cases reported is greater than normal. For many chronic diseases, for example, we are interested in long-term changes in the number of cases or in the rate of the condition. For other conditions, we may find it more revealing to look at the occurrence of the condition by season, month, day of the week, or even time of day. For a newly recognized problem, we need to assess the occurrence of the problem over time in a variety of ways until we discover the most appropriate and revealing time period to use.

Place

We describe a health event by place to gain insight into the geographical distribution of a problem. For place, we may use place of residence, birth-place, place of employment, school district, hospital unit, etc., depending on which may be related to the occurrence of the health event. Similarly, we may use large or small geographic units: country, state, county, census tract, street address, map coordinates, or some other standard geographical designation. Sometimes we may find it useful to analyze data according to place categories such as urban or rural, domestic or foreign, and institutional or noninstitutional.

Person

In descriptive epidemiology, when we organize or analyze data by "person" there are several categories available. We may use inherent characteristics of people (for example, age, race, sex), their acquired characteristics (immune or marital status), their activities (occupation, leisure activities, use of medications/tobacco/drugs), or conditions under which they live (socioeconomic status, access to medical care). These categories determine to a large degree who is at greatest risk of experiencing some undesirable health condition, such as becoming infected with a particular disease organism.

Analytic Epidemiology

With descriptive epidemiology we can identify several characteristics of persons with disease, and we may question whether these features are really unusual, but descriptive epidemiology does not answer that question. Analytic epidemiology provides a way to find the answer.

When we find that persons with a particular characteristic are more likely than those without that characteristic to develop a certain disease or experience a certain health event, the characteristic is said to be associated with the disease/health event. The characteristic may be a demographic factor such as age, race, or sex; a constitutional factor such as blood group or immune status; a behavior or act such as smoking or having eaten a specific food; or a circumstance such as living near a toxic waste site. Identifying factors that are associated with disease helps us identify populations at increased risk of disease; we can then target public health prevention and control activities. Identifying risk factors also provides clues that can direct research activities to the causes of a disease.

Thus, analytic epidemiology is concerned with the search for causes and effects, or the why and the how. We use analytic epidemiology to quantify the association between exposures and outcomes and to test hypotheses about causal relationships. It is sometimes said that epidemiology can never prove that a particular exposure caused a particular outcome. Epidemiology may, however, provide sufficient evidence for us to take appropriate measures for control and prevention.

CHAPTER SUMMARY

Epidemiology is the study of the distribution and determinants of health events in human populations. It is considered the basic science of public health, with good reason. Epidemiology is a tool for public health action to promote and protect public health based on science, causal reasoning, and practical common sense. Thus, epidemiology involves both science and public health practice. In this chapter we have:

- Defined epidemiology and behavioral epidemiology
- Summarized the historical evolution of epidemiology
- Discussed the primary applications of epidemiology in public health practice
- Discussed the epidemiologic triad
- Introduced the concept of natural history of disease and spectrum of disease
- Described different modes of transmission of communicable disease in a population
- Discussed key features and uses of descriptive epidemiology

KEY TERMS

epidemiology
behavioral epidemiology
epidemiologic triangle or triad
agent
natural history of disease
incubation period
latency period
infectivity
pathogenicity
virulence
reservoir
portal of exit
mode of transmission
portal of entry
host
chain of infection
carrier
asymptomatic carrier
incubatory or convalescent carrier
chronic carrier
zoonoses
direct transmission
direct contact
droplet spread
indirect transmission
vector
biologic transmission
vehicle
airborne transmission
dust

droplet nuclei
active immunity
passive immunity
herd immunity
endemic level
hyperendemic level
sporadic level
epidemic
outbreak
pandemic
common source outbreak
point source outbreak
propagated outbreak
mixed epidemic
public health surveillance
effectiveness
efficiency
case definition
sensitive
specific
rates
high-risk groups
risk factors
epidemiologic variables

REFERENCES

Brownson RC, Remington PL, Davis JR: *Chronic disease epidemiology and control.* Washington, DC: American Public Health Association, 1993.

Centers for Disease Control: Reduced incidence of menstrual toxic shock syndrome—United States, 1980–1990. *Morbidity and Mortality Weekly Report* 1990;39:421-423.

Centers for Disease Control and Prevention: *Principles of epidemiology: An introduction to applied epidemiology and biostatistics, 2d ed.* Atlanta, GA: CDC, 1992.

Centers for Disease Control and Prevention: Update: Dracunculiasis eradication—Ghana. *Morbidity and Mortality Weekly Report* 1993;42:93-94.

Chou JH, Hwang PH, Malison MD: An outbreak of type A foodbourne botulism in Taiwan due to commercially preserved peanuts. *International Journal of Epidemiology* 1988;17:899-902.

Dawber TR, Kannel WB, Lyell LP: An approach to longitudinal studies in a community: The Framingham study. *Annals of the New York Academy of Sciences* 1963;107:539-556.

Doll R, Hill AB: Smoking and carcinoma of the lung. *British Medical Journal* 1950;1:739-748.

Duncan DF: *Epidemiology: Basis for disease prevention and health promotion.* New York: Macmillan, 1988.

Elder JP, McGraw SA, Abrams DA: Organizational and community approaches to community-wide prevention of heart disease: The first two years of the Pawtucket Heart Health Program. *Preventive Medicine* 1986;15:107-115.

Farquhar JW, Fortmann SP, Maccoby N: The Stanford Five-City Project: Design and methods. *American Journal of Epidemiology* 1985;122:323-334.

Freedman DS, Chear CL, Srinivasan SR, Webber LS, Berenson GS: Tracking of serum lipids and lipoproteins in children over an 8-year period: The Bogalusa Heart Study. *Preventive Medicine* 1985;14:203-216.

Fox JP, Hall CE, Elveback LR: *Epidemiology: Man and disease.* New York: Macmillan, 1970.

Goldberger J, Waring CH, Tanner WF: Pellagra prevention by diet among institutional inmates. *Public Health Reports* 1923;38:2361-2368.

Goldsmith M: Critical moment at hand in HIV/AIDS pandemic, new global strategy to arrest its spread proposed. *The Journal of the American Medical Association* 1992;268:445-446.

Gordon T, Castelli WP, Hjortland MC, Kannel WB, Dawber TR: High-density lipoprotein as a protective factor against coronary heart disease: The Framingham Study. *American Journal of Medicine* 1977;62:707-714.

Green LW: *Community health* (sixth edition). St. Louis: Times Mirror/Mosby, 1990.

Hippocrates. *On airs, waters, and places.* Translated and republished in *Medical Classics* 1938;3:19-42.

Last JM: *Dictionary of epidemiology, 2d ed.* New York: Oxford University Press, 1988.

Lilienfeld AM, Lilienfeld DE: *Foundations of epidemiology, 2d ed.* New York: Oxford, 1980.

Lind J: *A treatise of the scurvy.* Edinburgh, Scotland: Sands, Murray, and Cochran, 1753.

MacMahon B, Pugh TF: *Epidemiology: Priniciples and methods.* Boston: Little, Brown, and Company, 1970.

Mann J, Tarantola D, Netter T: *AIDS in the world 1992.* Cambridge, MA: Harvard University Press, 1992.

Mausner JS, Kramer S: *Epidemiology: An introductory text, 2d ed.* Philadelphia: W. B. Saunders, 1985.

McAlister A, Puska P, Salonen JT, Tuomilehto J, Koskela K: Theory and action for health promotion: Illustrations from the North Karelia Project. *American Journal of Public Health* 1982;72:43-50.

Orenstein WA, Bernier RH: Surveillance information for action. *Pediatric Clinics of North America* 1990;37:709-734.

Schuchat A, Broome CV: Toxic shock syndrome and tampons. *Epidemiologic Reviews* 1991;13:99-112.

Stamler J, Wentworth D, Neaton JD: Is the relationship between serum cholesterol and risk of premature death from coronary heart disease continuous and graded? Findings in 356,222 primary screenees of the Multiple Risk Factor

Intervention Trial (MRFIT). *Journal of the American Medical Association* 1986;256:2823-2828.

Thacker SB, Berkelman RL: Public health surveillance in the United States. *Epidemiologic Reviews* 1988;10:164-190.

Winklestein W: Not just a country doctor: Edward Jenner, scientist. *Epidemiologic Reviews* 1992;14:1-15.

PROBLEMS

1. Tables 1.3, 1.4, 1.5, and 1.6 show *person* information about the cases of an unknown disease. Study the information in the tables and then describe how the disease outbreak is distributed by person factors.

TABLE 1.3 Incidence of the disease by age and sex in 24 villages surveyed for one year

	Males			Females		
Age Group (years)	*Population**	*# Cases*	*Rate per 1,000*	*Population**	*# Cases*	*Rate per 1,000*
<1	327	0	0	365	0	0
1	233	2	8.6	205	1	4.9
2	408	30	73.5	365	16	43.8
3	368	26	70.7	331	28	84.6
4	348	33	94.8	321	32	99.7
5-9	1,574	193	122.6	1,531	174	113.7
10-14	1,329	131	98.6	1,276	95	74.5
15-19	1,212	4	3.3	1,510	17	11.3
20-24	1,055	1	.9	1,280	51	39.8
25-29	882	1	1.1	997	75	75.2
30-34	779	4	5.1	720	47	65.3
35-39	639	4	6.3	646	51	78.9
40-44	469	10	21.3	485	34	70.1
45-49	372	7	18.8	343	18	52.5
50-54	263	13	49.4	263	12	45.6
55-59	200	5	25.0	228	6	26.3
60-64	164	9	53.6	153	3	19.6
65-69	106	4	37.7	105	2	19.1
≥70	80	6	75.0	114	2	17.5
Total	10,812	483	44.7	11,238	664	59.1

*As enumerated between May 1 and July 15

SOURCE: CDC, 1992.

TABLE 1.4 Incidence of the disease in women by marital status and age

	Married Women			Single Women		
Age Group (years)	*Population*	*# Cases*	*Rate per 1,000*	*Population*	*# Cases*	*Rate per 1,000*
16-29	1,905	89	46.7	1,487	16	10.7
30-49	1,684	98	58.2	141	4	28.4
≥50	387	4	10.3	26	0	0
Total	3,976	191	48.0	1,654	20	12.1

SOURCE: CDC, 1992.

TABLE 1.5 Incidence of the disease by occupation, age, and sex

Sex	*Mill Worker?*	*Age Group*	*Ill*	*Well*	*Total*	*Percent Ill*
Female	Yes	<10	0	0	0	—
		10-19	2	330	332	0.6
		20-29	4	194	198	2.0
		30-44	2	93	95	2.1
		45-54	0	9	9	0
		≥55	0	5	5	0
Female	No	<10	28	577	605	4.6
		10-19	5	200	205	2.4
		20-29	12	204	216	5.6
		30-44	16	220	236	6.8
		45-54	4	91	95	4.2
		≥55	1	92	93	1.1
Male	Yes	<10	0	0	0	—
		10-19	3	355	358	0.8
		20-29	1	361	362	0.3
		30-44	3	318	321	0.9
		45-54	0	93	93	0
		≥55	1	51	52	1.9
Male	No	<10	23	629	652	3.5
		10-19	4	161	165	2.4
		20-29	1	12	13	7.7
		30-44	0	10	10	0
		45-54	1	14	15	6.7
		≥55	4	26	30	13.3

SOURCE: CDC, 1992.

TABLE 1.6 Incidence of the disease by socioeconomic status in 24 villages* surveyed for one year

Family Socioeconomic Status	*Cases*	*Population*	*Rate per 1,000*
Stratum 1 (lowest)	99	796	124.4
Stratum 2	240	2,888	83.1
Stratum 3	260	4,868	53.4
Stratum 4	177	5,035	35.2
Stratum 5	132	5,549	23.8
Stratum 6	23	1,832	12.6
Stratum 7 (highest)	2	769	2.6
Total	933	21,737	42.9

*Restricted to cases developing after 30 days' residence.

SOURCE: CDC, 1992.

2. Use the Agent-Host-Environment model to describe the role of the human immunodeficiency virus (HIV) in AIDS.
   Agent:

   Host:

   Environment:

3. For each of the following outbreaks, choose the most likely epidemic pattern: a) point source, b) intermittent or continuous, or c) propagated.

   _______ a. Outbreak of salmonellosis traced to turkey cooked and held at an improper temperature and served at a potluck supper.

   _______ b. Outbreak of influenza among nursing home residents, new cases occurring over a 3-week period. (Hint: incubation period for influenza is less than 5 days.)

   _______ c. Episodic cases of Legionnaires' disease in hospitalized patients, traced to showers and the hospital's water supply.

4. In the definition of epidemiology, the terms "distribution" and "determinants" together refer to:

   a. frequency, pattern, and causes of health events
   b. dissemination of information to those who need to know
   c. knowledge, attitudes, and practices related to health
   d. public health services

5. When analyzing data by age, the categories should be:

   a. the same for all diseases
   b. <1 year, 1 to 4 years, 5 to 9 years, 10 to 14 years, 15 to 19 years, and 20 years for communicable diseases, but not necessarily for chronic diseases
   c. appropriate for each condition and narrow enough to detect any age-related patterns present in the data
   d. 5-year age groups for all diseases unless the data suggest the need for narrower categories to find a pattern or aberration

6. Because socioeconomic status is difficult to quantify, we commonly use all of the following measures EXCEPT:

   a. educational achievement
   b. family income
   c. occupation
   d. social standing

7. The functions of public health surveillance include which of the following? (Circle ALL that apply.)

   a. collection of health data
   b. analysis of health data
   c. interpretation of health data

d. dissemination of health data
e. disease control actions developed from the collection, analysis, and interpretation of health data

8. Direct transmission includes which of the following modes of transmission? (Circle ALL that apply.)

   a. Droplet spread
   b. Vehicleborne transmission
   c. Vectorborne transmission
   d. Airborne transmission

For Questions 9–11 describe the case-report pattern of disease X for three communities. The communities have the same size populations. Identify which term (a–d) best describes the occurrence of disease X.

a. Endemic
b. Epidemic
c. Hyperendemic
d. Pandemic

9. ______ Community A: usually 10 cases/week; last week, 28 cases

10. ______ Community B: 50–70 cases/week; last week, 55 cases

11. ______ Community C: usually 25 cases/week; last week 28 cases

12. An epidemic curve that follows the classic log-normal distribution pattern of sharp rise and more gradual decline is most consistent with which manner of spread?

    a. Continuous source
    b. Intermittent source
    c. Point source
    d. Propagated
    e. Mixed

ANSWERS

1. • Age distribution
     – no cases among infants (<1-year-olds)
     – increased incidence among children to 14 years of age
     – increased incidence among females aged 2 to 50 years
     – low incidence among males aged 15 to 40 years
     – increased incidence among males >50 years of age
   • Married women at greater risk than unmarried women at every age
   • Incidence inversely related to socioeconomic level
   • Mill workers at lower risk than non-mill workers

2. Agent: human immunodeficiency virus (HIV)

   Host:

   • behavioral factors that increase likelihood of exposure, such as intravenous drug use, men who have unprotected sex with men, and so on
   • biologic factors that determine whether an exposed person becomes infected, such as the presence of genital ulcers
   • biologic factors, largely unknown at present, that determine whether (or when) an infected person develops clinical AIDS

   Environment:

   • biologic factors, such as infected persons to transmit the infection
   • socioeconomic and societal factors, such as those that contribute to drug use

3. *point source* = a. Outbreak of salmonellosis traced to turkey cooked and held at an improper temperature and served at a potluck supper.

   propagated = b. Outbreak of influenza among nursing home residents, new cases occurring over a 3-week period. (Hint: incubation period for influenza is less than 5 days.)

   intermittent = c. Episodic cases of Legionnaires' disease in hospitalized patients traced to showers and the hospital's water supply.

4. a. "Distribution" refers to the frequency and pattern of health events in a population. "Determinants" refer to causes.

5. c.

6. d. Educational achievement, family income, and occupation are used because they are easy to measure. Social standing is not used.

7. The correct answers are a, b, c, and d. Public health surveillance includes the collection, analysis, interpretation, and dissemination of health data to be used for appropriate public health action, but surveillance does not include the action itself.

8. The correct answer is a, droplet spread. Airborne, vehicleborne, and vectorborne transmission are all types of **indirect transmission.**
9. b.
10. c.
11. a.
12. c, point source. Only a point source consistently produces the classic pattern described in question 12. Other modes of spread yield epidemic curves that are more spread out and irregular.

2 Epidemiologic Rates and Rate Adjustment

OBJECTIVES

On completion of this chapter, you will be able to:

- Recognize rates as basic tools in epidemiology practice
- Calculate and interpret the following: crude mortality, infant mortality, neonatal mortality, postneonatal mortality, and maternal mortality rates
- Explain the need to adjust rates for confounding variables
- Calculate rate adjustment by direct and indirect methods
- Calculate case-fatality rates, proportionate mortality rates, death-to-case ratios, and common natality rates
- Calculate prevalence rates
- Define years of potential life lost (YPLL) and years of potential life lost rate

What are rates and how are they calculated?

The most commonly used statistical tool in epidemiology is a **rate.** A rate is a statistical measure of the occurrence of a health event within a population group at a specified point in time or time period. Rates can be conceptualized as probability statements that estimate the frequency of occurrence of a health event in a group. Rates which describe the frequency of death in a population are **mortality rates.** Rates which describe the occurrence of disease in a population are **morbidity rates.** Using rates allows you to summarize a group's experience with a particular health event in a single expression, such as 18 deaths per 100,000 population.

Calculating rates requires being able to say whether an individual in the group of interest has or has not developed a particular disease or health event. The number experiencing the particular disease or health event of interest represents the **numerator** for the rate. The number in the population at risk of experiencing the health event is the **denominator** for the rate.

The form of a rate is as follows:

$$\frac{\text{Number of events (cases, births, deaths) during a specified time period}}{\text{Number at risk of experiencing the event}} \times K(10^n)$$

PROBLEM

Suppose that the population at risk of dying in the U.S. during 1989 was 248,762,000 (total U.S. population) and the number of deaths during that year was 2,155,000. How would you calculate the mortality rate from this information?

SOLUTION

The mortality rate for 1989 can be calculated by using the following formula:

$$\frac{\text{Number of deaths in 1989}}{\text{Number at risk of dying (total U.S. population)}} \times K(10^n)$$

Therefore:

$$\frac{2{,}155{,}000}{248{,}762{,}000} \times K(10^n)$$

2,155,000/248,762,000 = 0.008662. Because the probabilities when dividing denominators into numerators usually turn out to be very small numbers, they are multiplied by some constant (**K**) (typically a multiplier of 10, such as 100, 1,000, 10,000, or 100,000) to make numbers more understandable. For example, by multiplying the probability of 0.008662 by 100,000, we get 866.2, which represents the death rate per 100,000 persons in the U.S. for 1989.

Why are rates useful to public health?

Rates are useful in many ways. Using rates can help health professionals to identify groups in the community with an elevated risk of disease. These **high-risk groups** can be further assessed and targeted for special intervention; the groups can be studied to identify **risk factors** that are related to the occurrence of disease. Individuals can use knowledge of these risk factors to guide their decisions about behaviors that influence health (Centers for Disease Control and Prevention, 1992).

Because rates relate events or cases to a population base, they provide a basis for making valid comparisons of the health events in one population with the same events in another, by taking into consideration the number at risk (the denominator) of experiencing a particular event in each population. For instance, if the number of deaths among adolescents in three different communities were compared, the number of adolescent deaths in each community would probably differ only because the sizes of the populations of 13- to 19-year-olds would vary. The size effect can be removed by converting the number of adolescents to a rate that relies on a standardized denominator during a specified time period, such as per 1,000 or 10,000 adolescents 13 to 19 years of age.

There are three common types of rates. These are:

- crude rates
- specific rates
- adjusted rates

CRUDE RATES

What are crude rates and how are they calculated?

Crude rates are computed for an entire population. They disregard differences that often exist by race, age, gender, or other variables. An example of a crude rate is the **crude birth rate**. This rate is calculated by dividing the total number of births in an area by the total population living in the same area, and then multiplying the quotient by a factor of 10, say 1,000. The crude birth rate in the United States for 1990 was 16.7 live births per 1,000 population (National Center for Health Statistics, 1991) and was 16.2 live births per 1,000 population in 1991 (National Center for Health Statistics, 1992). The crude birth rate for 1992 (based on provisional data) is estimated to be 15.9 live births per 100,000 population (National Center for Health Statistics, 1993b).

The **crude death rate** includes the entire population (approximately 250 million) and is not reflective of any sub-population, such as only females or people aged 20 to 29. The crude death rate for the United States for 1990 was 861.9 deaths per 100,000 population (NCHS, 1991) and 854.0 deaths per 100,000 population in 1991 (NCHS, 1992). The crude death rate for 1992 (based on provisional data) is estimated to remain about the same as the 1991 rate (NCHS, 1993b).

PROBLEM

County X recorded 3,790 births and 1,257 deaths in 1992. The county's population was 183,000. What was the crude birth rate and crude death rate for County X in 1992?

SOLUTION

Crude birth rate = the number of live births in a given time interval divided by the total population living in a defined area

$$\frac{3,790}{183,000} \times 1,000 = 20.7 \text{ births per 1,000 population}$$

Crude death rate = the number of deaths in a given time interval divided by the total population living in a defined area

$$\frac{1,257}{183,000} \times 1,000 = 6.9 \text{ deaths per } 1,000 \text{ population}$$

Barring unusual circumstances such as wars or epidemics, which can cause an unusually high number of deaths, it is reasonable to apply mortality rates to future years for purposes of prediction. This is called **extrapolation.**

PROBLEM

How can you determine the population at risk when you want to calculate a rate?

SOLUTION

Determining the population at risk is not always a simple matter. For example, the number of persons exposed to the risk of dying (the denominator in the formula for calculating the U.S. crude death rate) includes the number of persons alive on January 1 of the particular year of interest plus all persons born in those states during that year, with adjustments made for persons who moved in or out of the U.S. or spent only part of the year in the U.S. A common solution to this complex problem of determining the population at risk is to estimate the population at the midpoint of the interval that the rate covers. For example, for 1992 the population at risk would be the population on July 1, 1992. Because the census is taken only once every 10 years, finding the population for intervening dates becomes a problem. Nevertheless, there are statistical techniques for estimating the population at any given time, provided the census data from recent years are available.

How useful are crude rates when comparing two or more populations?

Crude rates are not helpful when comparing two or more populations. Since populations differ in age distribution over time, especially in the proportion of the population that is elderly (over 64 years of age), and because age is related to death, with elderly people having the highest death rate, we cannot correctly compare the crude death rates until we make the population at risk comparable in age at the various points in time being considered. Manipulation is necessary because a population with a larger percentage of elderly people almost certainly will have a larger number of deaths than a population with a smaller percentage of elderly people, even though the total sizes of the two populations are the same. Obviously, the crude death rate will be higher for the population with the larger percentage of elderly people because elderly people are more likely to die than are younger people.

Therefore, group differences in age may confuse or confound our comparisons of two or more populations. Such confusing characteristics or variables are called **confounding variables.** Similarly, the crude death rate could be high in a country having few elderly people but a very high proportion of infants, who also have a relatively high age-specific death rate. This situation exists in many less-industrialized countries.

COMPARING RATES

How can we use rates to make populations comparable in characteristics such as age?

In order to make two populations comparable in age, we can do a statistical manipulation using various analytical methods to compare rates. In order to avoid having group differences in age confound our comparison of death rates, we must either control for age or adjust for age. In so doing, we are adjusting or controlling for compositional differences in the populations—in this example, for age. Once we have made the populations statistically similar in age, any differences we then observe with respect to death rates will not be due to age.

The overall principle is: If any two or more populations that are being compared differ on any characteristic that is related to the disease or health outcome being considered (in this instance, death) and to the exposure (or potential risk factor or cause), these differences must be taken into account when making comparisons.

If the populations being compared differ on any characteristic that is not related directly or indirectly to the disease or health status being considered, we can generally disregard the differences in this characteristic when making disease comparisons because the comparison being made would not be confounded by irrelevant characteristics. This suggests that in studying a disease or health event, we should know what characteristics, in addition to those being studied, are related to the event. A factor is potentially confounding if it is known to be associated with the outcome variable (effect) and the characteristic of the populations being studied. For example, if we are studying the association between obesity (exposure, cause, risk) and heart disease (effect), a potential confounding factor would be eating saturated fats since it is likely that obese people eat more saturated fats and eating saturated fats is associated with heart disease.

Knowledge about potential confounding variables allows more precision in associating disease (effect) with specific characteristics, unconfounded by other characteristics that are associated with disease but are not of interest in the study. Using available information, we can identify from other studies those factors which have been known to be associated with the health effect you are studying; these are potential confounders.

EFFECT MODIFIERS

What is an effect modifier?

The term **effect modifier** refers to a variable that modifies the effect (disease, outcome) and is often part of the causative network, in an interactive sense. For example, if we find that the risk of a disease is twice as great in obese persons compared with lean persons, then obesity is associated with the disease. But if we later find that this risk is four times greater in obese men than lean men, as compared with twice as great in obese women than lean women, the variable of sex appears to be modifying the effect measure—that is, the association of obesity and disease is different in the two sexes.

Other than age, what factors can modify health events?

As with age, there are other characteristics or variables in nature or the universe that modify many health events, including death. In studying most diseases or health events, these characteristics need to be considered when comparing groups that differ in them. Some characteristics or variables are related to most health happenings and may be considered as "universal" effect modifiers. Age, sex, ethnic group, social class status, marital status, and occupation are examples of such modifiers. That is why these characteristics—especially age, ethnic origin, and sex—are usually taken into account in making epidemiologic comparisons. For example, if there are usually differences in the occurrence of a health event between the sexes, and our two comparison groups differ in their proportions of males and females, then sex differences may confuse our attempts to show a relationship of another characteristic with the health event.

There are also group composition characteristics specifically related to certain diseases, causes of death, or health events. These characteristics must be considered in comparing population rates for only those specific diseases, causes of death, or other health events. These may be called "disease- or health event-specific" control or potentially confounding characteristics (or variables). However, in order for these group composition characteristics to be relevant to epidemiological considerations, they must be indirectly or directly related to the disease or health event being studied.

If we wish, for example, to find out whether height is related to lung cancer, we would have to consider whether short and tall people smoke similar amounts of cigarettes or have similar occupational exposures to cancer-producing agents. We would consider these variables because smoking and certain other exposures are known to be related to lung cancer. Age, sex, and perhaps other universal confounding variables would also have to be considered.

In this example, if we did not consider the cigarette smoking patterns of the two height groups, we might establish a relationship between height and lung cancer that might *not* be due to height but to the difference in the number of cigarettes the tall and short people smoked.

SPECIFIC RATES

How can specific rates be used to control for differences in population composition?

To nullify characteristics that are either directly or indirectly related to a disease or health outcome being considered in different populations, it is necessary to apply statistical manipulations either to control or adjust for these characteristics. The method most commonly used to control for differences in population composition is the calculation of specific rates. **Specific rates** consider the differences among subgroups computed by age, race/ethnicity, gender, or other variables of interest. For example, age-specific rates are often calculated as a basis for determining the rate of events in a particular age group, such as the rate of death among children aged 1 to 14. To calculate an age-specific death rate among children in this age category, divide the number of children in this age group who died by the total number of children in the same age group in the referent population. The resulting quotient is multiplied by a factor of 10.

This procedure was used to generate the rates presented in Table 2.1. These age-specific death rates confirm that death rates for various age categories are not equal to one another. As shown, the death rate for infants is high and that death rates decrease among those 1 to 4 years of age. The rates decrease even further for children 5 to 9 years of age. Hence, the relationship between age and death rate is nonlinear (not a straight line).

The U.S. and other industrialized nations are experiencing the "graying" of the population. More people are living to old age. Table 2.2 shows that as one moves to older age death rates go up. The older one gets, the higher the death rate, with a major increase in death rate starting at age 55.

TABLE 2.1 Age-specific death rates in the United States, first fifteen years of life

		Rate*		
Age	*Total Deaths*	*Both Sexes*	*Male*	*Female*
Under 1 year	38,891	1,032.1	1,152.7	905.8
1-4 years	7,480	52.0	57.9	45.8
5-9 years	4,082	23.6	27.5	19.5
10-14 years	4,706	28.4	36.1	20.3

*Per 100,000 population, 1986

SOURCE: U.S. Department of Health and Human Services: *Vital statistics of the United States*, Volume II, Mortality, Part A. U.S. Public Health Service, National Center for Health Statistics, 1986.

TABLE 2.2 Age-specific death rates in the United States, later years of life

		Rate*		
Age	*Total Deaths*	*Both Sexes*	*Male*	*Female*
50-54 years	68,746	631.3	816.9	457.9
55-59 years	110,323	978.8	1,291.0	695.7
60-64 years	168,706	1,539.1	2,023.8	1,118.0
65-69 years	218,649	2,263.0	2,984.1	1,665.8
70-74 years	266,890	3,479.7	4,661.6	2,601.3
75-79 years	293,520	5,206.1	7,012.9	4,049.9
80-84 years	281,629	8,230.0	10,838.7	6,846.2
85 and older	427,473	15,398.9	18,187.4	14,297.5

*Per 100,000 population, 1986

SOURCE: U.S. Department of Health and Human Services: *Vital statistics of the United States,* Volume II, Mortality, Part A. U.S. Public Health Service, National Center for Health Statistics, 1986.

It is interesting to note that the death rate for all age groups except those between 25 and 44 years of age declined between 1988 and 1989. Death rates for ages 25 to 44 increased. Contributing most to the increase for this age span were deaths due to human immunodeficiency virus (HIV) infection.

ADJUSTED RATES

What are adjusted rates?

Adjusted rates , also known as **standardized rates,** are derived from statistical procedures that adjust for differences in population composition (i.e., age, gender, race) that can increase or decrease the likelihood of death or disease in one or more of the populations under consideration and thereby influence the numerator and the rates. Rates are routinely adjusted for age because age is by far the most important attribute or characteristic related to death and disease.

The age-adjusted death rate for the United States, which eliminates the effects of the aging population, was 515.1 per 100,000 population for 1990 (NCHS, 1991). The age-adjusted death rate in 1991 was 507.9 per 100,000 population, which is the lowest rate ever recorded (NCHS, 1992). Provisional data for 1992 indicates that the age-adjusted death rate may be lower than the 1991 rate (NCHS, 1993b).

What is the "J-shaped" mortality curve?

The diversity of the age patterns of mortality for selected causes of death is illustrated in Figure 2.1, using death rates for 1988, which are similar to

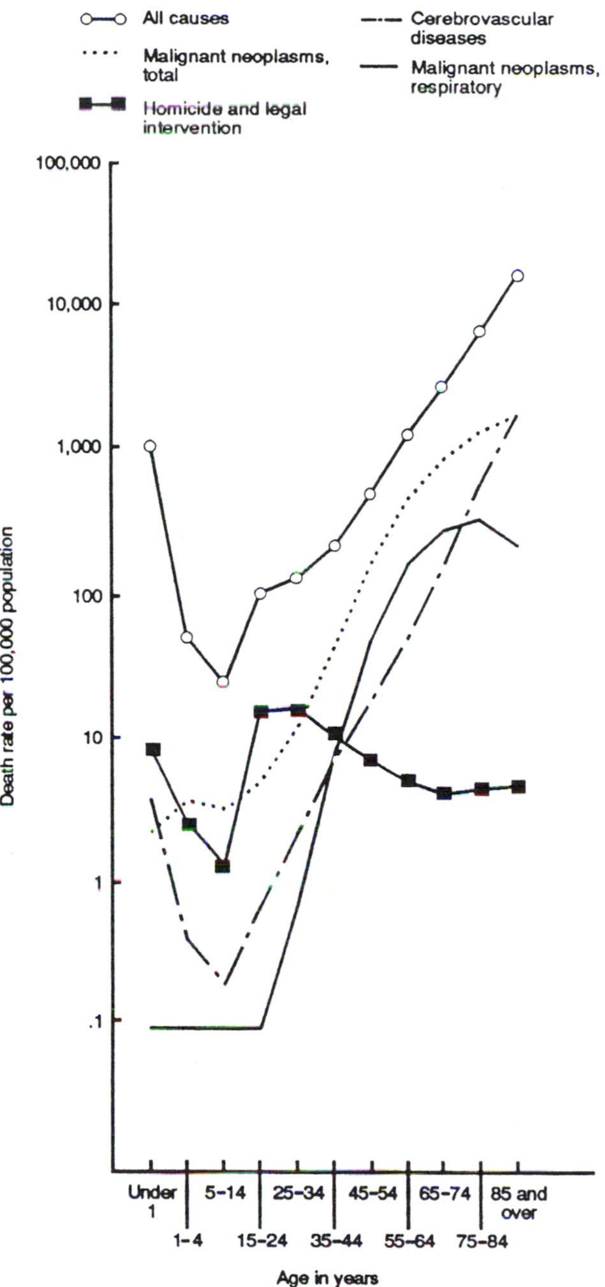

FIGURE 2.1 *Death rates by age for selected causes of death: United States, 1988*

those for other years. For all causes of death combined, the age schedule of mortality shows the well-known "J-shaped" pattern with slightly elevated rates for infants, lowest rates at ages 5 to 14 years, and gradual increases beyond 14 years. This general pattern is characteristic of most "natural" causes of death, in contrast to those caused by external trauma such as accidents, homicides, and suicides, in which the age pattern of mortality reflects predominately social and behavioral factors rather than biological factors related to aging (Rosenberg, Curtin, Maurer, and Offutt, 1992).

METHODS OF RATE ADJUSTMENT

How do we adjust rates to control for differences in characteristics between groups?

Direct Method of Rate Adjustment

The most commonly used method of statistical adjustment for factors such as age is the **direct method of adjustment**. It should be noted that the use of stratification as depicted in Table 2.2 is only one method of controlling for the differences in characteristics between groups being compared. These specific rates (such as age- or sex-specific rates) compare groups who are similar by excluding everyone but a selected group (an age or sex group, for example). In this way, differences that we observe cannot be explained on the basis of the "specific characteristic" since the groups are similar regarding this factor. However, as shown by Table 2.2, comparing specific rates for just two variables (age and sex) was challenging both to one's attention and to one's eyes. Imagine the difficulties involved in making comparisons in a table with four or more variable-specific rates that have to be examined.

To some extent we can avoid these difficulties by using a standard population and examining what would happen if population A's death rates apply. By repeating this process using the same standard population, we can apply population B's rates. The calculated expected rates would be comparable and not influenced by age differences between A and B because we would be using the same standard population. Furthermore, this would give us one adjusted rate to compare for each population instead of several specific rates. The total population as enumerated in 1940 is used as the standard population by the National Center for Health Statistics in the calculation of official U.S. age-adjusted rates (Curtin, 1992; Patterson, 1992).

The process of adjusting rates using the direct method of adjustment is illustrated in the following example. The first step in this example is to calculate the age-specific and the crude death rates for communities A and B and complete Table 2.3. When you have completed Table 2.3, it should resemble Table 2.4. Note that the crude rate in community A is twice as high as that in community B. The age-specific rates, however, are not very different; in the older age groups and in the under-1-year group, B's rates are higher than A's.

It is apparent that the disparity between the comparison of crude rates and age-specific rates is due to the larger percentage of elderly people (over 64 years) in A; 40% of community A, but only 15% of community B, is 65 years of age or older.

It must be stressed that the problem of differences in ages of populations can be avoided by using a standard population. If we use a standard population (the age distribution is standard), we can apply A's age-specific rates and find out how many deaths we would expect in A and then repeat the process for population B. We can use any population we choose to be a standard. We can even use the combined population of A and B.

TABLE 2.3 Calculating crude death rates: Two communities compared

	COMMUNITY A			COMMUNITY B		
Age (years)	*Population*	*Deaths*	*Death Rate (per 1,000)*	*Population*	*Deaths*	*Death Rate (per 1,000)*
Under 1	1,000	15	______	5,000	100	______
1-14	3,000	3	______	20,000	10	______
15-34	6,000	6	______	35,000	35	______
35-54	13,000	52	______	17,000	85	______
55-64	7,000	105	______	8,000	160	______
Over 64	20,000	1,600	______	15,000	1,350	______
Totals	50,000	1,781	______	100,000	1,740	______

SOURCE: From Slome et al., 1986 (p. 19).

TABLE 2.4 Crude death rates: Two communities compared—Results

	COMMUNITY A			COMMUNITY B		
Age (years)	*Population*	*Deaths*	*Death Rate (per 1,000)*	*Population*	*Deaths*	*Death Rate (per 1,000)*
Under 1	1,000	15	15.0	5,000	100	20.0
1-14	3,000	3	1.0	20,000	10	0.5
15-34	6,000	6	1.0	35,000	35	1.0
35-54	13,000	52	4.0	17,000	85	5.0
55-64	7,000	105	15.0	8,000	160	20.0
Over 64	20,000	1,600	80.0	15,000	1,350	90.0
Totals	50,000	1,781	35.6	100,000	1,740	17.4

SOURCE: From Slome et al., 1986 (p. 21).

To continue the process of direct rate adjustment, complete Table 2.5 by writing the age-specific rates for community A in the third column, and for community B in the fifth column (previously calculated in Table 2.3). Calculate for each age category the number of deaths expected in the standard population if A's age-specific death rates apply (write numbers in the fourth column) and again if B's rates apply (sixth column).

Divide the total expected deaths for A and for B by the population in the standard (150,000) to get the age-adjusted rate. The completed table should look like Table 2.6.

Let's work through this process once again. There are 6,000 persons under 1 year of age in the standard population. At A's age-specific death

TABLE 2.5 Standard population by age, calculating age-specific death rates: Two communities (A and B) compared

Age (years)	Standard Population (A and B)	Death Rate in A (per 1,000)	Expected Deaths at A's Rates	Death Rate in B (per 1,000)	Expected Deaths at B's Rates
Under 1	6,000	______	______	______	______
1-14	23,000	______	______	______	______
15-34	41,000	______	______	______	______
35-54	30,000	______	______	______	______
55-64	15,000	______	______	______	______
Over 64	35,000	______	______	______	______
Totals	150,000	______	______	______	______
Age-adjusted death rate		______		______	

SOURCE: From Slome et al., 1986 (p. 21).

TABLE 2.6 Standard population by age, age-specific death rates: Two communities (A and B) compared—Results

Age (years)	Standard Population (A and B)	Death Rate in A (per 1,000)	Expected Deaths at A's Rates	Death Rate in B (per 1,000)	Expected Deaths at B's Rates
Under 1	6,000	15.0	90	20.0	120
1-14	23,000	1.0	23	0.5	11.5
15-34	41,000	1.0	41	1.0	41
35-54	30,000	4.0	120	5.0	150
55-64	15,000	15.0	225	20.0	300
Over 64	35,000	80.0	2,800	90.0	3,150
Totals	150,000	35.6	3,299	17.4	3,772.5
Age-adjusted death rate		22		25	

SOURCE: From Slome et al., 1986 (p. 22).

rate (15 per 1,000), we would expect 90 deaths in this age group. At B's death rate, in this age group we would expect 120 deaths. Adding all of the expected deaths at A's rate yields 3,299 deaths; adding them at B's rate yields 3,772.5 deaths. (The 0.5 death is a statistical reality, not 0.5 of a body!) Dividing each of the expected number of deaths by the standard population (150,000) gives an age-adjusted rate of 22 per 1,000 for A and 25 per 1,000 for B.

In this example we used the direct method to adjust rates for age. As mentioned earlier, rates are routinely adjusted for age because age is by far the most important attribute or characteristic related to death and disease. It may be necessary—and it is possible—to use the direct method to adjust for additional variables, such as race and gender. To adjust for age we need age-specific rates for the populations being studied. A standard population is always available. In our example we used the combined populations as our standard population; some researchers use the U.S. population of a given census year. The world standard population may also be used. Remember, the standard population is used for comparative purposes only. One cannot use two different standard populations in adjusting rates.

How should age-adjusted rates be interpreted?

Next, we discuss the interpretation of the age-adjusted rates. Recall that the crude death rates for communities A and B were 35.6 per 1,000 and 17.4 per 1,000, respectively. It *appeared* that community A had a disproportionate number of deaths than community B. However, noting that community A had a much larger proportion of elderly people than community B, we calculated the age-adjusted death rates for each community—22 per 1,000 for A and 25 per 1,000 for B. The age-adjusted death rates are fairly similar; in fact, the rate is slightly higher in community B. The difference between the adjusted rates of 22 and 25 cannot be due to age differences in the two populations since we have adjusted (or controlled statistically) for age. The difference may reflect an actual difference in death rates in the two populations, or it may be due to some other confounding factor or variable (such as gender or race) for which we have not adjusted.

Indirect Method of Rate Adjustment

Is there another method of rate adjustment?

The other method of adjustment that we will consider is the reverse of the direct method. Instead of using a standard population and specific rates from the comparison populations, we use standard rates and apply them to our comparison populations. This is called the **indirect method** of rate adjustment.

Let us work through another example to learn how to apply the indirect method in rate adjustment. We begin by calculating the expected number of deaths in community A, if the standard rates apply (we are using B's rates as standard), to complete Table 2.7.

In Table 2.3 there were 1,781 deaths observed (called O) in community A. This compares to 2,032.5 expected deaths (called E) in community A (see Table 2.8).

TABLE 2.7 Population and expected deaths in Community A by age, and standard rates of age

Age (years)	*Population in "A"*	*Standard Death Rate (per 1,000)*	*Expected Deaths in "A" at Standard Rates*
Under 1	1,000	20.0	________
1-14	3,000	0.5	________
15-34	6,000	1.0	________
35-54	13,000	5.0	________
55-64	7,000	20.0	________
Over 64	20,000	90.0	________
Totals	50,000	17.4	________

SOURCE: From Slome et al., 1986 (p. 24).

TABLE 2.8 Population and expected deaths in Community A by age, and standard rates of age—Results

Age (years)	*Population in "A"*	*Expected Deaths in "A" at Standard Rates*
Under 1	1,000	20.0
1-14	3,000	1.5
15-34	6,000	6.0
35-54	13,000	65.0
55-64	7,000	140.0
Over 64	20,000	1,800.0
Totals	50,000	2,032.5

SOURCE: From Slome et al., 1986 (p. 25).

Compare the number of deaths observed (O) in community A with the number expected (E) by calculating the **Standardized Mortality Ratio** (SMR), the ratio of observed deaths in community A to expected deaths in A (O/E). By way of review, the 20 expected deaths for the under-1-year age category is obtained by multiplying 1,000 × 20/1,000, and the 1.5 expected deaths for young people 1 to 14 years of age is obtained by multiplying 3,000 × 0.5/1,000.

The expected (E) number of deaths in community A at standard rates is 2,032.5. Hence, the SMR for community A is 1,781/2,032.5 = 0.876, or 88%. Thus, A has fewer deaths than expected, if we assume that community B's age-specific death rates apply in community A.

To use the indirect method to compare two populations, calculate an SMR for each population and compare the two. The SMR for community A is 0.876. The SMR for community B will be 1.00, since the standard rates are the age-specific death rates for community B. In comparing 0.876 to 1.00, the death rate (adjusted for age) is slightly lower in community A.

Summary of Rate Adjustment

It is important to understand age adjustment, a basic statistical technique often used in epidemiology. Some important points to remember about this technique are:

1. Age-adjusted rates, using either method, permit a comparison of rates while controlling any confounding due to age. To see the association of age with death or the effect being studied, compare the age-specific rates.

2. **Adjusted rates** are not rates that describe an actual occurrence, but hypothetical rates that would occur given certain assumptions.

3. Age adjustment provides one rate per population to compare and is preferable to several age-specific comparisons.

4. The direct method of age adjustment uses a standard population and applies the age-specific rates of the populations being compared in order to determine the expected number of events (deaths) in the standard population. This method requires that the age-specific rates be available for each of the populations to be compared and that they be based on numbers that are not too small (a general guideline is at least five deaths or events per age category).

5. The indirect method of age adjustment is used if the number of observed deaths or events per age category is small or if age-specific rates are not available. With this method standard rates are applied to the populations being compared in order to calculate the expected number of deaths. The ratio of the observed number of events to the expected number of events is called a **standardized** (we have used standard rates) **mortality** (or morbidity if sickness, not death, is being studied) **ratio**, or **SMR**.

INFANT AND MATERNAL MORTALITY RATES

What are some other important death rates in epidemiology?

Infant mortality rates are the most commonly used rates for measuring the risk of dying during the first year of life. These rates are some of the most frequently used measures for comparing health services among nations. High infant mortality rates are a reflection of poor economic conditions, unmet health care needs, and other unfavorable environmental factors. They are calculated by dividing the number of infant deaths in a calendar year by the number of live births registered for the same time period. Infant mortality rates are presented as rates per 1,000 or per 100,000 live births.

In 1991, there were 36,500 deaths of infants under 1 year of age compared to 39,655 in 1989. The infant mortality rate for the United States

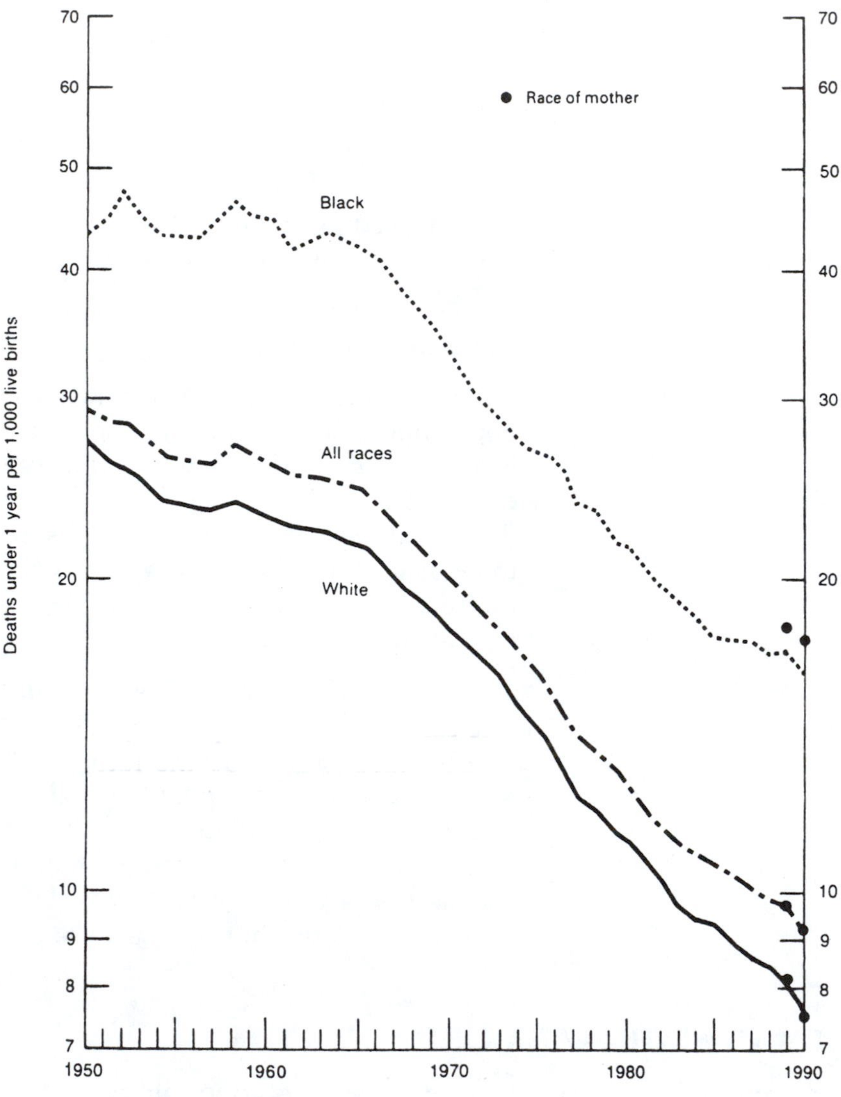

NOTE: Infant deaths are classified by race of decendent. Beginning in 1989, live births are classified by race of mother; from 1950 to 1989, by race of child.

SOURCE: Advance report of final mortality statistics, 1990. National Center for Health Statistics. *Monthly Vital Statistics Report*. 1993:41(7).

FIGURE 2.2 *Infant mortality rates by race: United States, 1950–90*

in 1991 was 8.9 infant deaths per 1,000 live births. The 1991 infant mortality rate was the lowest infant mortality rate ever recorded for the United States, and provisional data from 1992 has been used to estimate an infant mortality rate of 8.5 for that year. The infant mortality rate for black infants is nearly 2.4 times the rate for white infants. The infant mortality rate for Hispanic infants is about 8% higher than for non-Hispanic white infants (National Center for Health Statistics, 1993a). Figure 2.2 shows how infant mortality rates have declined for black and white infants in the past 40 years.

Neonatal mortality rates are an index of the risk of dying in the first 28 days of life. The numerator is the number of deaths in one year for children younger than 28 days of age. The denominator is the number of live births in the same year. In 1990, the neonatal mortality rate for the U.S. was 5.8 deaths per 1,000 live births. Between 1989 and 1990, the neonatal mortality rate declined from 6.2 to 5.8 deaths for infants under 28 days old per 1,000 live births.

The **postneonatal mortality rate** is an index of the risk of death in infants aged 28 days to 11 months. The numerator is the number of deaths in one year for children 28 days old through the age of 11 months. The denominator is the number of live births in the same year. The postneonatal mortality rate in 1990 was 3.4 per 1,000 live births. The rate in 1989 was 3.6 for the fourth consecutive year.

Another important death rate is the **maternal mortality rate.** The numerator is expressed as the number of deaths in a year from puerperal causes (complications of pregnancy, childbirth, and the puerperium). The denominator is the number of live births in the same year. Notice that the denominator does not include all pregnancies, but is the number of live births. Because there is no system for gathering information regarding all pregnancies, the closest useful measure is the number of live births. Because maternal mortality is much less common than infant mortality, the maternal mortality rate is usually expressed per 100,000 live births. From the early 1960s to the present, the U.S. maternal mortality rate has decreased markedly. In 1960 the rate was 37.1; in 1990, the rate had declined to 8.3 maternal deaths per 100,000 live births.

OTHER MORTALITY MEASURES USED IN EPIDEMIOLOGY[1]

Death-to-Case Ratio

The **death-to-case ratio** is the number of deaths attributed to a particular disease during a specified time period divided by the number of new cases of that disease identified during the same time period:

---

[1]This section is adapted from Centers for Disease Controland Prevention, *Principles of epidemiology: An introduction to applied epidemiology and biostatistics 2d ed*. Atlanta, GA: Centers for Disease Control and Prevention, 1992.

Death-to-case ratio =

$$\frac{\text{number of deaths of particular disease during specified period}}{\text{number of new cases of the disease identified during same period}} \times 10^n$$

The figures used for the numerator and denominator must apply to the same population. The death figures in the numerator are not necessarily included in the denominator, however, because some of the deaths may have occurred in persons who developed the disease before the specified period.

For example, in 1987, there were 22,157 new cases of tuberculosis reported in the United States. During the same year, 1,755 deaths occurred that were attributed to tuberculosis. Presumably, many of the deaths occurred in persons who had initially contracted tuberculosis years earlier. Thus, many of the 1,755 deaths in the numerator are not among the 22,517 new cases in the denominator. Therefore, the death-to-case ratio is a ratio but not a proportion. The tuberculosis death-to-case ratio for 1987 is:

$$\frac{1{,}755}{22{,}517} \times 10^n$$

The number of deaths per 100 cases can be calculated by dividing the numerator by the denominator (10^n = 100 for this calculation):

$$1{,}755/22{,}517 \times 100 = 7.8 \text{ deaths per 100 new cases}$$

Alternatively, the number of cases per death can be calculated by dividing the denominator by the numerator (10^n = 1 for this calculation):

$$22{,}517/1{,}755 = 12.8$$

Therefore, there was 1 death per 12.8 new cases. It is correct to use either expression of this ratio.

PROBLEM

In 1980-1989 there were 3 diphtheria-associated deaths in the United States and 27 new cases of diphtheria (Centers for Disease Control, 1989). How does the death-to-case ratio (per 100 new cases) differ from 1970-1979 (1,956 new cases and 90 deaths) and 1960-1969 (3,679 new cases and 390 deaths).

SOLUTION

The death-to-case ratio in 1980-1989 was 3/27 × 100 or 11.11 per 1,000. The death-to-case ratio in 1970-1979 was 90/1,956 × 100 = 4.60. The ratio in 1960-1969 was 390/3,679 × 100 = 10.60 per 100. Thus, the death-to-case ratio has fluctuated over the past 30 years.

Case-Fatality Rate

The **case-fatality rate** is the proportion of persons who die from a particular condition (cases). The formula is:

$$\text{Case-fatality rate} = \frac{\text{number of cause-specific deaths among the incident cases}}{\text{number of incident cases}} \times 10^n$$

Unlike the death-to-case ratio, which is simply the ratio of cause-specific deaths to cases during a specified time, the case-fatality rate is a proportion and requires that the deaths in the numerator be limited to the cases in the denominator. Thus, if 11 newborns were to develop listeriosis and 2 of these newborns died as a result, the case-fatality rate would be:

$$\text{Case-fatality rate} = 2 \text{ deaths}/11 \text{ cases} = 18.2\%$$

Proportionate Mortality

Proportionate mortality describes the proportion of deaths attributable to different causes in a specified population over a period of time. Each cause is expressed as a percentage of all deaths, and the sum of the causes must add to 100%. These proportions are not mortality rates, since the denominator is all deaths, not the population in which the deaths occurred. For a specified population over a specified period,

$$\text{Proportionate mortality} = \frac{\text{deaths due to a particular cause}}{\text{deaths from all causes}} \times 100$$

Table 2.9 shows the distribution of primary causes of death in the United States in 1987. The data are grouped into two age groups. The first group includes persons of all ages, and the second group includes only persons 25 to 44 years old. For the first group, the number of deaths, proportionate mortality (indicated as a percentage), and rank value for each cause of death are listed.

In Table 2.9 we find that cerebrovascular disease was the third leading cause of death among the population as a whole ("all ages"), with a proportionate mortality of 7.1%. Among 25- to 44-year-olds, however, cerebrovascular disease accounted for only 2.6% of the deaths.

Sometimes we compare the proportionate mortality in one age group or occupational group to the entire population, either for deaths from all causes or from a specific cause. The resulting ratio is called a **proportionate mortality ratio**, or **PMR**.

PROBLEM

Using the data in Table 2.9, calculate the missing proportionate mortalities (PMR) and ranks for persons aged 25 to 44 years.

TABLE 2.9 Distribution of primary causes of death, all ages, and ages 25 to 44 years, United States, 1987

	All Ages			*Ages 25 to 44 Years*		
Cause	*Number*	*Percent*	*Rank*	*Number*	*Percent*	*Rank*
Heart disease	760,353	35.8	1	15,874	____	____
Cancer	476,927	22.5	2	20,305	____	____
Cerebrovascular disease	149,835	7.1	3	3,377	2.6	8
Accidents, adverse effects	95,020	4.5	4	27.484	____	____
Chronic pulmonary disease	78,380	3.7	5	897	0.7	<10
Pneumonia & influenza	69,225	3.3	6	1,936	1.5	9
Diabetes mellitus	38,532	1.8	7	1,821	1.4	10
Suicide	30,796	1.5	8	11,787	____	____
Chronic liver disease	26,201	1.2	9	4,562	3.5	7
Atherosclerosis	22,474	1.1	10	53	<0.1	<10
Homicide	21,103	1.0	<10	10,268	____	____
HIV infection	13,468	0.6	<10	9,820	____	____
All other	341,009	16.1	—	22,980	17.5	—
Totals (all causes)	2,123,323	100.0		131,164	100.0	

SOURCE: From National Center for Health Statistics, 1990, as cited in CDC, 1992.

SOLUTION

Heart disease, PMR = 12.1%; rank is 3rd.
Cancer, PMR = 15.5%; rank is 2nd.
Accidents, PMR = 21.0%; rank is 1st.
Suicide, PMR = 9.0%; rank is 4th.
Homicide, PMR = 7.8%; rank is 5th.
HIV infection, PMR = 7.5%; rank is 6th.

Years of Potential Life Lost

Years of Potential Life Lost (YPLL) is a measure of the impact of premature mortality on a population. It is calculated as the sum of the differences between a predetermined end point and the ages of death for those who died before that end point. The two most commonly used end points are age 65 and average life expectancy. Because of the way in which YPLL is calculated, this measure gives more weight to early deaths.

The **Years of Potential Life Lost Rate** represents years of potential life lost per 1,000 population below the age of 65 years (or below average life expectancy). YPLL rates should be used to compare premature mortality

TABLE 2.10 Frequently used measures of natality

Measure	*Numerator (x)*	*Denominator (y)*	*Expressed per Number at Risk (10^n)*
Crude birth rate	# live births reported during a given time interval	Estimated total population at mid-interval	1,000
Crude fertility rate	# live births reported during a given time interval	Estimated number of women aged 15–44 years at mid-interval	1,000
Crude rate of natural increase	# live births minus # deaths during a given time interval	Estimated total population at mid-interval	1,000
Low birth weight ratio	# live births under 2,500 grams during a given time interval	# live births reported during the same time interval	100

SOURCE: CDC, 1992.

in different populations since YPLL does not account for differences in population sizes.

NATALITY AND MORBIDITY RATES

In addition to mortality rates, rates dealing with natality (birth) and morbidity (illness and injury) are valuable epidemiologic tools. Prevalence rates are discussed in the following section and incidence rates are covered in Chapter 3. Natality rates are especially useful in the area of maternal and child health. Table 2.10 shows a summary of some frequently used measures of natality.

CHAPTER SUMMARY

The basic tools of epidemiology are the rates that can be used to describe the distribution and determinants of health events in groups of people rather than individuals. Methods for calculating common types of mortality rates have been presented in this chapter. In addition, this chapter provided a detailed explanation of the need to adjust rates for confounding variables and how to calculate such adjustments. We also introduced commonly used mortality measures—proportionate mortality, case-fatality rate, death-to-case ratios, years of potential life lost, and years of potential life lost rate. Morbidity and natality rates were also introduced.

The rates and rate adjustment methods covered in Chapter 2 are fundamental to the practice of epidemiology. It is essential to understand the following points before proceeding to the next chapter:

1. General form and definition of rates
2. Key points about how to examine and interpret rates in tables
3. Purposes of calculating rates
4. Calculation, interpretation, and limitations of crude rates
5. Calculation and interpretation of characteristic-specific rates (such as age/sex-specific death rates) and their relevance in comparing health experiences of groups
6. Controlling for the effects of confounding characteristics such as age in making group comparisons either through control tables or adjustment

KEY TERMS

rate
mortality rate
morbidity rate
numerator
denominator
high-risk group
risk factors
crude rates
crude birth rate
crude death rate
extrapolation
confounding variables
effect modifier
specific rate
adjusted or standardized rate
direct method of rate adjustment
indirect method of rate adjustment
standardized mortality ratio
infant mortality rate
neonatal mortality rate
postneonatal mortality rate
maternal mortality rate
death-to-case ratio
case-fatality rate
proportionate mortality
proportionate mortality ratio
years of potential life lost (YPLL)
years of potential life lost rate

REFERENCES

Centers for Disease Control: Summary of notifiable diseases, United States 1989. *Morbidity and Mortality Weekly Report* 1989;38(54).

Centers for Disease Control and Prevention: *Principles of epidemiology: An introduction to applied epidemiology and biostatistics, 2d ed.* Atlanta, GA: CDC, 1992.

Curtin LR: A short history of standardization for vital events. In M Feinleib, AO Zarate (Eds.), Reconsidering adjustment procedures, *Vital and Health Statistics*. DHHS Publication No. (PHS) 93-1466, Series 4(29):11-28, 1992.

National Center for Health Statistics: Annual summary of births, marriages, divorces, and deaths: United States, 1990. *Monthly Vital Statistics Report*, 1991;39(13):August 28.

National Center for Health Statistics: Annual summary of births, marriages, divorces, and deaths: United States, 1991. *Monthly Vital Statistics Report*, 1992;40(13):September 30.

National Center for Health Statistics: Advance report of final mortality statistics, 1990. *Monthly Vital Statistics Report*, 1993a;41(7):January 7.

National Center for Health Statistics: Births, marriages, divorces, and deaths for 1992. *Monthly Vital Statistics Report*, 1993b;41(12):May 19.

Patterson JE: Age adjustment in National Center for Health Statistics mortality data: Implications of a change in procedure. In M Feinleib, AO Zarate (Eds.), Reconsidering adjustment procedures, *Vital and Health Statistics*. DHHS Publication No. (PHS) 93-1466, Series 4(29):71-72, 1992.

Rosenberg HM, Curtin LR, Maurer J, Offutt K: Choosing a standard population: Some statistical considerations. In M Feinleib, AO Zarate (Eds.), Reconsidering adjustment procedures, *Vital and Health Statistics*. DHHS Publication No. (PHS) 93-1466, Series 4(29):29-67, 1992.

Slome C, Brogan D, Eyres S, Lednar W: *Basic epidemiological methods and biostatistics: A workbook*. Boston: Jones and Bartlett, 1986. Figures and tables used with permission.

PROBLEMS

1. Using the information in the following table, calculate the crude death rates, age-specific death rates, and adjusted death rates for Populations X and Y. Use the direct approach for age-adjusted rate calculation.

Age	Population (X)	Deaths (X)	Age-specific Death Rate in X per 1,000	Population (Y)	Deaths (Y)	Age-specific Death Rate in Y per 1,000
<5	20,000	200		20,000	250	
5-14	10,000	20		20,000	25	
15-24	10,000	50		30,000	200	
25-34	10,000	25		20,000	75	
35-44	25,000	100		10,000	35	
45-64	25,000	200		10,000	350	
65+	50,000	4,000		10,000	450	
	150,000			120,000		

2. Waterville County vital statistics records indicated that there were 3,790 live births in 1992, compared to 3,334 live births in 1990. In 1992 there were 10 more neonatal deaths and 17 more infant deaths than in 1990. In 1990 there were 70 neonatal deaths and 80 infant deaths. Calculate neonatal and infant mortality rates (per 1,000) for Waterville County for 1990 and 1992.

3. Use the following standard death rates to calculate standardized mortality ratios (SMRs) for Green City and Red City. How do standardized mortality ratios compare to crude death rates for Green City and Red City? There were 4,050 deaths in Green City and 30,025 deaths in Red City.

Age	Standard Death Rates	Population Green City	Expected Deaths Green City	Population Red City	Expected Deaths Red City
<1	15.0	6,000		50,000	
1-4	1.0	7,000		75,000	
5-14	2.0	7,000		25,000	
15-24	1.5	7,000		30,000	
25-34	1.0	10,000		70,000	
35-44	2.5	10,000		25,000	
45-54	8.0	13,000		20,000	
55-64	10.0	15,000		20,000	
65+	60.0	25,000		20,000	
		100,000		335,000	

4. Rates are adjusted (standardized) to:

   a. remove the bias of dissimilar age group distribution between populations

b. minimize the health problems of a community as compared with a standard
c. determine how well a community compares with acceptable national birth, death, and disease rate standards
d. allows valid comparisons between populations with similar age distributions but different race and sex makeup
e. "b" or "d" above

5. Multiplying the age-specific death rate of a population of interest by the number of persons in the standard age group and dividing by 1,000 yields:

   a. age-specific death rate of the standard population
   b. index death rate
   c. expected deaths in the standard population
   d. adjusting factor
   e. adjusted rate for the population of interest

6. If the population of a standard age group is 2,700 and the death rate for a study population age group is 1.4 per 1,000, the number of expected deaths for this age group is approximately:

   a. 2
   b. 4
   c. 38
   d. 193
   e. none of the above

7. Of the following mortality rates, which use the same denominator? (Circle all that apply)

   a. infant mortality rate
   b. neonatal mortality rate
   c. postneonatal mortality rate
   d. maternal mortality rate

8. Use the following data for Community A and Community B to calculate crude death rates and age-adjusted death rates for the two communities.

Age	*Population in Community A*	*Deaths in Community A*	*Population in Community B*	*Deaths in Community B*
Under 1	1,000	15	5,000	100
1-14	3,000	3	20,000	10
15-34	6,000	6	35,000	35
35-54	13,000	52	17,000	85
55-64	7,000	105	8,000	160
65+	20,000	1,600	15,000	1,350

9. A total of 2,121,323 deaths were recorded in the United States in 1987. The mid-year population was estimated to be 243,401,000. HIV-related mortality and population data by age for all residents and for black males are shown in Table 2.11. Use these data to calculate the following four mortality rates:

a. Crude mortality rate
b. HIV-(cause)-specific mortality rate for the entire population
c. HIV-specific mortality among all 35- to 44-year-olds
d. HIV-specific mortality among 35- to 44-year-old black males

TABLE 2.11 HIV mortality and estimated population by age group overall and for black males, United States, 1987

	All Races, All Ages		*Black Males*	
Age Group (years)	*HIV Deaths*	*Population (× 1,000)*	*HIV Deaths*	*Population (× 1,000)*
0-4	191	18,252	47	1,393
5-14	47	34,146	7	2,697
15-24	492	38,252	145	2,740
25-34	5,026	43,315	1,326	2,549
35-44	4,794	34,305	1,212	1,663
45-54	1,838	23,276	395	1,117
≥55	1,077	51,855	168	1,945
Unknown	3		1	
Totals	13,468	243,401	3,301	14,104

SOURCE: From National Center for Health Statistics, 1990, as cited in CDC, 1992.

10. Using the data in Table 2.9 (see page 68), calculate the ratio of homicide proportionate mortality among 25- to 44-year-olds to the homicide proportionate mortality among all ages.

ANSWERS

1. The crude death rate for population X is 4,595/150,000 × 1,000 or 30.6. The crude death rate for population Y is 1,385/120,000 × 1,000 or 11.5.

   The following table shows the age-specific death rates for populations X and Y.

Age	Population in X	Deaths (X)	Age-specific Death Rate in X per 1,000	Population in Y	Deaths (Y)	Age-specific Death Rate in Y per 1,000
<5	20,000	200	10.0	20,000	250	12.5
5-14	10,000	20	2.0	20,000	25	1.25
15-24	10,000	50	5.0	30,000	200	6.66
25-34	10,000	25	2.5	20,000	75	3.75
35-44	25,000	100	4.0	10,000	35	3.5
45-64	25,000	200	8.0	10,000	350	35.0
65+	50,000	4,000	80.0	10,000	450	45.0
Totals	150,000	4,595		120,000	1,385	

   Combine populations X and Y to create a standard population. Then apply the age-specific rates for each age group to determine the expected death rates as shown below.

Age	Standard Population (X and Y)	Death Rate in X per 1,000	Expected Deaths at X's Rate	Death Rate in Y per 1,000	Expected Deaths at Y's Rate
<5	40,000	10.0	400	12.5	500
5-14	30,000	2.0	60	1.25	37.5
15-24	40,000	5.0	200	6.66	266.4
25-34	30,000	2.5	75	3.75	112.5
35-44	35,000	4.0	140	3.5	122.5
45-64	35,000	8.0	280	35.0	1,225
65+	60,000	80.0	4,800	45.0	2,700
Totals	270,000		5,955		4,963.9

   To calculate the age-adjusted death rate for population X, divide the total expected deaths for X (5,955) by the total population in the standard population (270,000). Then multiply by 1,000. This gives the age-adjusted death rate for population X, which is 22.0 per 1,000.

   To calculate the age-adjusted death rate for population Y, divide the total expected deaths for Y (4,963.9) by the total population in the standard population (270,000). Once again, multiply by 1,000. The age-adjusted death rate for Y is 18.4 per 1,000.

2. The infant mortality rate for 1990 was 80/3,334 × 1,000 = 24.0 per 1,000 live births. The neonatal mortality rate for 1990 was 70/3,334 × 1,000 = 21.0 per 1,000 live births.

The infant mortality rate for 1992 was 97/3,790 × 1,000 = 25.6 per 1,000 live births. The neonatal mortality rate for 1992 was 80/3,790 = 21.1 per 1,000 live births.

3. The crude death rate for Green City is 4,050/100,000 × 1,000 or 40.5 per 1,000. The crude death rate for Red City is 30,025/335,000 × 1,000, or 89.6 per 1,000.

   The following table shows the expected deaths in Green City and Red City at the Standard Death Rates. The total expected death rates in the two cities can then be used to calculate standardized mortality rates.

Age	*Standard Death Rates*	*Population in Green City*	*Expected Deaths in Green City*	*Population in Red City*	*Expected Deaths in Red City*
<1	15.0	6,000	*90*	50,000	*750*
1-4	1.0	7,000	*7*	75,000	*75*
5-14	2.0	7,000	*14*	25,000	*50*
15-24	1.5	7,000	*10.5*	30,000	*45*
25-34	1.0	10,000	*10*	70,000	*70*
35-44	2.5	10,000	*25*	25,000	*62.5*
45-54	8.0	13,000	*104*	20,000	*160*
55-64	10.0	15,000	*150*	20,000	*200*
65+	60.0	25,000	*1,500*	20,000	*1,200*
Total		100,000	*1,910.5*	335,000	*2,612.5*

The standardized mortality ratio (observed deaths divided by expected deaths) for Green City is 4,050/1,910.5, or 2.1. The standardized mortality ratio for Red City is 30,025/2,612.5 or 11.5. Therefore, Red City has a higher death rate (more deaths are observed than were expected) than Green City. The higher crude death rate in Green City reflects the fact that there is a higher proportion of elderly people in Green City than in Red City. Yet, the higher standardized mortality ratio in Red City indicates that this city experiences more deaths among all age groups.

4. The correct answer is a, remove the bias of dissimilar age group distribution between populations.

5. The correct answer is c, expected deaths in the standard population.

6. The correct answer is c, 38 expected deaths.

7. a, b, c, and d all have the same denominator, the number of live births during a specified time period.

8. The crude death rate for Community A is 1,781/50,000 × 1,000 = 35.6 per 1,000. The crude death rate for Community B is 1,740/100,000 × 1,000 = 17.4 per 1,000.

Age	*Population in Community A*	*Deaths in Community A*	*Population in Community B*	*Deaths in Community B*
Under 1	1,000	15	5,000	100
1-14	3,000	3	20,000	10
15-34	6,000	6	35,000	35
35-54	13,000	52	17,000	85
55-64	7,000	105	8,000	160
65+	20,000	1,600	15,000	1,350
Totals	50,000	1,781	100,000	1,740

The information in the table above can be used to calculate age-specific and expected death rates for the two communities. When using the direct method of rate adjustment, we can combine the two populations to create a standard population.

Age	*Standard Population (A and B)*	*Death Rate in A per 1,000*	*Expected Deaths at A's Rate*	*Death Rate in B per 1,000*	*Expected Deaths at at B's Rate*
<1	6,000	15.0	*90*	200	*120*
1-14	23,000	1.0	*23*	0.5	*11.5*
15-34	41,000	1.0	*41*	1.0	*41*
35-54	30,000	4.0	*120*	5.0	*150*
55-64	15,000	15.0	225	20.0	*300*
65+	35,000	80.0	*2,800*	90.0	*3,150*
Totals	150,000		*3,299*		*3,772.5*

The age-adjusted death rate for Community A is 3,299/150,000 × 1,000, or 22.0 deaths per 1,000. The age-adjusted death rate for Community B is 3,772.5/150,000 × 1,000, or 25.1 deaths per 1,000.

Community B had a lower crude death rate than Community A; yet when age was controlled (adjusted for), Community B had a higher death rate. Community A had a higher proportion of elderly people than did Community B.

9. a. Crude mortality rate for 1987 was 2,121,323/243,401,000 × 100,000 = 872.4 deaths per 100,000.
   b. HIV-(cause)-specific mortality rate for the entire population is calculated by dividing the number of HIV deaths by the number in the total population × 10^n. Therefore, 13,468/243,401,000 × 100,000 = 5.5 HIV-related deaths per 100,000 population.
   c. HIV-specific mortality rate among 35- to 44-year-olds is calculated by dividing the number of HIV deaths in 35- to 44-year-olds by the population of 35- to 44-year-olds × 10^n. Therefore, 4,794/34,305,000 × 100,000 = 14.0 HIV-related deaths per 100,000 35- to 44-year-olds.
   d. HIV-related mortality rate among 35- to 44-year-old black males is calculated by dividing the number of HIV deaths in 35- to 44-year-old black males by the number in the population of 35- to 44-year-old black males × 10^n. Therefore, 1,212/1,663,000 × 100,000 = 72.9.

10. $$\frac{\text{Homicide proportionate mortality among 25- to 44-year-olds}}{\text{Homicide proportionate mortality among all ages}}$$

is calculated by:

$$\frac{\text{Number of homicide deaths in 25- to 44-year-olds/all deaths in 25- to 44-year-olds}}{\text{Number of homicide deaths, all ages/all deaths for all ages}}$$

Therefore:

$$\frac{10{,}268/131{,}164}{21{,}103/2{,}123{,}323} = \frac{.078}{.010} = 7.8 \text{ to } 1$$

REVIEW QUESTIONS—CHAPTERS 1 AND 2

1. What is epidemiology and what is its purpose in community and public health?
2. To what type of health events has epidemiology been applied in recent years?
3. Describe the uses of epidemiology in terms of community health assessment, individual decisions, and clinical medicine.
4. What are mortality and morbidity rates?
5. Discuss what is represented in the numerator and the denominator of epidemiologic rates.
6. What is the purpose of expressing health events as rates?
7. How do crude rates differ from age-specific and age-adjusted rates?
8. What are confounding variables? How can the presence of confounding variables make comparisons between two or more populations inappropriate?
9. What does the term "effect modifier" mean?
10. What are some group composition characteristics associated with certain health events, such as particular diseases or death?
11. What does it mean to say that the relationship between age and death rate is nonlinear?
12. In what age group have death rates recently increased? What seems to account for this increase?
13. How does the direct method for adjusting rates differ from the indirect method?
14. What is the standard population used by the National Center for Health Statistics in the calculation of official U.S. vital statistics?
15. What is the Standardized Mortality Ratio? How is it calculated?
16. Differentiate between infant mortality rate, neonatal mortality rate, and postneonatal mortality rate.
17. What is used as the denominator in the calculation of maternal mortality rate? Why is this particular measure used in the denominator?

3 Epidemiologic Research

OBJECTIVES

On completion of this chapter, you will be able to:

- Recognize the usefulness and relative advantages and limitations of cross-sectional, case-control, cohort, and experimental studies in epidemiology
- Provide examples of cross-sectional, case-control, cohort, and experimental study methods
- Explain how the Behavioral Risk Factor Survey is conducted
- List advantages and disadvantages of telephone surveys
- List factors in epidemiologic studies that can potentially lead to bias
- Recognize why it is not possible to establish antecedent-consequent relationships from cross-sectional and case-control studies
- Calculate incidence rates, incidence density, and cumulative incidence and list factors which influence incidence
- Interpret the meaning of relative risk, attributable risk, and population attributable risk from prospective epidemiologic data
- Describe what a historical cohort study is
- Discuss ethical considerations in experimental studies
- Describe the concept of internal validity
- Describe how random allocation of subjects is accomplished
- Discuss the importance of the element of control in experimental epidemiologic studies
- State what placebo effect is
- Identify what a clinical trial is
- Define quasi-experimental

Epidemiologic research is concerned with the search for causes and effects, the *why* and the *how*. Epidemiologic research can be used to quantify the association between exposures and outcomes and to test hypotheses about causal relationships. Findings from epidemiologic research often provide evidence for appropriate disease control and prevention measures (CDC, 1992).

In this chapter we review the four major types of epidemiologic research studies:

- Cross-sectional
- Case-control
- Cohort
- Experimental

CROSS-SECTIONAL STUDIES

Cross-sectional epidemiology is a way of describing the distributions (or frequency of distributions) of health characteristics in populations and the associations of health characteristics with other variables. This type of study allows us to determine which groups of people experience more or less of certain disorders, vital events (e.g., births, deaths), or health behaviors of interest. By identifying groups of people at highest risk of acquiring a particular health condition, cross-sectional epidemiologic studies provide important clues to the causes of diseases and other health conditions.

Paffenbarger (1988) describes cross-sectional studies as "snapshot" studies. This type of study might be compared to a still photograph because it describes particular groups of people at a single hypothetical point in time.

What is the value of the cross-sectional method in epidemiology?

Cross-sectional epidemiologic studies cannot tell *why* any observed health differentials exist, but are valuable in indicating that such differentials in health events exist. Rather than determine actual causes of disease, cross-sectional studies generate hypotheses about the causes of disease. The hypotheses generated from cross-sectional studies often provide foundations for future epidemiologic research studies which seek to delineate specific cause-and-effect relationships.

Data generated from cross-sectional studies can be used by health planners and administrators to initiate and evaluate effective health services and programs. For example, knowing the number of people with a certain health condition can suggest the number of hospital beds, clinics, health care providers, and medications that a geographic area may need.

EXAMPLE

Cross-sectional Surveys: The National Health and Nutrition Examination Surveys

The National Health and Nutrition Examination Survey (NHANES) provides a classic example of a nationally representative cross-sectional survey. NHANES includes data from in-person interviews and medical examinations. The third National Health and Nutrition Examination Survey (NHANES III) began in 1988 and will be completed in 1994. The first NHANES began in 1960. These surveys allow for current estimates of prevalence for health parameters such as lipoprotein levels and trends in the prevalence of parameters. For example, studies by Sempos et al. (1993) and Johnson et al. (1993) describe the prevalence of high blood cholesterol during various phases of the Health and Nutrition Examination Survey and the declining trends in serum total cholesterol levels among U.S. adults.

Why are cross-sectional studies sometimes referred to as "snapshot" studies?

Cross-sectional studies can be compared to a "snapshot" or still photograph because they provide a cross-sectional observation at a single hypothetical point in time. A "snapshot" study describes the prevalence of health events at a particular point in time.

In a cross-sectional study, each subject is assessed only once at one point in time. Theoretically, a cross-sectional study should be completed within a short period of time if there are many observers. In reality, such studies may take months or even years to complete. But each person is assessed only once, and at that point the existence of the disease and other characteristics are evaluated in that person.

Suppose researchers from a local university examined a representative sample of 1,000 adults residing in a particular community to determine risk factors for coronary heart disease. In the study, each sample member had blood pressure, blood cholesterol, body composition, and aerobic fitness level tested and evaluated in a single evaluation by the researchers. Taking nearly six months to complete the examinations of all 1,000 sample members, researchers determine the prevalence of hyperlipidemia, hypertension, obesity, and physical inactivity at a particular point in time.

In this cross-sectional study, researchers would also be able to determine whether sample members with observable coronary heart disease symptomatology differed with respect to the prevalence of these risk factors from those who were symptom-free (adjusting for potentially confounding variables such as age, gender, and race/ethnicity). Observing a higher prevalence of risk factors in those with disease would *suggest* the possibility of certain risk factors as causes of coronary disease. However, such determinations would require much more intensive epidemiologic research to show cause-and-effect relationships.

Considerations in Conducting Cross-sectional Studies

Both the general public and health professionals have subjective impressions about the frequency of particular health events. For example, it is not uncommon to hear declarations such as "We have a very high rate of teenage pregnancy in our community" or "There is a high rate of bladder cancer and I believe it is due to the pollution coming from the manufacturing plant outside of town." Such assertions may be founded on good information; on the other hand, they may result from biased opinions, misinformation, or simply hunches. Nevertheless, hunches about the frequency of health events have often motivated important health actions and research activity in communities. Before any health action, however, it is imperative to confirm accurately and scientifically whether such statements are valid for the community.

Why should we be cautious when using data obtained from health care facilities and health care providers?

At first glance, it would seem that obtaining data from health facilities would allow us to make accurate determinations about health events such as disease frequency in communities. However, many sick people diagnose and treat themselves and never appear at health facilities; others go to physicians who may not write down their diagnosis or may write it illegibly; other people are treated by nurses, pharmacists, chiropractors, ministers of religion, parents, grandparents, or herbalists who are not affiliated with a health facility. Therefore, data obtained from health facilities or providers of health services may yield incorrect or incomplete information about the community.

What can we do if the population of interest is too large to examine or interview everyone?

It would be ideal to examine or interview everyone in the population of interest to determine whether they suffer from the "common" disorder. Yet, if the population is large, it is not feasible in terms of time and money to examine every person in the population. In many cases, a representative sample of the population is selected, even though it is much smaller than the population. A **sample** is defined as a selected subset of a population.

It is important to realize that the inferences and generalizations possible from any sample are directly related to the method used to select the sample. If there is doubt about sampling techniques and their uses, experts in sampling strategies should be consulted.

Why is it often difficult to discern people with a disease from people without a disease?

The presence of a disease or disorder must be discernible by ethical scientific methods if the frequency of the disorder is to be documented systematically. However, some chronic diseases have clinical remissions—periods of freedom from any signs or symptoms. During these periods, persons with such diseases ("cases") may be called "noncases." Studies of conditions with remissions, such as arthritis, peptic ulcer, and asthma, require special attention.

An important consideration is to define the condition under study (the condition of interest may be any health event of interest, including health-relevant behaviors). This definition must be practical, feasible, measurable, ethically derived, and the best available. Reading material published in scientific journals is helpful in this respect. Once such considerations are satisfied, the number of persons in the population (or in the sample selected) who fulfill the criteria defined for the condition can be counted.

EXAMPLE

Cross-sectional Study: Youth Risk Behavior Survey

The national school-based Youth Risk Behavior Survey is a component of the Centers for Disease Control and Prevention's Youth Risk Behavior Surveillance System that periodically measures the prevalence of priority health-risk behaviors among youth through representative national, state, and local surveys. A three-stage sample design was used to obtain a representative sample of 11,631 students in grades 9-12 in the 50 states, the District of Columbia, Puerto Rico, and the Virgin Islands. We report some of the findings obtained from this cross-sectional survey that pertain to selected sexual behaviors that increase risk for HIV infection.

Of all students in grades 9 to 12, the median age of reported first intercourse was 16.1 years of age for male students and 16.9 years of age for female students. About one-third (33.5%) of male students and 20.0% of female students initiated sexual intercourse before age 15 years. Nearly two-thirds (64.8%) of male students and 52.4% of female students initiated sexual intercourse before age 17 years.

Of all students, 19.0% reported having had four or more sex partners during their lifetime. Male students (26.7%) were significantly more likely than female students (11.8%) to report having had four or more sex partners. Black male students (60.4%) were most likely to report having had four or more sex partners. The percentage of students who had four or more sex partners increased significantly by grade, from 12.4% and 14.8% in 9th and 10th grades, respectively, to 28.6% in 12th grade.

Among students who reported sexual intercourse during the 3 months preceding the survey (i.e., were currently sexually active), 44.9% reported that they or their partners had used a condom at last sexual intercourse. Male students (49.4%) were significantly more likely than female students (40.0%) to report condom use at last sexual intercourse. Students who had four or more sex partners were significantly less likely to have used a condom at last sexual intercourse (40.6%) than were students with fewer sex partners (48.3%).[1]

Point Prevalence Rates

In Chapter 2, we learned that using rates allows us to account for the different sizes of groups at risk, thus making comparisons possible. By way of review, in order to calculate rates, we need to know the number of persons who have the health condition or disease of interest, and we need to know the size of the group or **population at risk** (PAR). **Prevalence** is a measure of the number or proportion of cases or events or conditions in a given population. **Prevalence rates** express the proportion of persons who have a particular disease or attribute at a specified point in time or over a specified period of time in a given population.

Point prevalence rates are obtained by conducting a prevalence or cross-sectional study. A cross-sectional study describes the existence of the condition studied, and the extent to which it prevails in various groups at the time of assessment. It is, in fact, a point-in-time prevalence, much like a "snapshot" of a community's health state, as contrasted with a movie or video film that takes a picture over time.

Why are point prevalence rates useful in epidemiology?

Point prevalence rates serve many useful functions. Prevalence rates indicate which groups to look at for cases, if one needs to find cases for care, which groups need what sort of health care, and the differential need among groups for staff and budget. Thus, point prevalence rates indicate priority groups for health and medical services, including case finding. If a health program aims to reduce the burden of illness in a community, point prevalence rates will serve as baseline indices for subsequent evaluations of health and medical care services in the groups served.

Prevalence rates are probability statements. A prevalence rate expresses the likelihood of cases existing in certain groups. In planning epi-

[1]From Centers for Disease Control and Prevention: Selected behaviors that increase risk for HIV infection among high school students—United States, 1990. *Morbidity and Mortality Weekly Report*, 1992;41(14):231, 237-240.

demiologic studies, prevalence rates can tell us how many people, on the average, would have to be examined to find a desired number of cases for study. Thus, if we wished to carry out a study on 100 cases of a particular disease, and we know the point prevalence rate is 2%, we would need to examine at least 5,000 people to be reasonably sure of obtaining 100 cases of the disease.

How do we calculate point prevalence rates?

To calculate a point prevalence rate, divide the number of cases with the disease at a specified point in time by the number of persons in the population at risk, and multiply by a factor of 10. Use the following formula:

$$\frac{\text{Number of cases of disease/condition}}{\text{Number in population at risk*}} \times K$$

What factors influence point prevalence rates?

Let's examine some factors that could raise or lower point prevalence rates. The numerator (number of cases) can be increased by adding in the occurrence of new cases (incidence) or by keeping cases alive longer through improved care. Curing cases, however, will reclassify cases as "noncases." Similarly, a rise in deaths from the disease reduces the number of cases prevailing (found living) and thus reduces the point prevalence rate. If cases migrate in or out of the study area, point prevalence rates will be affected. Out-migration of cases decreases the point prevalence rate; conversely, in-migration of cases increases the numerator, thus raising the point prevalence rate.

The denominator can also be affected. Because healthy immigrants inflate the denominator and not the numerator, they decrease the point prevalence rate. As shown in Figure 3.1, factors influencing the point prevalence rate are presented as a balance.

Period Prevalence Rates

In addition to point prevalence rates, period prevalence rates are frequently used in epidemiology. **Period prevalence** is the number or rate of cases found during a specified period of time, for example, one or more years. Cases are counted for period prevalence even if they die, migrate, or recur during the period. Thus, if a case is found in the population in January and dies, departs, or is cured by March, it is counted in the year's

*where the number in the PAR are those persons eligible to be in the numerator

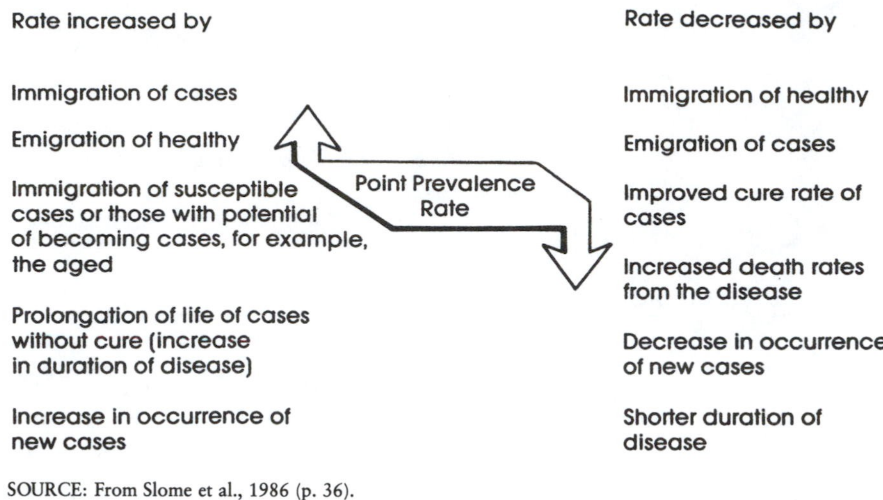

SOURCE: From Slome et al., 1986 (p. 36).

FIGURE 3.1 *Logical balance of a point prevalence rate*

period prevalence, but that case would not be included in the point prevalence in June of that year. Similarly, period prevalence includes cases current during the specified period, regardless of when they became a case or ceased to be a case.

Thus, at the start of the time period, period prevalence will equal point prevalence and all new or nearly identified cases (incidence) during the period, divided by the average midyear population during the period. Period prevalence, then, gives the amount of illness in a group over a period of time.

Period prevalence is not used as often as point prevalence in epidemiologic literature. Use of the term "prevalence" suggests point prevalence, unless otherwise indicated.

Application of Cross-sectional Methodology

Suppose that a 1990 cross-sectional epidemiologic study in Hometown, Idaho (fictitious location) generated the findings in Table 3.1 from examinations of the population aged 40 to 74 years. The entire population (not a sample) was measured.

From these data, it is possible to calculate the point prevalence rate of coronary heart disease (CHD) among persons 40 to 74 years old in Hometown in 1990. The point prevalence rate is the number cases found, divided by the population at risk (PAR), that is, those eligible to be cases. The point prevalence rate (PPR) for CHD is calculated as follows:

$$\text{PPR} = \frac{130}{2{,}216} \times 1{,}000 = 58.6 \text{ per } 1{,}000$$

TABLE 3.1 Cases of CHD, population 40 to 74 years old, Hometown, Idaho, 1992

Number Examined	*Cases of CHD**	*Persons Free from CHD*
2,216	130	2,086

*CHD = coronary heart disease. Cases include "definite," "probable," and "possible" cases of CHD.

SOURCE: From Slome et al., 1986.

TABLE 3.2 Age distribution of cases of CHD, white males, 40 to 74 years old, Hometown, Idaho, 1992

	Age (years)	*Cases of CHD**
	40-49	12
	50-59	19
	60-69	29
	70-74	11
Totals	40-74	71

*CHD = coronary heart disease. Cases include "definite," "probable," and "possible" cases of CHD.

SOURCE: From Slome et al., 1986.

The determination of the PPR tells us the size of the burden of CHD in Hometown. This may allow health care planners to estimate facilities and funding needed and to determine the extent of employment disability. It could also indicate whether CHD is more prevalent than other disorders in Hometown and thereby contribute information to set priorities for decisions regarding health services.

Further, the PPR indicates the likelihood of finding a case. If we know that in Hometown, in 1990, an epidemiological study of CHD needed 30 cases for its sample, we would have to examine about 500 persons in the age category of 40 to 74 years.

Also, if a program is instituted to reduce the number of cases of CHD in Hometown over the next few years, and if it is successful, a repeat cross-sectional study years later among persons 40 to 74 years old should find CHD at a point prevalence rate of less than 58.6 per 1,000. However, a reduction in prevalence should occur because of "good" things happening that reduce PPR (fewer new cases) and not "bad" things (increased death rates). Figure 3.1 reviews factors which increase and decrease prevalence rates.

Table 3.2 shows that the number of cases of CHD increases with age up to 69 years, but the population of each age category might also increase. Not knowing the population of each age category, no statement can be made of an age association with CHD prevalence until we calculate age-specific rates. Comparisons of groups or categories (e.g., age) demand the use of rates, not the number of cases (numerator data) only.

What is meant by an association between two variables?

An **association** between two variables implies that as one variable (characteristic) changes, there is a concomitant or resultant change in the quantity or quality of the other variable. In this instance, an association of age with CHD would mean different rates of CHD for different age groups. In order to determine whether there is an association, we need to know how many persons were examined in each age category, that is, the PAR in each age category. Table 3.3 provides us with this information and Table 3.4 shows the calculation of age-specific prevalence rates.

From an inspection of the age-specific prevalence rates in Hometown, it is apparent that age-specific rates increase with age, a **positive association** of age with CHD prevalence rates. Note also that the rates of CHD do not increase steadily; there is a substantial difference in the rates

TABLE 3.3 Age distribution of white males, 40 to 74 years old, Hometown, Idaho, 1992

	Age (years)	*Persons*
	40-49	254
	50-59	219
	60-69	139
	70-74	52
Totals	40-74	664

SOURCE: From Slome et al., 1986.

TABLE 3.4 Age-specific prevalence rates, white males 40 to 74 years old, Hometown, Idaho, 1992

	Age (years)	*Rate per 1,000*
	40-49	(12/254) × 1,000 = 47.2
	50-59	(19/139) × 1,000 = 86.7
	60-69	(29/139) × 1,000 = 208.6
	70-74	(11/52) × 1,000 = 211.5
Totals	40-74	71/664 × 1,000 = 106.9

SOURCE: From Slome et al., 1986.

TABLE 3.5 Prevalence of CHD among white male farm owners, 40 to 74 years old, by physical activity of work, Hometown, Idaho, 1992

Category of Activity	*Persons Examined*	*Cases of CHD*	*Prevalence Rate (per 1,000)*	*Age-adjusted Prevalence Rates (per 1,000)*
Not physically active	89	14	157.3	126
Physically active	90	3	33.3	36

SOURCE: From Slome et al., 1986.

of the two older-age categories compared to the younger-age ones. Because age is associated with CHD prevalence, age modifies CHD prevalence and is therefore a potential confounder in all prevalence studies of CHD. Once the confounding effect of age is confirmed, all subsequent analyses of CHD must control or adjust for age differences in groups being compared. We thus avoid erroneously interpreting differences between two or more groups that, in fact, may differ only in their age composition.

For example, if we want to see whether obese men have higher CHD rates than non-obese men, we must ensure comparability of age in the two weight groups before we are able to test or establish an association of obesity with CHD.

The researchers in the hypothetical community of Hometown wanted to determine whether there was an association of CHD with physical activity. They compared the prevalence rates of CHD among white male farm owners who did their own farm work with those who did not. The results are listed in Table 3.5.

The CHD prevalence rate is greater among the *not* physically active category. In fact, the rate is almost five times as great as among those in the physically active category. The differences in the crude point prevalence rates could be due to age differences. However, in Table 3.5, the age-adjusted rates which control or adjust for age differences also differ in the same way. The adjusted rates make the two comparison groups statistically similar in age. Thus, the difference in CHD rates by activity groups is not explained by age.

The total population prevalence rate of CHD in Hometown was 58.6 per 1,000. The prevalence rate of CHD in white male farm owners, from Table 3.5, is 17/179 = 95.0 per 1,000. The rate among white male farm owners (95.0 per 1,000) is higher than the prevalence rate in the total population (58.6 per 1,000).

Because the white male farm owners had a higher prevalence rate than the total population, other categories must have had lower rates (e.g., white non-farm owners, females, non-whites). Another consideration is that the age distribution may be different in farm owners as compared to the total population. Also, other CHD-relevant differences may exist among farm owners compared with other groups in the population (for example, they may smoke more cigarettes than other groups).

What are dependent and independent variables?

The **dependent variable** refers to the disease or health state being studied epidemiologically. In this application it is CHD. The **independent variable** refers to all other characteristics of groups or environments that we are attempting to associate with the occurrence of the dependent variable. In this case, the independent variable is physical activity. These terms are used because we want to see whether the occurrence of the disease or health state is dependent on other characteristics.

What conclusions can we make from the application of a cross-sectional study of physical work and CHD?

In this application, we cannot conclude that physical work prevents CHD. This example merely provides us with cross-sectional rates of CHD at a given time. We know neither when the CHD began nor when the physical activity occurred. It is apparent that CHD can cause inactivity as much as inactivity can cause CHD. As a result, these types of data do not permit cause-effect interpretation. Thus, in cross-sectional studies, we can only make statements about associations; for example, that having a particular characteristic is associated with the occurrence of a disease. However, associations generate hypotheses or suggest areas for further study, both highly worthwhile outcomes of cross-sectional/prevalence studies.

Relative Advantages/Disadvantages of Cross-sectional Studies

The following are relative advantages of the cross-sectional/prevalence type of study:

1. It is quick, requiring only a "one-time" examination/interview.
2. It is less expensive than some other study designs.
3. Because it indicates case loads and priorities for care, it is helpful in program planning, designing and locating hospitals and clinics, budgeting for drugs and medical equipment, and determining types of health services.

4. It is useful in determining associations between variables of interest, thereby generating hypotheses.
5. Its descriptions of the relative distributions of health and disease in populations can direct case-finding priorities.

The following are relative disadvantages of a cross-sectional study:

1. It does not separate cause-effect relationships in the associations established; it merely points out relationships between characteristics and health attributes.
2. Being cross-sectional at a point in time, it deals only with survivors and those surviving to be found as cases.
3. It is not useful when rare health conditions are being considered. If the prevalence rate of a disease is small, such as 5 per 100,000, and one wishes to establish the association of the disease with gender, age, or any other characteristic, one would have to examine at least 200,000 persons to find 10 cases—a lot of work for little return. For rare events, other strategies are available.
4. It is not useful in describing the load of cases or health events when the cases are recurrent and not countable at the "point" of the study. For studying conditions such as school or industrial absences, acute recurrent illness, and seasonal variations in illness, period prevalence studies are more appropriate.
5. It does not identify risk or future likelihood of the occurrence of the disease from a given characteristic. Therefore, it cannot predict future health event happenings.
6. It has limited usefulness for explosive epidemics or acute, short duration illnesses such as measles or upper respiratory infections; a point prevalence study may miss an epidemic that occurs and subsides rapidly.

Behavioral Risk Factor Survey—An Example of the Cross-sectional Method

Since 1981, the Centers for Disease Control and Prevention has helped states survey adults by telephone about their health behaviors.[2] By 1991, 47 states and the District of Columbia were participating in the Behavioral Risk Factor Surveillance System (BRFSS). The BRFSS is now a monthly telephone survey for which participants use a standard protocol and standard interviewing methods. Staff from each state complete more than 100 to 300 interviews each month during an 8- to 14-day period.

The interviewing instrument used for the BRFSS consists of the core questionnaire, the standard modules, and state-specific questions. The

---

[2]This section is adapted from Frazier EL, Franks AL, Sanderson LM: Behavioral risk factor data. In Centers for Disease Control, *Using chronic disease data: A handbook for public health practitioners*. Atlanta, GA: Centers for Disease Control and Prevention, 1992.

TABLE 3.6 Selected core questions* by category, BRFSS

Category	*Question*
Smoking status	Have you smoked at least 100 cigarettes in your lifetime? Do you smoke cigarettes now?
Cholesterol screening and awareness	Have you ever been tested for blood cholesterol? Do you know your blood cholesterol level?
Alcohol use	Have you recently had any beer, wine, or other alcoholic beverages? How many times did you drink during the last month? How many drinks did you have on the average? How many times did you drink and drive?
Blood pressure screening and treatment	Have you ever been told that you have high blood pressure? Have you been told more than once that your blood pressure was high? Is any medicine currently prescribed for your high blood pressure?
Obesity	How tall are you? How much do you weigh?
Sedentary lifestyle	Did you exercise in the past month? What type of exercise did you spend the most time doing? How many times did you exercise during the month?
Preventive health practices (women only)	Have you ever had a mammogram? Have you ever had a Pap smear?

*Paraphrased from the 1991 questionnaire

core questionnaire is a set of questions asked by all participants; it deals primarily with recent or current behaviors that are risk factors for disease. The topics covered by the core questionnaire have remained nearly the same since the BRFSS program began and concern behaviors related to physical activity, blood pressure, diet, body weight, smoking, alcohol consumption, and use of preventive services. Table 3.6 provides abbreviated descriptions of several core questions.

Responses to certain core questions are used to define the risk factor variables that classify respondents as either at risk or not at risk for adverse health events. For example, in the 1989 BRFSS, all interviewees were asked, "Have you ever been told by a doctor, nurse, or other health professional that you have high blood pressure?" The response to this question is coded for the variable hypertension. The variables are used for estimating the prevalence of risk factors in the general population. Table 3.7 gives examples of several risk factor variables.

The standard modules are sets of questions developed by the CDC on specific topics suggested by participants. Participants decide which (if any) standard modules they will include each year. State-specific questions are developed and used by individual participants. Over the years, topics covered by standard modules and by state-specific questions have included screening for cervical, breast, and colorectal cancer; health care visits; health insurance; smoke detector use; smoking cessation; perceived health problems; and sources of health information.

TABLE 3.7 Characteristics of respondents at risk for chronic disease, by variable

Variable	*Characteristic*
Hypertension	Reported having been told that their blood pressure is high.
Overweight	At or above 120% of their ideal weight, based on reported height and weight.
Current smoker	Reported currently smoking cigarettes and having smoked at least 100 cigarettes in their lifetime.
Sedentary lifestyle	Reported no physical activity or less than 20 minutes of physical activity less than three times per week.

In 1993, the structure of the BRFSS was changed so that more information can be collected from all states. The core questionnaire consists of a fixed set of questions, considered important to ask every year, and a rotating core of questions to be asked during specified years.

Survey Methodology

Although the main purpose of the BRFSS is to estimate the prevalence of behavioral risk factors in the general population, interviewing each person in the general population is not economically feasible. Thus, a probability (random) sample is selected in which all persons have a known chance of selection. Such population surveys usually use one of three types of sampling design: simple random sampling, stratified random sampling, or cluster sampling. The BRFSS uses a special type of probability cluster sampling—the multistage-cluster-design procedure, based on random-digit dialing.

Below is a description of the three stages that constitute the sampling methodology. This description does not present all the information necessary to actually construct a sample but introduces the main aspects of the sampling procedure.

Stage 1. Sample banks of telephone numbers are randomly selected from a list of area codes and prefixes for each participant. Each bank consists of 100 telephone numbers with the same area code, prefix, and first two digits of the suffix—for example, 100 numbers beginning with (312) 377-77. These banks of telephone numbers are called primary sampling units (PSUs) because they are basic blocks from which a sample is constructed.

Stage 2. The first number from each PSU is dialed; for the example above, the number might be (312) 377-7733. If it is a nonworking number or if it reaches a business or institution, the entire PSU is rejected; no numbers in that bank are used in the sample. If the telephone call reaches a residence, the PSU is accepted into the sample; the caller apologizes for having disturbed the respondent and hangs up.

Stage 3. Interviewers begin to call the numbers from each PSU accepted into the sample. If someone answers the telephone and confirms that the call has reached a residence, the interviewer asks how many men and how many women reside at the household. One adult (aged 18 or older) from the household is randomly selected and interviewed.

This process continues until the predetermined cluster size—three completed interviews for each accepted PSU—is reached, all the numbers in the cluster have been used, or the interviewing period ends (as at year end).

Weighting

As used here, unweighted data are the actual responses of each respondent. By weighting the data, the responses of persons in various subgroups are adjusted to compensate for overrepresentation or underrepresentation of these persons in the survey sample. Factors that are adjusted for include the following:

- The number of telephone numbers per household
- The number of adults in a household
- The number of interviews completed per cluster
- The demographic distribution of the sample

The first three factors address the problem of unequal selection probability, which could result in a biased sample—one that does not really represent the population. For example, an interviewee in a one-adult household has four times the chance of being selected for an interview as does an adult in a four-adult household. A household with two telephone numbers has twice the chance of being dialed as a household with one telephone number. If three interviews per PSU are not completed, compensation must also be made for the missing ones. The first three factors are combined to compute a raw (or unadjusted) weight.

Data are then weighted further. Poststratification is the method used to adjust the distribution of the sample data so the distribution reflects the total population of the sampled area. The poststratification factor is calculated by computing the ratio of the age, race, and sex distribution of the state population divided by that of the survey sample. This factor is then multiplied by the raw weight to compute an adjusted, or final-weight, variable.

Thus, weighting adjusts not only for variation in selection and sampling probability, but also for demographic characteristics. If the data were not weighted, projections could not be made from the sample to the general population.

Data Reporting

Three types of standard reports are supplied to participants each year. Portions of these reports are illustrated in the tables that follow.

TABLE 3.8 Cross-tabulation* of hypertension† variable and demographic characteristics of respondents, New Mexico, BRFSS, 1990

	Yes		*No*		*Unknown*		*Total****	
	N	%	*N*	%	*N*	%	*N*	%
Sex								
Male	78	14.6	444	85.4		—	522	100.0
Female	120	17.2	546	82.7	1	0.1	667	100.0
Age Group								
18-24	4	2.9	131	97.1	—	—	135	100.0
25-34	13	5.2	252	94.8	—	—	265	100.0
35-44	29	11.6	223	88.4	—	—	252	100.0
45-54	31	18.9	156	81.1	—	—	187	100.0
55-64	43	31.3	107	68.4	1	0.4	151	100.0
65+	78	39.4	117	60.6	—	—	195	100.0
Unknown/Refused	—	—	4	100.0	—	—	4	100.0
Total***	198	15.9	990	84.0	1	0.0	1189	100.0

*Of weighted data.
†Defined as ever having been told that blood pressure is high.

The cross-tabulation report, which is available by June of each year, presents the prevalence of risk factor variables by demographic characteristics. Because weighted data are presented in the report, projections can be made to the general population. Table 3.8 illustrates the information as it appears in this report for the variable of hypertension.

From this example, we can estimate that in New Mexico 14.6% of men and 17.2% of women have hypertension, and the highest percentage of people with hypertension are in the 65-or-older age group (39.4%). The report includes similar tabulations for other risk factor variables.

The prevalence report, which is also available each June, helps answer two questions about each risk factor:

- Does prevalence differ between men and women?
- Does prevalence differ by race?

Table 3.9 illustrates the types of tables that appear in the prevalence report. Prevalence is displayed first by sex and race and then for combined race/sex groups. The first half of the report allows for comparisons; in the other half differences between groups are given and evaluated.

The following definitions may help in the interpretation of Table 3.9.

Sample size is the number of persons who responded to the specific BRFSS question.

Variance expresses the spread of individual data points around the mean value for the sample.

TABLE 3.9 Prevalence of hypertension,[†] Georgia, BRFSS, 1990

	Total	*Males*	*Females*	*Nonwhites*	*Whites*
Sample size	1801	802	999	421	1380
Prevalence	20.0%	18.5%	21.4%	26.7%	17.6%
Standard error	1.05	1.55	1.4	2.4	1.1
95% C.I.	(18.0,22.1)	(15.4,21.5)	(18.6,24.2)	(21.9,31.5)	(15.4,19.9)

	Nonwhite Males	*White Males*	*Nonwhite Females*	*White Females*
Sample size	168	634	253	746
Prevalence	27.0%	15.6%	26.5%	19.5%
Standard error	3.9	1.55	3.0	1.55
95% C.I.	(19.2,34.8)	(12.4,18.7)	(20.5,32.5)	(16.4,22.7)

	Absolute Difference	*95% C.I. for Difference*	*Z-statistic for Difference*	*Prevalence Ratio*	*95% C.I. for Prevalence Ratio*
Males/Females					
Total	3.0%	(0.0,7.2)	1.40	0.86	(0.70,1.06)
Nonwhite	0.6%	(0.0,10.4)	0.11	1.02	(0.71,1.48)
White	4.0%	(0.0,8.4)	1.76	0.80	(0.62,1.03)
Nonwhites/Whites					
Total	9.1%	(3.7,14.4)	3.32*	1.52	(1.19,1.94)**
Males	11.4%	(3.0,19.9)	2.66*	1.73	(1.16,2.60)**
Females	6.9%	(0.1,13.7)	1.99*	1.35	(1.00,1.82)**

*Difference is significant at alpha = 0.05.
**1.0 is not in the confidence interval.

[†]Defined as ever having been told that blood pressure is high.

Standard error is the square root of the variance divided by the sample size. Although the mean tells where the values for a group are centered, the standard error tells how widely dispersed the values are around the center. The smaller the number, the less dispersed the values.

Confidence interval (C.I.) expresses the range of values within which the true prevalence is believed to be. A 95% confidence interval indicates that if the survey were repeated many times, the true value would be expected to fall within the range 95% of the time. The confidence interval is displayed as the lowest value followed by the highest value of the range.

Absolute difference is the difference in the prevalence for a risk factor between two groups. In the lower section of the report, the differences are given for males and females and for nonwhites and whites.

Z-statistic is computed to test the statistical significance of the difference between two prevalences. The value is compared by statistical software to a calculated z-value to determine whether the difference is significant at the 5% level of significance—that is, that the probability of the difference occurring by chance is less than 1 in 20. When the z-statistic is significant at the 5% level, the value in the report is followed by an asterisk. Thus, for example, we conclude that the absolute difference in the prevalence estimates for nonwhite and white women (6.9%) is statistically significant (z-statistic = 1.99).

Prevalence ratio is the prevalence for a risk factor for one group divided by that for another group. In the lower section of the report, the prevalence for males is divided by that for females, and the prevalence for nonwhites is divided by that for whites.

Reports that compare the prevalence of risk factors among participants are sent to each participant by October of each year. Table 3.10 illustrates this report. The column labeled "Percent" provides the prevalence. As an example, using New Mexico data from 1,189 persons who responded to the question "Have you ever been told that your blood pressure is high?", we estimate that approximately 15.9% of the state's population has hypertension. The estimated confidence interval for this prevalence is 13.55 to 18.29, and the standard error is 1.21.

Advantages and Disadvantages of Telephone Surveys

For several reasons, the BRFSS uses telephone interviewing for collecting information about behavioral risk factors.

- Surveys based on telephone interviews are much faster to complete than surveys based on in-person interviews. In one hour, an experienced telephone interviewer can handle busy numbers, calls not answered, and refusals to participate, and still successfully complete 1 1/2 interviews. In contrast, in one day of in-person interviewing, many miles of travel might be required, and only a few interviews may be completed.
- Telephone interviews are less expensive to conduct than in-person interviews. In 1991, almost 92,000 BRFSS interviews were completed at an average cost of about $50 each. In contrast, an in-person interview costs at least twice as much.
- Supervision and administration are simpler for telephone interviews than for in-person interviews. All calls can be made from one central location, and supervisors can monitor interviewers for quality control.

One main limitation, however, applies to telephone surveys. Because only about 93% of all U.S. households have telephones, approximately 7% of the population cannot be reached. Persons of low socioeconomic status are less likely than persons of higher socioeconomic status to have telephones and therefore are undersampled. Also, the percentage of households with a telephone varies by region. However, prevalence estimates from the BRFSS correspond well with the findings from surveys based on

TABLE 3.10 Statewide prevalence of hypertension* among participants, BRFSS, 1990

Participant	*Sample Size*	*Percent*	*Standard Error*	*95% Confidence Interval*
Alabama	2140	22.88	1.02	(20.88, 24.88)
Arizona	1500	19.02	1.13	(16.81, 21.23)
California	2701	20.65	0.88	(18.93, 22.37)
Colorado	1725	16.67	0.96	(14.79, 18.55)
Connecticut	1865	23.60	1.13	(21.39, 25.81)
Delaware	1503	22.38	1.11	(20.20, 24.56)
District of Columbia	1493	16.95	1.08	(14.83, 19.07)
Florida	2143	24.23	1.03	(22.21, 26.25)
Georgia	1801	20.02	1.05	(17.96, 22.08)
Hawaii	1870	19.47	1.10	(17.31, 21.63)
Idaho	1800	19.30	1.01	(17.32, 21.28)
Illinois	1796	18.09	1.04	(16.05, 20.13)
Indiana	2413	24.89	0.96	(23.01, 26.77)
Iowa	1512	21.35	1.09	(19.21, 23.49)
Kentucky	1800	22.79	1.04	(20.75, 24.83)
Louisiana	831	16.54	1.37	(13.85, 19.23)
Maine	1260	22.06	1.36	(19.39, 24.73)
Maryland	1668	20.54	1.12	(18.34, 22.74)
Massachusetts	1296	19.14	1.24	(16.71, 21.57)
Michigan	2388	23.43	0.94	(21.59, 25.27)
Minnesota	3420	20.33	0.73	(18.90, 21.76)
Mississippi	1581	28.23	1.33	(25.62, 30.84)
Missouri	1508	20.68	1.14	(18.45, 22.91)
Montana	1188	18.64	1.16	(16.37, 20.91)
Nebraska	1612	20.02	1.05	(17.96, 22.08)
New Hampshire	1500	19.54	1.09	(17.40, 21.68)
New Mexico	1189	15.92	1.21	(13.55, 18.29)
New York	1399	21.11	1.29	(18.58, 23.64)
North Carolina	2130	22.44	1.00	(20.48, 24.40)
North Dakota	1620	19.92	1.13	(17.71, 22.13)
Ohio	1319	18.70	1.23	(16.29, 21.11)
Oklahoma	1375	20.35	1.12	(18.15, 22.55)
Oregon	3308	20.12	0.74	(18.67, 21.57)
Pennsylvania	2468	23.36	0.96	(21.48, 25.24)
Rhode Island	1805	22.62	1.11	(20.44, 24.80)
South Carolina	2236	20.89	0.98	(18.97, 22.81)
South Dakota	1799	19.32	1.02	(17.32, 21.32)
Tennessee	2697	23.24	0.93	(21.42, 25.06)
Texas	1497	20.12	1.16	(17.85, 22.39)
Utah	1793	20.17	1.02	(18.17, 22.17)
Vermont	1111	19.68	1.32	(17.09, 22.27)
Virginia	1764	16.37	0.97	(14.47, 18.27)
Washington	2101	22.63	0.99	(20.69, 24.57)
West Virginia	2372	24.80	0.96	(22.92, 26.68)
Wisconsin	1260	22.62	1.27	(20.13, 25.11)

*Defined as ever having been told that blood pressure is high.

in-person interviews, including studies conducted by the National Institute on Alcohol Abuse and Alcoholism, the CDC's National Center for Health Statistics, and the American Heart Association.

Some inaccuracy is expected from any survey based on self-reported information. For example, respondents are known to underreport their weight and inaccurately recall dietary habits. The potential for bias must always be kept in mind when self-reported data is interpreted.

Summary of the Cross-sectional Method

The cross-sectional or prevalence study method is probably the most commonly used strategy in epidemiology. The following are the main methodological points that were considered in our discussion of this study method.

1. The meaning and description of any rate
2. The identification and use of the correct numerators and denominators in rates
3. The meaning of an association between two variables
4. The need to control or adjust for differences in the groups being compared
5. The usefulness of prevalence rates in epidemiology
6. Differences between point and period prevalence rates
7. Factors that affect prevalence rates
8. The contribution of control tables in controlling other variables
9. Relative advantages and disadvantages of the cross-sectional method

CASE-CONTROL STUDIES

We have discussed how the cross-sectional study design does not allow us to determine which came first, a characteristic (e.g., high serum cholesterol) or a condition of interest, such as coronary heart disease. Instead of contributing to the identification of cause and effect in the interpretation of association, the cross-sectional study describes what exists at the time a study was conducted.

In an effort to support hypotheses about supposed antecedents, we may also look retrospectively by asking people who have the health outcome (or effect) at the time of the study about their past in order to find out about supposed causes. These people are considered "cases," because they have the condition or health outcome of interest (e.g., people diagnosed with CHD). Next, we also select a group of individuals as "controls" (people who are free of CHD) who do *not* have the health condition, and ask about their history of contact with or exposure to the supposed causes (e.g., high serum cholesterol). This retrospective approach is referred to as the **case-control method** because we compare cases and controls for the presence of the presumed antecedent. The method is also called **retrospective** (from the Latin, *retro spicere*, "to look back") because one is looking back in time to see whether the presumed antecedent occurred.

Paffenbarger (1988) refers to the case-control study as a "flashback" study. Unlike the "snapshot" (cross-sectional) study, the "flashback" study includes the passage of time. The case-control method uses a flashback (historical) technique to assess past characteristics or exposures in two groups of people—cases and controls.

Selecting Cases and Controls

To conduct a case-control study, one must find cases of the supposed effect (e.g., disease) and obtain *from* them or *about* them the history of the assumed antecedent or cause (exposure). It is also necessary to find control persons similar in those characteristics which are known to be related to the effect (potential confounders), such as age or gender but *without* the supposed effect, and obtain histories of the exposure from or about them. A control or comparison group is needed to ensure that cases had a higher frequency or greater degree of exposure than noncases. Epidemiology is a science of comparison of groups or aggregates.

Cases must differ from controls by having the health effect; the controls *must not* have the effect. This raises the question of what is a case and what is not a case. Some of the difficulties one could face in accurately defining cases are, for example, one who died, one who was dissatisfied with the medical care given, one who developed postoperative complications, one who developed schizophrenia, etc. Sometimes there is disagreement among health professionals in how to define cases of specific conditions or diseases. This underscores the importance in an epidemiologic study of establishing objective criteria for the identification of cases and applying the criteria rigidly.

How should cases and controls be selected?

Cases and controls should come from a similar population. The case-control study is one way the observational scientist tries to support causal associations by showing that people who developed the disease were similar to other people in the community *except* for the supposed antecedent. Thus, we are looking for differences in the frequency with which a supposed antecedent appears among the cases versus the controls. If our controls are well chosen, the *only* antecedent difference between cases and controls will be in the level of a characteristic that is related causally to the development of the disease. Using the comparison group strategy, we are controlling for many other characteristics that may confound our ability to show an association between a supposed antecedent and the disease. Hence, the use of the term "control" in case-control studies. The selection of controls is not easy and is never perfect, but there are ways of selecting controls that help us considerably in making comparisons.

To make comparisons, we have to be able to gather "the evidence." The investigation will certainly fail if we can get information only about the supposed antecedent for the cases and not for the controls, or vice versa. Thus, we must have access to information in a similar way for cases and controls, and the quality of the information must be especially good for cases and controls.

What is "matching" and of what value is it in case-control studies?

Suppose that we were interested in conducting a case-control study to determine whether lung cancer was linked to cigarette smoking. In a case-control study, we start with information about the health outcome (lung cancer) and look retrospectively at the extent of smoking (presumed antecedent) among cases and controls to see whether this explains why cases developed lung cancer and controls did not. We know that age is related to smoking histories and that age is related to cancer of the lung. The confounding effect of age can be avoided by selecting cases and controls of the same age group or by **matching** the two groups for age. Known associations (i.e., race, gender) with the disease under study are the bases for matching the cases and controls. Matching provides for the cases and controls to be similar with respect to the variable for which subjects are matched.

In matching, we try to control for confounding variables. If we do *not* match for a confounding variable, we can eliminate it by subject selection (e.g., by studying only males to eliminate gender as a confounding variable). Another way is through statistical control during data analysis, as in the adjustment of rates as discussed in Chapter 2.

Matching sounds easier than it really is. The more variables to be matched, the greater the universe we need from which to draw control patients. The problem is that if one is matching for age, sex, and socio-economic class, the control person has to be similar to the case in all three characteristics, not just in two or one. Homogeneous "captive" populations (such as students or persons in the armed services) are usually excellent sources for matching, but these populations are not relevant to the study of many diseases.

Application of the Case-control Method

Clinical observations/hunches and hypotheses generated from cross-sectional research studies frequently lead to case-control studies. For example, case reports led to studies which later confirmed associations between diethylstilbestrol (DES) in pregnancy and cancer of the vagina in

TABLE 3.11 Smoking histories of select male patients and controls

Group	*Total*	*% Nonsmokers*
Male patients with lung cancer	82	14.6
Male patients with cancer of sites other than lungs, larynx, pharynx and lips	522	23.9

Note: Age distributions of both groups are similar

SOURCE: Adapted from Schrek R, Baker L, Ballard G, et al.: *Cancer Research*, 1950; 10:49-58.

offspring, and to studies which confirmed associations between rubella in pregnancy and congenital abnormalities.

In research linking cigarette smoking and lung cancer the same was true; observations from clinicians and cross-sectional studies laid an important foundation for our present state of knowledge by showing that lung cancer was associated with cigarette smoking. The case-control method was then applied by epidemiologists to investigate this supposition of hypotheses of smoking as a presumed antecedent of lung cancer.

An example of a case-control study from an early stage in smoking–lung cancer research shows how to apply this method. The study was carried out by Robert Schrek and others in 1950 in the United States. A summary of their findings is presented in Table 3.11.

The particular control group that was selected in this study was chosen to see whether smoking histories are associated with all cancers or only cancer of the lung. Such control groups are often chosen on the basis of the *same* pathology in *different* sites to separate site (local) specificity of cause and effect, or on the basis of *different* pathologies in the same site to separate specificity of pathology. In this instance, a control group of non-cancerous tumors of the lungs or chronic bronchitis cases would be examples of the latter sort of control group. Choosing the comparison group from patients admitted to the same hospital also minimizes the selective differences that bring people into a particular hospital.

What are some factors that could bias or invalidate findings in a case-control study?

There are many things to consider in a study that could potentially bias or lead to invalid findings. For example, having cancer of the lung may make patients overreport smoking (due to guilt, knowledge, selective memory). Having cancer of other sites, or being healthy, may produce underreporting because of non-concern with remembering smoking or belief in a non-association. There could be biased reporting of the antecedent when the bias is produced by the disease (or effect).

Various forces of subject selection might also be a source of inaccurate findings. Case-control studies are often carried out on patients attending treatment facilities. Those who are selected for a particular facility might differ from controls on some important variables (e.g., less financially able to purchase cigarettes, live in air-polluted cities). For this reason, controls may be chosen from admissions to the same facility. Thus they may share some of the same characteristics as cases attending the facility.

As in cross-sectional studies, case-control studies are often limited to including only those cases who have survived to that time. If cases who never smoked died more quickly than those who smoked, there will be more cases who smoked available for study. This is another example of selective survival.

Figure 3.2 provides us with a flow diagram of the case-control study investigating smoking as a suspected characteristic or antecedent of lung cancer. Using this information, we can prepare a table (Table 3.12) that shows the number of cases and controls who were smokers and nonsmokers.

Inspection of Table 3.12 reveals that 85.4% of lung cancer cases were smokers, and 76.1% of the controls were smokers. Since cases and controls were unequally exposed to smoking, with *more* cases exposed, this may help to support the hypothesis of an association between smoking and lung cancer.

Calculating the Odds Ratio: An Estimate of Relative Risk

At this point we have information about the disease state (lung cancer) and are looking backward in time for evidence of differences between cases and controls in the antecedent or supposed cause (smoking). The problem is, however, that we do not know whether the cases developed lung cancer and then started smoking or whether smoking started before their lung cancer. That is, we are unable to establish antecedent-consequent (cause-effect) relationships from the case-control study.

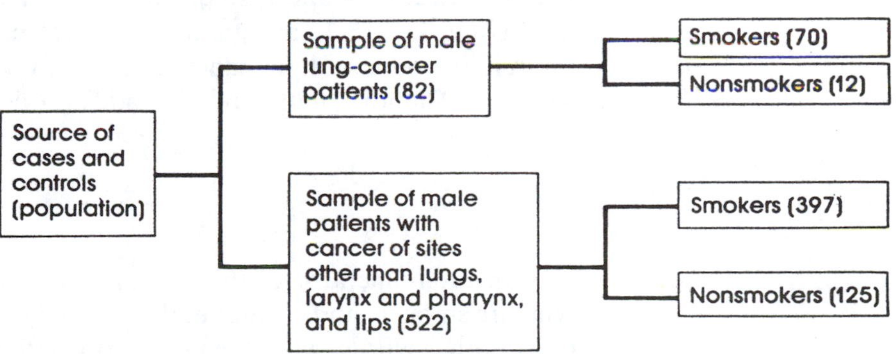

SOURCE: From Slome et al., 1986 (p. 79).

FIGURE 3.2 *Smoking histories in male patients and controls in a case control study*

TABLE 3.12 Distribution of smoking history among male cases of lung cancer and controls

Smoking History	*Case*	*Control*	*Total*
Smoker	70 (85.4%)	397 (76.1%)	467
Nonsmoker	12 (14.6%)	125 (23.9%)	137
Totals	82	522	604

SOURCE: From Slome et al., 1986 (p. 81).

TABLE 3.13 Frequency of cases and controls, by smoking history

Smoking History	*Case*	*Control*	*Total*
Smoker	a	b	a + b
Nonsmoker	c	d	c + d
Totals	a + c	b + d	a + b + c + d

SOURCE: From Slome et al., 1986 (p. 82).

However, we are eager to quantify the risk among smokers of developing lung cancer, compared with (relative to) nonsmokers. The optimal way to do this is to start studying smokers and nonsmokers *before* they have cancer of the lung and then quantify the ratio of the rate of occurrence of new cases of lung cancer in these groups. This ratio is called **relative risk.** In case-control studies it is not possible to calculate relative risk. (The reason for this is that you cannot calculate incidence rates, which reflect risks of developing a health effect (disease), from case-control/retrospective studies. We will discuss how to calculate incidence rates and relative risk later in this chapter.) However, there is a technique for estimating relative risk even though the data were derived from a case-control study. This estimate is called the **odds ratio** or **relative odds.** The technique has a solid mathematical base and is frequently used in case-control studies.

Using Table 3.13 as a guide, we can calculate an odds ratio to estimate the relative odds of lung cancer among smokers as compared with nonsmokers. The formula for relative odds (odds ratio) is:

$$\frac{a \times d}{b \times c}$$

In the numerator of this formula, **a** represents the number of cases who are smokers and **d** signifies the number of controls who are nonsmokers. In other words, what the numerator reflects is in accordance with our hypotheses: those with lung cancer are likely to be smokers and conversely, those with no lung cancer are likely to be nonsmokers. The denominator, on the other hand, reflects the situations in our study that are at odds with our hypotheses. Therefore, in the denominator, **b** denotes the number of controls who are smokers and c the number of cases who are nonsmokers. We can now calculate the odds ratio for our example from the data in Table 3.12:

$$\frac{a \times d}{b \times c} \text{ or } \frac{70 \times 125}{397 \times 12} = 1.84$$

This means that in this study, smokers had a risk of lung cancer 1.84 times that for nonsmokers. Methods are also available for calculating a confidence interval relative to the risk estimate. A **confidence interval** is a statistical method to determine in what ranges the true risk is likely to be. Confidence intervals surrounding risk estimates are statistically significant when they do not include 1.0 within the interval. For example, if the confidence interval for the relative risk estimate above (1.84) was 1.5 to 2.2, the estimate would be significant (meaning that the risk is significantly greater than in the nonexposed reference group).

EXAMPLE

Case-control Study: Baldness and Heart Attacks?

The relationship between male pattern baldness and the risk of myocardial infarction (heart attack) was evaluated in a hospital-based, case-control study involving men under 55 years of age (Lesko, Rosenberg, and Shapiro, 1993). Cases were men admitted to a hospital for a first nonfatal myocardial infarction, and controls were men admitted to the same hospitals for reasons other than cardiovascular disease. After relative risk estimates were adjusted for age, the relative risk estimate for frontal baldness compared with no hair loss was 0.9 (95% confidence interval, 0.6 to 1.3), for baldness involving the vertex scalp the relative risk was 1.4 (95% confidence interval, 1.2 to 1.9). Risk of heart attack increased as the degree of vertex baldness increased; for severe vertex baldness the relative risk was 3.4 (95% confidence interval, 1.7 to 7.0).

Relative Advantages/Disadvantages of Case-control Studies

The following are relative advantages of case-control studies:

1. Cases are easily available. This is the method of choice for less common or rare conditions and for studies done in clinical situations as opposed to community situations.
2. The case-control study is relatively quick and inexpensive and can be conducted by clinicians in clinical facilities.
3. Studies using this method tend to support, but not prove, causal hypotheses by establishing associations.
4. Historical data are often available from clinical records of patients, so it is possible to do secondary analyses (analyses of existing data)

without having to obtain more information from the cases or controls themselves.

5. The number of subjects needed to test the hypothesis of association is small compared to a cross-sectional design or a cohort design.

The following are disadvantages of the case-control method:

1. Information regarding the antecedent is often dependent on memory, and thus is potentially biased. Also, data from clinical records may be inadequate or incomplete.
2. Criteria used in the diagnoses of cases may not be the same among health care providers or researchers, so that "case groups" may not be homogeneous.
3. The chosen cases are selective survivors. The histories of the deceased cases may be selectively different from the cases who survive in the study. Thus, cases at one point in time do not represent a universe of cases.
4. Nonrepresentativeness of cases also occurs because often hospital or clinic cases are used in studies, and these cases may be selectively different from cases who have *not* presented themselves for treatment, or from cases who went to a different facility. This restricts the generalizability of the findings to other populations. Making such generalizations from hospital or clinical samples to the general population, therefore, may be erroneous. Such a fallacy is called **Berkson's fallacy**, after the statistician who first demonstrated it.
5. The occurrence of the assumed antecedent in the history is obtained from selected cases and controls. Thus, the "antecedents" are not obtained from a universe of all antecedents, so we cannot know what the association would be for all or for a representative sample of all people having the antecedent.

EXAMPLE

Case-control Study: Smoking and Residential Fires

To investigate whether tobacco, alcohol, and their combined use are important risk factors for fire injuries, Ballard et al. (1992) analyzed data from a population-based case-control study in King County, Washington, between 1986 and 1987. Cases (n = 116) were households with at least one reported fatal or nonfatal intentional residential fire injury from 1984 through 1985. Random digit dialing was used to select controls (n = 256). After adjusting for education, household size, and other possible confounders, the following odds ratios were determined relative to households with no smokers:

- 1.5 (confidence interval, 0.6 to 4.2) for households whose members collectively smoked 1-9 cigarettes per day;

- 6.6 (confidence interval, 2.5 to 17.5) for households whose members smoked 10-19 cigarettes per day; and
- 3.6 (confidence interval, 1.9 to 7.2) for households whose members smoked 20 or more cigarettes per day.

Summary of the Case-control Method

The case-control method is often used because it is easy, quick, and permits health professionals to test their hunches. It is usually chosen for select clinical or other similar situations, when the disease is rare, or when there is not time, money, or inclination to launch a community study or long-term follow-up study.

Here are some of the main points covered in our discussion of the case-control method:

1. How to conduct case-control studies
2. Considerations in selecting a control group wisely
3. Control of possible confounding variables by sampling or matching at the design stage
4. Calculation and interpretation of odds ratios (relative risk estimates) from data generated from case-control studies
5. Relative advantages and disadvantages of the case-control method

COHORT STUDIES

By way of review, the cross-sectional study provides a "snapshot" view of a representative sample or total population of a community in order to determine concurrent associations of a health condition and other group characteristics. The case-control study starts with a determination of the health state (or condition) and looks backward in time (retrospectively) for the history of the presumed antecedent characteristic—"flashback" view. In these study designs, association may be supported, but the antecedent-consequent relationship cannot be confirmed. Both designs fail to establish that the hypothesized cause (characteristic or risk factor) precedes the development or appearance of the effect (condition or health outcome).

The next type of study we discuss is the **cohort study**, also known as the **prospective study** or **incidence study**. This method meets the need to confirm the causal association, the definite time/entity relationship missing in cross-sectional or case-control methods. It establishes time (secular) relationships between presumed antecedents and presumed effects, and in so doing, ensures knowing which came first. It is the preferred method for epidemiological predictions and prognoses because it can best determine the magnitude of risks for future events in those groups with specified characteristics. By establishing future outcomes, it provides health service personnel with knowledge about which antecedents to alter in order to prevent disease or promote health and the amount of reduction of disease such action can be expected to produce. Clearly, such a contribution is important in planning and evaluating any program related to the prevention of disease or complications of disease.

This method is the most powerful one available for use in analytic epidemiology. As opposed to retrospective techniques, the cohort, or prospective, study is a forward-looking strategy. With this technique we can identify more directly specific characteristics of groups or environments associated with a high risk or probability of future health events.

Health planners and administrators can capitalize on these findings in terms of predicting future health needs by knowing which characteristics precede disease. Cohort/prospective studies do confirm risk (or causal) factors and so present health promoters and educators with the health characteristics or behaviors that need modification to prevent illness in communities.

Paffenbarger (1988) refers to cohort/prospective studies as "motion picture" studies. This study method follows groups of individuals free from disease through a period of time in "motion picture" fashion to determine whether disease develops.

EXAMPLE

Prospective Cohort Study: Body Fat Distribution and Five-year Risk of Death in Older Women

Folsom et al. (1993) conducted a study to test the hypothesis that both body mass index (ratio of weight in kilograms per height in meters squared) and the ratio of waist circumference to hip circumference are positively associated with mortality risk in older women. This was a prospective cohort study of 41,837 Iowa women aged 55 to 69. After these women were "followed" for the five-year period, 1504 deaths occurred. Body mass index (an index of relative weight) was found to be associated with mortality in a J-shaped fashion; rates were elevated in the leanest and in the most obese women. In contrast, waist/hip circumference ratio was strongly and positively associated with mortality in a dose–response manner. A 0.15-unit increase in waist/hip circumference ratio was associated with a 60% greater relative risk of death (after adjustment for age, body mass index, smoking, educational level, marital status, estrogen use, and alcohol use). It was concluded by the researchers that waist/hip circumference ratio is a better marker than body mass index of risk of death in older women. Health care professionals should measure waist/hip circumference as part of routine surveillance and risk monitoring.

Considerations in Conducting Cohort Studies

In conducting a cohort/prospective/incidence study, one starts with persons having the presumed cause (antecedent or exposure) *but free from the effect* (disease) and then waits for them to develop the effect. The comparison group (which is central to prospective epidemiology) must also be a group of persons free from the disease, but who, in addition, *do not have* the presumed cause. These persons are watched for the same period of time to see whether the new disease or effect develops. In both groups, we await "new" effects or cases or incidents, because we know these events were not manifest at the beginning of the study. Therefore, we can call this study the prospective, incidence, or cohort study method.

What is a cohort? What are examples of cohorts?

A **cohort** is a group or aggregate of persons who have presumed antecedent characteristics in common and who are followed so that we may observe the development or nondevelopment of a given health outcome. Examples of a cohort might include all new employees to a factory during a certain year, all the gall-bladder patients who were operated on in a given hospital during a certain period of time, or all the first-year students in a university during a certain year. The essence of a cohort study is (1) being able to define who is in the group and who is not and (2) putting some time bounds on the time period we are considering in observing our group or cohort of interest. An additional consideration required for a cohort to be used in an incidence study is that all the members of the group to be followed must be free of the health outcome at the start of the follow-up period. Only in this way can we look for "new" cases or incident cases of the health outcome of interest.

Why is it essential that epidemiologists determine who is free from disease?

It is essential that epidemiologists ascertain those who are free from the disease (effect) at the beginning of a study. To achieve this, all persons in a selected sample or population have to be examined to find out who has, or does not have, the effect (e.g., blood clots) and also the presumed antecedent (e.g., oral contraceptive use or non-use). The prospective study is confined to those free from the disease or health outcome under study. Those with the condition are excluded from the study.

Clearly, one has to be free of something in order to be at risk of becoming a *new* something in the future. An exception is being at risk of repeated episodes. For instance, a person is only at risk of a first stroke if he/she has never had a previous stroke. But she/he must have had a first stroke to be eligible for a second one. And the antecedents of the first stroke may be different from the antecedents of a second one.

To review, when we begin a cohort study, we start off with a prevalence or cross-sectional study to identify cases and noncases in the study

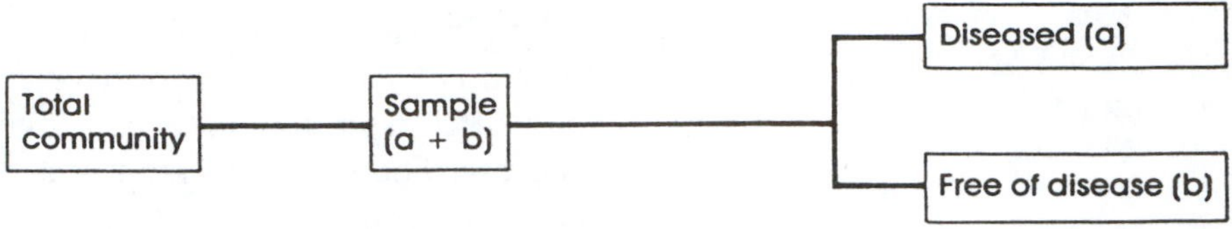

SOURCE: From Slome et al., 1986 (p. 96).

FIGURE 3.3 *Finding the cohort*

population, and we ascertain the presence or absence of the antecedent of interest. The cohort of interest is those persons who are free of the disease at the start of the study and thus are eligible to become new cases. This is diagrammed in Figure 3.3.

Incidence Rates

In discussing the cross-sectional (prevalence) study design, we looked at a population and counted the number of persons in the group who had the disease at the time of the prevalence study. Those persons who already had the disease were available for counting or enumerating. The prevalence rate (PR) is

$$\text{PR} = \frac{\text{Existing cases at a given point in time}}{\text{Persons eligible or "at risk" of being a case (size of sample or population)}} \times \text{K}$$

What does incidence measure?

Incidence, however, establishes that everyone in the group who is eligible to develop the disease is also free of the disease at the beginning of the incidence study. Thus, the incidence rate (IR) measures the frequency of developing new cases.

$$\text{IR} = \frac{\text{New cases over a given time period}}{\text{Persons at risk of becoming a new case (free of the disease at the start of the study)}} \times \text{K}$$

The numerator is the number of new cases or incidents over a time period. The denominator is **PAR (population at risk)**, *those free* from the disease or event at the start. Multiply by a constant (in this case 1,000) and express the rate per 1,000 persons per time period.

What factors can influence incidence rates?

Because incidence represents new cases, factors associated with the development or prevention of new cases produce strong influences on incidence rates. An increase in the proportion of the population who have the risk factors of a disease (antecedents, exposures) will often raise the incidence. For example, if the proportion of smokers in a population increases, lung cancer incidence will increase. Also, if preventive measures are known and applied, we would expect a decreasing incidence of a particular disease (e.g., application of a vaccine and a resulting decrease in incidence of a childhood infectious disease).

In general, treatment of cases (cure or care) does not influence the incidence rate of the same disorder. Treatment of disease occurs "after the horse is out of the barn"—cure influences prevalence rates but not incidence rates. Once a disease has appeared to warrant treatment, it is no longer possible to prevent it in that person. The exception, of course, is that treatment of a disease such as hypertension, which is a risk factor for stroke and coronary heart disease, may reduce the incidence rates of complications. But treatment of hypertension will not reduce the rate of occurrence of new cases of hypertension itself. This, in part, applies to infectious diseases too, for transmission is often effected before treatment is instituted. Similar considerations apply to chronic diseases.

Cumulative Incidence and Incidence Density

Often the period for calculating incidence rates is one calendar year, but this is arbitrary. One can express the rate for four-year or ten-year periods, or one can collect the new events over a number of years and express the rate as an average annual incidence rate. However, rates may change over time, so the longer the time period used, the more likely that we are putting different rates into the average. In so doing, we may mask important secular variations (changes over time) in the rates or change the relationship of antecedent to effect. Obviously the longer the period covered by the rate, the greater its magnitude. Therefore, when comparing incidence rates resulting from different studies, it is essential to ensure that the time periods being compared are the same, or that average annual rates are used. Average incidence rates are termed **cumulative incidence.**

What is incidence density? What are person-years?

Often in cohort studies people are followed for different lengths of time. Some drop out or come into the study at different times. In such cases, the denominator will not be the number of people, but the accumulated periods of time each person is in the study—that is, **person-years.** The term **incidence density** is sometimes applied to such an incidence rate.

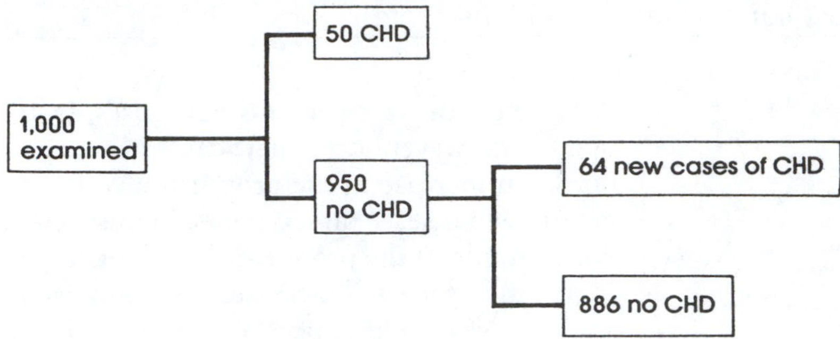

SOURCE: From Slome et al., 1986 (p. 98).

FIGURE 3.4 *Cohort study of CHD, men 30-59 years (1980-1990)*

The person-years approach has been an effective method of utilizing information about each member of the cohort, even if the period of follow-up of that person is short. Incidence density is useful in that it uses all the data on participants in the follow-up study, even if they enter the study early or late. It still demands that persons on entry to the study be free from the effect (disease) and be classified as to the exposure variable.

Calculating Incidence and Prevalence Rates in Cohort Studies

For purposes of illustration let us examine a hypothetical cohort study (see Figure 3.4) of coronary heart disease (CHD). In 1982, 1,000 men aged 30 to 59 years were examined. Of those, 50 had detectable CHD. Of those free from CHD in 1982, 64 developed CHD during the period 1983-1990.

From these data, we can see that the point prevalence rate of CHD in 1982 was 50/1,000, or 50 per 1,000 men 30 to 59 years old. This rate tells us the frequency of existing cases among those who were examined.

To calculate the eight-year (cumulative) incidence rate of CHD we use the following formula:

$$\text{IR} = \frac{\text{New cases of CHD during 1983-1990}}{\text{PAR}}$$

Included in the PAR must be only those free from the disease at the beginning of the time interval, so PAR = 950, *not* 1,000 men 30 to 59 years old. Those CHD cases found in 1982 are not at risk of becoming *new* cases; they already have the disease.

Hence, the eight-year incidence rate of CHD is 64/950 × 1,000 or 67.4 per 1,000 men 30 to 59 years old. In Figure 3.4, note that in each case the PAR, or denominator, is in the part of the diagram from which the numerator flows. This rate (67.4 per 1,000) tells us the probability or risk of development of CHD among males aged 30 to 59 over the eight-year period. In other words, 67.4 of 1,000 men aged 30 to 59 will develop CHD in an eight-year time period, or 67.4/8 each year.

Suppose there were no deaths, no cures, and no migration between 1982 and 1990. The population would remain steady at 1,000 because there were no deaths or migration. The point prevalence rate of CHD in 1990 among this cohort of men (now aged 38 to 67) would be 114 per 1,000. The numerator is all existing cases in 1990, and with no deaths, cures, or migration of cases, it must equal 50 (the existing cases in 1982) plus 64 (the new cases developed 1983-1990).

$$\text{PR in 1990} = \frac{\text{All cases of CHD prevalent in 1990}}{\text{PAR in 1990}} \times 1{,}000$$

$$= \frac{\text{50 old cases and 64 new cases}}{1{,}000} = \frac{114}{1{,}000}$$

It is possible, but unlikely, to find during eight years that none of a population migrated and that all the cases survived for that period. This example reinforces the point, however, that prevalence represents an accumulation of cases that survived, regardless of time of occurrence. In contrast, incidence rates pertain only to *new* cases during a time interval among a population initially free of disease.

Relative Risk

To learn how to calculate relative risk we will use data from a classical cohort study as an example. This study, the Framingham (Massachusetts) Heart Study, assessed among other study objectives serum cholesterol as being associated with CHD. The results from this prospective study of CHD (figures were approximated for ease of calculation) are presented in Table 3.14.

From these data we are able to calculate the prevalence rate of CHD in 1950 and the eight-year incidence rate of CHD for 1951-1958 by applying the formulas presented earlier in this chapter. Prevalence rates indicate existing cases, but incidence rates indicate new cases. The results of applying these formulas for prevalence and incidence rates for the low cholesterol group, high cholesterol group, and total group are presented in Table 3.15.

TABLE 3.14 Coronary heart disease cases, white men, aged 30-59, Framingham, 1950 and 1951-1958, by levels of cholesterol

Serum Cholesterol Level (1950)	*Population*	*CHD Cases 1950*	*New CHD Cases 1951-1958*
Low cholesterol	1,120	20	66
High cholesterol	1,127	27	135
Totals	2,247	47	201

SOURCE: Kannel W, Dawder T, Kagan A, et al.: The Framingham study. *Annals of Internal Medicine*, 1961;55:33-50.

TABLE 3.15 Prevalence rates per 1,000 in 1950, and incidence rates per 1,000, 1951-1958, of coronary heart disease by levels of cholesterol among white males, aged 30-59, Framingham

	Prevalence Rate of CHD (1950)			*Incidence Rate of CHD (1951-1958)*		
	Population	*Cases*	*Rates*	*Population*	*Cases*	*Rates*
Low cholesterol	1,120	20	17.9	1,100	66	60.0
High cholesterol	1,127	27	24.0	1,100	135	122.7
Totals	2,247	47	20.9	2,200	201	91.4

SOURCE: From Slome et al., 1986 (p. 102).

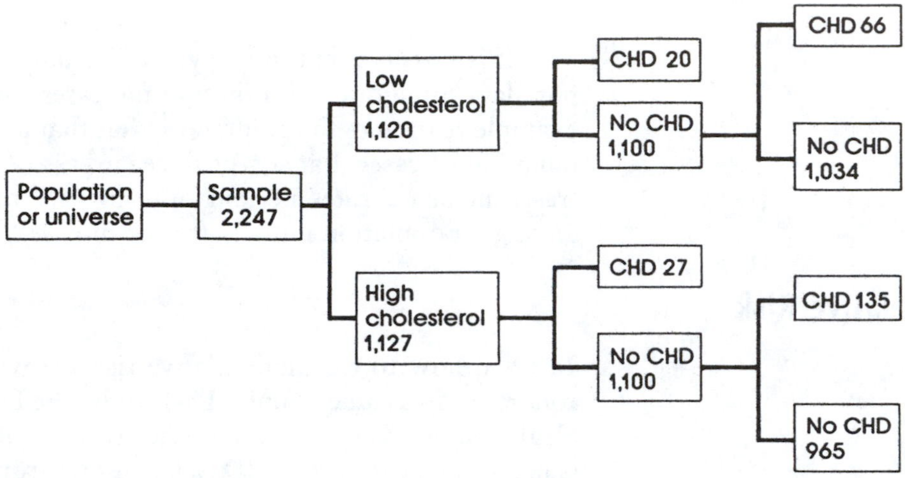

SOURCE: From Slome et al., 1986 (p. 103).

Figure 3.5 *Cohort study of CHD, men 50-59 years (1980-1991)*

The prevalence rate (PR) is slightly higher in the high cholesterol category (24.0 per 1,000) than in the low cholesterol category (17.9 per 1,000). The incidence rate (IR) is twice as great in the high cholesterol category (122.7 per 1,000) as in the low cholesterol category (60.0).

A flow diagram (Figure 3.5) of this study may be helpful. In each cholesterol category, "new CHD" cases can arise only from the "no CHD" (free from CHD) categories of the 1950 prevalence study. For example, 20 of the population at risk had CHD in 1950 and thus are not at risk of being *new* cases. Therefore, they are excluded from the PAR (denominator) of the incidence rate.

What is relative risk? How do we interpret relative risk?

Because this is a prospective study, we can make risk assessments. The **relative risk** is calculated by dividing the incidence rate in one group (those exposed) by the incidence rate in the other group (those not exposed). In this case the relative risk is calculated by dividing the incidence rate in the high cholesterol category by the incidence rate in the low cholesterol category: 122.7/60 = 2.04. As its name suggests, the ratio indicates relative degrees of risk. Thus, in this study, white men with high cholesterol were 2.04 times more likely to develop CHD than white men with low cholesterol. This study provides substantial evidence that high cholesterol is associated as an antecedent with the probability of developing CHD. This conclusion assumes that other potential confounding variables were evaluated and controlled.

The relative risk tells us the ratio of the risk in one group or aggregate compared to the risk in another group. This ratio is useful to those in search of causative associations, but the size of the relative risk in no way indicates the magnitude of the incidence rates in the exposed and non-exposed groups. For example, a relative risk of 4.0 can be obtained from incidence rates for the following two diseases: (4 per million/1 per million) and (400 per 1,000/100 per 1,000). The first disease is relatively rare, even in the exposed group, whereas the other disease is very common. One may decide that the rare disease affects so few people that no preventive action is warranted, even though the relative risk is 4.0.

However, relative risk helps to compare the relative contributions of risk factors, no matter how much of the disease exists. Its size helps in deciding whether the association between the antecedent risk factor and the disease is a likely part of the cause. If the relative risk is very large, regardless of the respective incidence rates, a causative association is more likely.

EXAMPLE

Prospective Cohort Study: Vasectomy and Prostate Cancer

To examine prospectively the relationship between vasectomy and prostate cancer, a prospective cohort study of health professionals was conducted (Giovannucci, Ascherio, Rimm, Colditz, Stampfer, and Willett, 1993). The cohort consisted of 10,055 male members of the Health Professionals Follow-up Study, aged 40 to 75 years, who had had a vasectomy, and 37,800 members who had not had a vasectomy at the time of study entry in 1986. These participants provided detailed information on various lifestyle variables including diet. The outcome measure was diagnosis of prostate cancer; between 1986 and 1990, 300 new cases were diagnosed among participants who were initially free of diagnosed cancer. Vasectomy was associated with an elevated risk of prostate cancer (age-adjusted relative risk, 1.66; 95% confidence interval, 1.25 to 2.21). The risk of prostate cancer was even higher among men who had a vasectomy at least 22 years in the past (relative risk, 1.85; 95% confidence interval 1.26 to 2.72). The researchers controlled for diet, level of physical activity, smoking, alcohol consumption, educational level, body mass index, and geographical area of residence. These results support evidence from case-control studies that vasectomy increases the risk of prostate cancer.

Attributable Risk

Based on the data from the Framingham study, it is appropriate to try to reduce cholesterol levels in all men to a "low" level in order to prevent new cases (incidence) of CHD. If everyone in the study had low cholesterol, the rate for the total population would be 60 per 1,000. Let us theoretically examine the effect that would be seen if a community intervention was successful in lowering all high cholesterol levels to low cholesterol levels. If IR_e is the incidence rate for the exposed group (high cholesterol) and IR_o is the incidence rate for the non-exposed group (low cholesterol), then $IR_e = 122.7$ per 1,000 and $IR_o = 60$ per 1,000. Therefore, the expected reduction in the CHD rate is 122.7 minus 60, or 62.7 per 1,000 men with high cholesterol. This is the amount of risk we can attribute to having a high cholesterol level.

We derived this risk assessment by *subtracting* the incidence rate in the low cholesterol (without risk or non-exposed) group from the incidence rate found in the high cholesterol (with risk or exposed) group. Epidemiologists call this the **attributable** (individual-based) **risk** (or risk difference).

Next, let's examine by what proportion we would reduce the disease rate in the whole population if we successfully reduced all high cholesterol levels to low cholesterol levels. A measure of this benefit in the population is derived by modifying a risk factor known as the **population attributable risk proportion**, also called *population attributable risk fraction*. This is the proportion (or fraction) of the disease rate in *the whole population* that the rate in the exposed group represents. The total population rate minus the rate in the non-exposed group is the amount contributed by the exposed persons; that as a proportion of the total rate gives us the population attributable risk proportion (a percentage, if multiplied by 100, or a fraction if left as it is).

Let's calculate the population attributable risk percent (PARP) from the data in Table 3.15. The incidence rate for the total population is 91.4 per 1,000. The rate in the non-exposed (low cholesterol) group is 60.0. Therefore, the *population attributable risk* is $91.4 - 60.0 = 31.4$ per 1,000. This is different from the simple (individual) *attributable risk*, which is $IR_e - IR_o$ or $122.7 - 60.0 = 62.7$.

As a proportion of the total population rate, the population attributable risk is 31.4/91.4, or 0.0314/0.0914 = 0.345, or 34.5%. This means that 34.5% of the new cases of CHD in Framingham men could be prevented if all the men had low cholesterol levels.

What does population attributable risk percent or etiological fraction tell us?

Population attributable risk percent (also called an etiologic fraction) tells us what reduction in the disease or outcome (effect) variable we can expect if the exposure (risk factor) is removed. Because many diseases have more than one risk factor, we can calculate the PARP for each and evaluate whether their relative values offset the cost and feasibility of reducing or removing the risk, and the reduction in cost that follows the reduction in the disease. The population attributable risk percent can also be used to evaluate a preventive program.

What are other methods for deriving the population attributable risk percent or etiological fraction?

There are other methods for deriving the etiologic fraction (population attributable risk percent); three are presented below.

Method 1:

1. Calculate the simple attributable risk (AR), $IR_e - IR_o$.
2. Multiply this by the prevalence (P) of the risk factor, $AR \times P = AR_p$ (population attributable risk).
3. Divide this by the incidence rate of the disease in the total population (RT) or $(AR_p/RT) \times 100$, which equals the population attributable risk percent calculated earlier.

Method 2:
This method uses the relative risk (RR), IR_e/IR_o.

1. Multiply the prevalence of the risk factor (P) by (relative risk−1).
2. Divide this by the same entity + 1,

$$\frac{P(RR - 1)}{P(RR - 1) + 1} = PARP$$

Method 2, using RR, is the most useful because with this method we can derive estimates of relative risk from both case-control studies and cohort studies (this method is called the odds ratio for case-control studies). Since we cannot calculate the true attributable risk in case-control studies, method 2 applies to both case-control and cohort studies.

Method 3:
By subtracting the disease incidence rate for the non-exposed group (IR_o) from the total rate of the disease (RT), a population attributable risk is established for that disease and that exposure in that population. The population attributable risk is $(RT - IR_o)$. To obtain the PARP, divide this difference by the rate in the total population (RT) and then multiply by 100. In brief, this method would be:

$$PARP = \frac{(RT - IR_o)}{RT} \times 100$$

What do the various measures of attributable risk tell us?

The various measures of attributable risk (simple attributable risk, population attributable risk, and population attributable risk percent, or proportion or fraction) all indicate the proportion of incidence that can be attributed to the antecedent cause of the disease. These measures can be used to estimate the *maximal* reduction of a disease rate in a community if the antecedent (or exposure) is eliminated. Since more than one exposure is often involved in the causative network, we may have to eliminate many antecedents. The maximal reduction is obtained only if everyone in the community has the antecedent and there is only one cause (antecedent). The smaller the percentage of community people who have the antecedent (the prevalence of the risk factor), and the smaller the risk attached to that antecedent, the smaller the rate reduction produced by eliminating the antecedent of the disease. For that reason, a highly prevalent risk factor (e.g., smoking or hypertension) plus a high simple attributable risk (e.g., risk of lung cancer in heavy smokers or of heart disease in hypertensives) provide a large population attributable risk proportion, and thus a large potential reduction in these diseases.

Inferences from Cohort Studies: Secular Trends

Cohort/prospective/incidence studies do not give conclusive proof that an antecedent causes a health outcome. However, they infer more evidence to support causal hypotheses than do cross-sectional or retrospective studies. Prospective studies help to establish that a hypothesized cause (characteristic or risk factor) precedes the development or appearance of the effect (condition or health outcome). The prospective method establishes time (secular) relationships between presumed antecedents and presumed effects, and in so doing, ensures knowing which came first. At this point, it is important for us to examine the inferences that are possible and not possible from comparing rates over time (secular trends). Table 3.16 shows some hypothetical prevalence and incidence rates.

Notice that the prevalence rate remains steady over time and that the incidence rate declines. The proportionately fewer new cases may be due to a successful prevention program or to antecedents of the disease dis-

TABLE 3.16 Prevalence and incidence rates per 1,000 (hypothetical)

Year	*Prevalence Rate*	*Annual Incidence Rate*
1970	70	15
1980	71	8
1990	69	4
2000	70	1

SOURCE: From Slome et al., 1986 (p. 119).

appearing or decreasing. But why is the prevalence rate steady during the same time period?

Cases may be receiving better care so that there is longer survival with the disease and lower death rates of cases. An increased cure ratio is not occurring because that would cause the prevalence rate to decline. Another possibility is that the cure ratio went up but was balanced by immigration of "old" cases who kept the prevalence rate steady but were not included as new cases in incidence.

Thus, the interplay of incidence and prevalence is related to case fatality or cure ratios—those forces which determine the presence of cases in the prevalence "pool." Prevalence varies with incidence and duration. Four patterns of secular trends of point prevalence rates and incidence rates are represented in Figure 3.6 and interpreted below.

Pattern I—The incidence rate has increased over time, but the prevalence rate has remained steady. Possible explanations are that (1) the cure ratio might be improving and/or (2) the case-fatality ratio might be increasing, so duration of disease is shortened. With a secular increase in the incidence rate, the prevention program clearly is less effective.

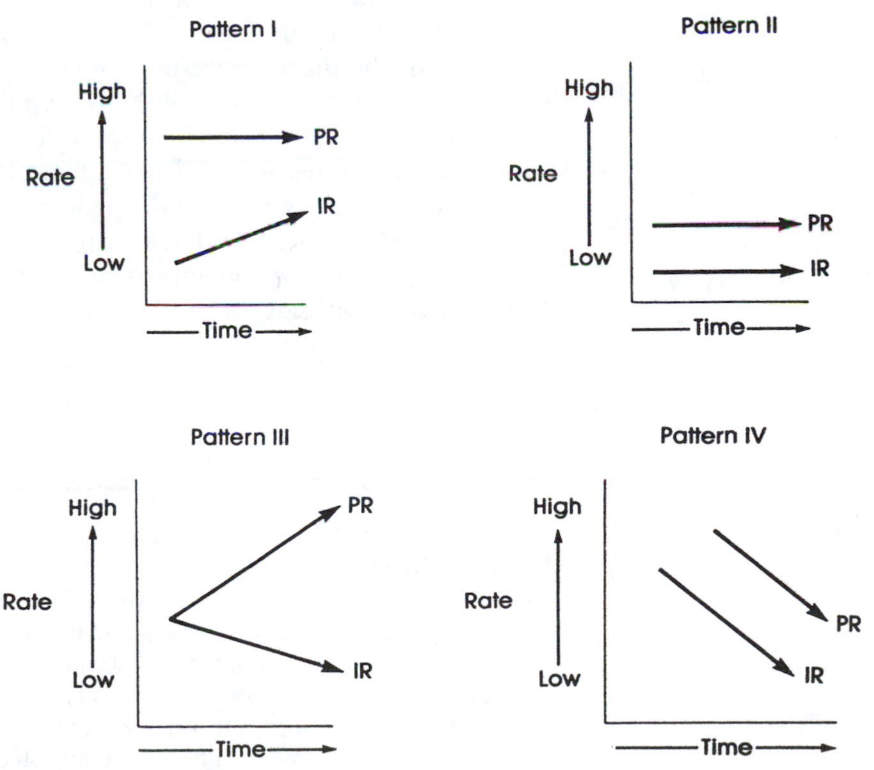

SOURCE: From Slome et al., 1986 (p. 120).

FIGURE 3.6 *Different patterns of incidence and prevalence rates*

Pattern II—There is no change in either rate over time. The case cure ratio and case-fatality ratio have been steady with no migration of cases or healthy people.

Pattern III—Although the incidence rate has declined, the prevalence rate has increased. The cure ratio may have decreased over time, or care improved, and more cases are surviving longer and are still available to be counted as cases. Thus, over time, the case-fatality ratio decreased.

In this pattern, either the prevention program is successful, the antecedents are decreasing (perhaps by migration of high risk persons), or the antecedents are not as harmful because of other changes, such as the development of immunity or resistance.

Pattern IV—Both incidence and prevalence have decreased. Declining incidence, again, may be due to a diminishing occurrence of risk factors or to better prevention. The fact that prevalence has also decreased indicates that the case indices (death and cure ratios) have remained fairly constant.

Inferences from Cohort Studies: Dose–Response Relationships

The likelihood of an association between a characteristic and a disease being causal is enhanced if a stronger "dose," or more of the antecedent, produces higher rates of disease; that is, a "dose–response" relationship is shown. Thus, the more cigarettes one smokes, the greater should be the risk of lung cancer or chronic obstructive pulmonary disease (COPD).

Table 3.17 depicts a dose–response relationship between cholesterol level and CHD incidence from Framingham Heart Study data. The higher the cholesterol level, the higher the incidence rate. The "very high" category has an exceptionally high CHD incidence rate. The relative risks for the "very high" category are approximately three times that for the "low" category, two times that for the "moderate" category, and 1.7 times that for the "high" category.

EXAMPLE

Prospective Cohort Study: Physical Fitness and All-cause Mortality

This study tested the relationship between physical fitness and risk of all-cause and cause-specific mortality among 10,224 men and 3,120 women. Physical fitness was measured by a maximal treadmill exercise test, and the average follow-up period was just over 8 years—a total of 110,482 person-years of observation. Subjects were categorized according to fitness quintiles ranging from highest fitness to lowest fitness. Age-adjusted all-cause mortality declined across fitness quintiles for both men and women. For example, the least fit men experienced 64.0 deaths per 10,000 person-years, compared to 18.6 deaths per 10,000 person-years among the most fit men. The least fit women had 39.5

deaths per person-years, compared to only 8.5 deaths per person-years among the highest fitness group of women. These declines in death rates remained after statistically controlling for such factors as age, smoking, serum cholesterol, blood pressure, blood glucose, and parental history of coronary heart disease. Low physical fitness was determined to be an important risk factor from attributable risk estimates. Declines in all-cause mortality in fit men and women appear to be due to lowered rates of cardiovascular disease and cancer (Blair, Kohl, Paffenbarger, Clark, Cooper, and Gibbons, 1989).

TABLE 3.17 Ten-year CHD incidence rates per 10,000 white men, aged 30-59 at entry, Framingham study, by starting cholesterol level

	Cholesterol Level			
	Low	*Moderate*	*High*	*Very High*
CHD incidence rate	514	708	914	1,553

SOURCE: Kannel W, Dawder T, Kagan A, et al.: The Framingham study. *Annals of Internal Medicine*, 1961; 55:33-50.

The Historical Cohort Study

One disadvantage of the cohort/prospective study is the time it takes to wait for outcomes to happen. For example, the Framingham Heart Study has been in progress for more than 40 years.

Any time one identifies a cohort of persons who are known to be free of the health outcome of interest, on whom measures of the antecedent characteristic can be obtained, and who can be followed forward in their time, they can be utilized in a cohort/prospective study. When investigators do their research today on a cohort defined in the past, the study is similar to a prospective study even though the cohort was formed in the past. Just as with the usual cohort study (starting in the present), this type of study requires persons to be free of the disease, to be stratified on the basis of the antecedent characteristic, and followed forward in time. The period of follow-up may have ended in the past (before the present), if data are available about the occurrence of new events over a period of time. The follow-up may also continue into the present or future. This study design has been given many names, however, the most useful is **historical cohort study**.

EXAMPLE

Historical Cohort Study: Vasectomy and Prostate Cancer

In questionnaires administered in 1976 and 1978, 14,607 married female participants of the Nurses' Health Study reported vasectomy as the couple's form of contraception. In 1989, researchers contacted these 14,607 women and 14,607 age-matched participants whose husbands had not had a vasectomy before 1978 to ascertain their husband's disease status between 1976 and 1989 (Giovannucci, Tosteson, Speizer, Ascherio, Vessey, and Colditz, 1993). During the study period (1976-1989), 96 new cases of prostate cancer were diagnosed in the cohort. Vasectomy was associated with an increased risk of prostate cancer (age-adjusted relative risk, 1.56; 95% confidence interval, 1.03 to 2.37). The relative risk of prostate cancer increased over time after vasectomy. For example, in men who had a vasectomy 20 or more years before, the relative risk was 1.89. The elevated risk of prostate cancer among vasectomized men persisted after the data were adjusted for smoking, alcohol consumption, educational level, body mass index, and geographical area of residence.

What are some settings in which historical cohort studies have occurred?

The historical cohort study has been widely used in studies in occupational settings where population registers (e.g., payroll records) are available historically and medical records are accessible for the period of study follow-up. Most countries record birth certificates for everyone, and prenatal records, examinations of school children or army inductees may be available on past cohorts who could be reassessed for likely outcomes. There are many other examples—survivors of the atomic bomb explosions and their offspring are still being followed up; children of mothers who took diethylstilbestrol (DES) years ago during pregnancy also represent past cohorts available now.

EXAMPLE

Historical Cohort Study: Black–White Differences in Fracture Rates

To compare the incidence of all nonvertebral fractures between elderly blacks and whites, Griffin, Ray, Fought, and Melton (1992) conducted a retrospective (historical) cohort study among Tennessee Medicaid enrollees aged 65 or older from 1987-1989. Among the 6,802 enrollees there were 7,645 new nonvertebral fractures. The incidence of fractures in blacks was only half that of whites. This finding (relative risk = 0.4 (95% confidence interval, 0.4 to 0.5) persisted after adjustment for sex, age, and nursing home residence. Fracture incidence rates were consistently lower in blacks than whites for each of the 13 different fracture sites examined.

Relative Advantages/Disadvantages of Cohort Studies

The following are relative advantages of the cohort study method:

1. Cohort studies help confirm causes of disease because they extend over a long time period.
2. Risk statements can be produced from data generated from cohort studies. In other words, the magnitude of the effect of a causative (risk) factor can be quantified.
3. Cohort studies provide baseline rates for new cases of disease against which prevention programs can be evaluated.
4. Cohort studies provide health services planners with an estimate of the number of prevalent cases at the beginning point in the study, and estimates of the new cases that will require attention. They also provide planners with the number and proportion of cases they can expect to prevent if they are successful in reducing the risk factors.
5. Cohort studies allow for analytical testing of hypotheses concerning cause and effect, and enable an estimate of the relative contributions of different causes to the occurrence of the effect (disease or outcome).
6. Factors of information bias are reduced. Selective recall/memory does not occur as a manifestation of the disease or health state. Those responsible for classifying the subjects at the start of the study cannot know who will eventually have the disease and so cannot consciously or unconsciously introduce information bias in categorizing the antecedent.
7. Bothersome selection factors are minimized because "disease-free" representative samples of a cohort with and without the presumed causal characteristics are followed over time. Thus, incidence rates are not influenced selectively by the presence of the effect (outcome, disease) at the beginning of the study.

The relative disadvantages of the cohort study method are:

1. The time required to achieve answers is longer for a cohort/prospective study, especially if the determination or latent period between the antecedent characteristic and the effect (outcome) is extensive.
2. Some participants leave the geographic area of the study and cannot be traced; some die with no known cause or lose interest in participating; some are inevitably "lost" to follow-up for the effect, despite intensive efforts to track them. This introduces selection bias.
3. Because of the time and effort involved in tracking down participants for follow-up, and because more than one

examination of subjects is required for the presence of the disease, cohort studies are expensive.

4. Participation rates in cohort studies are lower than those in cross-sectional studies because they require a longer time of participant cooperation.
5. Unexpected changes in the environment or culture that occur during the follow-up period may influence the associations of the disease and the antecedent over time. It is hoped that these events or behaviors equally affect the comparison groups, but they may not. For example, participants may change their attendance for health care or their exposure to the antecedent (i.e., a nonsmoker beginning to smoke during the study period).
6. For diseases of relatively low incidence cohort studies are not feasible because none or very few persons in the sample may actually manifest the disease. Usually an estimate of the expected incidence is required before a cohort study is begun. The investigators need to know how many cases can be expected among subgroups and how long they will need to follow them to get answers to the questions of association.

Summary of the Cohort Method

The main points covered in our discussion of the cohort method include:

1. Following a cohort of healthy individuals forward in time and observing the incidence of disease among those with a suspected risk factor along with those without the risk factor. This method involves comparing the incidence of disease between the groups to determine possible association between risk factors and disease.
2. Relating incidence and prevalence rates
3. Calculating, using, and interpreting:
   a. relative risk
   b. attributable risk, or simple attributable risk
   c. population attributable risk
   d. population attributable risk percent or population attributable fraction (etiologic fraction)
   e. estimates of community impact of health programs
4. Making inferences from cohort studies
5. Realizing advantages and disadvantages of the cohort study design.

EXPERIMENTAL STUDIES

We have examined the three common study designs used in epidemiologic research, including their strengths and weaknesses. In terms of confirming causal (antecedent) associations of health outcomes, the cohort method is the preferred choice. An extension of the cohort method would be an

experiment to see whether the expected outcome is found in a group receiving the antecedent (or exposure) compared with a control group not receiving the same antecedent. Similarly, we could conduct a **natural experiment** by following up cohorts exposed to a natural phenomenon of health consequence and compare the health effects in the exposed population with those not exposed to the phenomenon.

These sorts of studies are referred to as **experimental epidemiology.** They are often applied as **clinical trials** to assess the efficacy of some intervention procedure—medicine, education, surgical technique, type of facility, or type of health service.

EXAMPLE

Natural Experiment: Hip Fractures and Fluoridation in the Elderly

The incidence of hip fractures or fractures of the femoral neck in patients 65 years of age or older was compared in three communities in Utah, one with water fluoridated to 1 ppm and two without fluoridation. The outcome measure in the study was the rate of hospital discharge for hip fracture. The relative risk for hip fracture for women in the fluoridated area was 1.27 (95% confidence interval, 1.08 to 1.46) and for men was 1.41 (95% confidence interval, 1.00 to 1.81) relative to the nonfluoridated areas. The results of this study show a small but significant increase in the risk of hip fracture in both men and women exposed to a fluoridated water supply at 1 ppm. This suggests that low levels of fluoride may increase the risk of hip fracture in the elderly (Danielson, Lyon, Egger, and Goodenough, 1992).

What are some examples of experimental epidemiologic studies?

Here are several examples of epidemiologic studies that would classify as experimental epidemiology:

- All prophylactic vaccines, such as those against measles and rubella (German measles), diphtheria, and polio, tested on populations of children to prove the efficacy of the vaccines in preventing the diseases
- Prophylaxis with drugs such as penicillin to prevent episodes of rheumatic fever or isoniazid hydrochloride (INH) in the prevention of active tuberculosis
- Antihypertensive drugs, proven effective in clinical trial experiments, to reduce blood pressure and prevent complications such as stroke
- Testing various forms of health service delivery, such as comparing family practitioner services with physician specialty services

- Health effects of radiation following the atom bomb explosions
- Treating a group of cancer patients with a drug and comparing the group's survival or cure ratio with a similar group of cancer patients not given the same drug
- Impact on health-related behavior (e.g., smoking rates, participation in aerobic physical activity) and coronary heart disease rates in response to community-wide heart disease prevention interventions

Why are experiments often referred to as the "Supreme Court" of epidemiologic research?

Experiments can be viewed as the "Supreme Court" of epidemiologic research because they provide the strongest possible evidence of disease causation. Using experimental study designs, epidemiologists are able to rule out with greater certainty factors that may confound potential cause-and-effect relationships. By eliminating the possibility of several confounding factors (or alternative explanations for an association) a researcher increases the **internal validity** of a study. The degree of internal validity in a study depends on the study design's ability to determine whether an antecedent causes an effect (or outcome).

EXAMPLE

Experimental Trial: Nonpharmacologic Interventions and Blood Pressure

The short-term efficacy of seven nonpharmacologic interventions in persons with high normal diastolic blood pressure (80-89mm) was tested in randomized control multicenter trials. 2182 men and women were randomized into three lifestyle groups (weight reduction, sodium reduction, stress management) and four nutritional supplementation groups (calcium, magnesium, potassium, and fish oil). Each lifestyle group was compared with unmasked nonintervention controls over 18 months. Each of the four nutritional supplement groups were compared singly, in double-blind fashion, with placebo controls for a period of at least 6 months. Weight reduction intervention and sodium reduction intervention produced significant decreases in diastolic and systolic blood pressure. Despite high compliance, neither stress management intervention nor nutritional supplements reduced blood pressure significantly (The Trials of Hypertension Prevention Collaborative Research Group, 1992).

Hallmark of Experiments: The Element of Control

What is the key distinguishing factor between experimental strategies and other research strategies?

The key distinguishing factor between experimental studies and the other strategies we have discussed (cross-sectional, case-control, cohort) is the element of control. In experimental epidemiology, the investigator usually decides what the experimental factor will be, which participants will receive it, and which will not. This type of research gives the investigator more control than in cases in which the participants themselves decide whether they have the antecedent (e.g., smoke cigarettes, use oral contraceptives, or take a certain drug).

What is a quasi-experimental research situation?

There are **quasi-experimental** (literally, "as if experimental") situations in which the investigator does not have as much control as to who receives the experimental factor (e.g., experiments of "nature" such as earthquakes or famines). These situations, however, expose a large number of persons to a factor and give opportunities for epidemiologic pursuits. Many epidemiological observations of the health effects of natural occurrences have led astute observers to great discoveries (e.g., John Snow to cholera, Joseph Goldberger to pellagra).

EXAMPLE

Quasi-experimental Study: Improved Cholesterol Levels after a Worksite Nutrition Education Program

Of 80 management-level male employees who participated in a company-sponsored comprehensive physical examination, 70 had a triglyceride level above 5.17 mmol/L. These 70 men were invited to participate in a nutrition education program. Thirty-three of those who chose to participate served as the intervention group; the other 37 served as the control group. Thus, the design of the study was not random. Subjects completed 3-day dietary records before and after the nutrition education program. The intervention consisted of a year-long program of individualized instruction, group sessions, and telephone follow-up. Men in the intervention group decreased their dietary intake of calories, cholesterol, and percentage of energy from total fat and protein, and increased their consumption of carbohydrate and dietary fiber. Significant reductions in total plasma cholesterol, triglycerides, body weight, and body fat were observed in the intervention group. This study provides limited evidence that worksite nutrition education programs can decrease risk factors associated with coronary heart disease (Baer, 1993).

Ethical Considerations in Conducting Experiments

A difficult but important issue in human experimentation is ethics. Human experimentation is ethical when *without* dangerous or severely unpleasant side effects there is no effective treatment available, no animal model for testing, or when a new treatment has an acceptable chance (perhaps based on animal experimentation) of success. However, experimentation is not ethical when a treatment is potentially hazardous and satisfactory treatments are available. Moreover, *not* to experiment, when new treatments are available before an adequate trial has been carried out (e.g., new treatments for patients with HIV disease), may sometimes be considered unethical.

It is ethical for a control group to receive no treatment only if the withdrawal or withholding of treatment is in no way detrimental to the life and well-being of subjects, and the subjects are fully informed. For example, withholding treatment in an experimental trial of a new common cold remedy would be reasonable, as would be substituting a placebo for the cold remedy. A **placebo** is a treatment that the investigator believes has no effect but the subject may believe to be effective. (The word is derived from the Latin, meaning "shall be pleasing.") However, comparing the new treatment with the best available treatment is a better option for certain diseases than using a placebo.

The participant in a trial sometimes can be his or her own control by providing before use and after use information. This applies especially in drug trials in which the drug action is temporary and the individual inevitably returns to his or her original state. In this case, drugs can be assessed for effects on a before use and after use basis. The advantage is that experimental variability is reduced. However, there are only a few circumstances to which these conditions pertain; usually we want to see whether a drug affects the natural history of an illness. A before-and-after trial with only an experimental group might be used to investigate the prevention of motion sickness, alleviation of chronic, unremitting symptoms, or a change in some usually stable physiological measure.

Other aspects, such as cost, side effects, and clinical indications affect choice of treatments, but they are only partly epidemiological. Therefore it is imperative that all participants, even volunteers, be fully informed before they give written consent to participate in the trial.

In recent years, increased professional and public sensitivity to the issues involved in research with human participants has arisen for all types of study designs, not only those with an experimental element. In an effort to protect study participants, substantial local and federal guidelines have been formulated to regulate research activities. (Because these regulations vary by locality and change rapidly, it is impossible to present them here.)

Anyone who plans to undertake an epidemiological or other kind of study should be familiar with local and federal procedures for "human subjects." It is important to remember that in studying the health of humans scientific progress can only be made in a social context. Where guidelines do not exist, local professional and community leaders should be consulted regarding the acceptability of the intended trial and the conditions under which it can be carried out.

Conducting Experimental Trials

To show effective treatment, the improvement rate in a treated group (TI/T) should be greater than the improvement rate in an untreated group (NTI/NT), and the differences in rates should be unlikely to be due to chance (see Figure 3.7). The control group should be similar to the treatment group in all characteristics associated with the expected outcome (recovery), but should not receive the treatment under study. Under certain circumstances the control group may be deprived of treatment, receive the prevailing standard of care, or receive a placebo.

Placebos are given to "control" the nonbiological or nonpharmaceutical effect of the test treatment (e.g., attention being paid to the subject). (However, placebos sometimes have an effect—referred to as "placebo effect.")

A frequently used way to obtain comparable research subjects is to take all participants eligible for a clinical trial according to the study criteria (e.g., all males with third-stage prostatic cancer) and assign them to treatment or control groups at random. This is called randomizing the allocation of subjects. **Random allocation** means that each subject has an equal chance of being assigned to any group. Randomization procedures

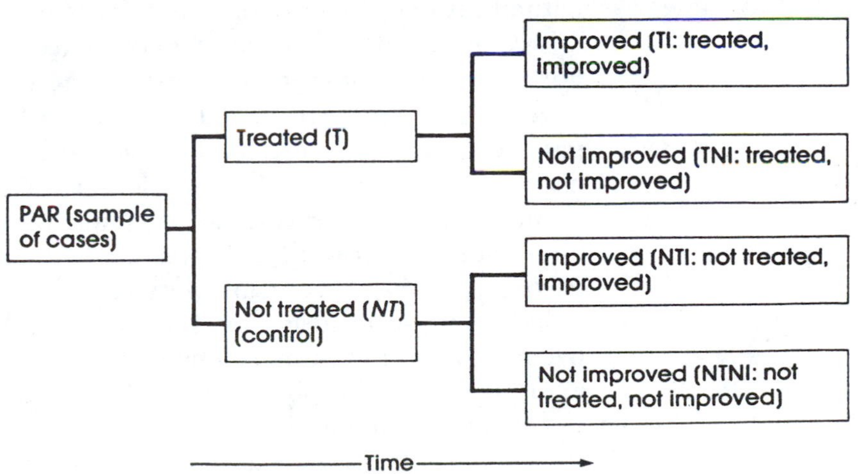

SOURCE: From Slome et al., 1986 (p. 137).

FIGURE 3.7 *Flow diagram for an experimental epidemiological study*

should produce two or more groups similar in all characteristics not controlled by other methods such as subject selection.

How is random allocation accomplished?

Random allocation can be done in many ways, from tossing a coin to using a table of random numbers, found in many statistics books and texts. The researcher decides which random scheme to use for allocating groups. Random allocation of subjects is preferable because it is an acceptable method for obtaining comparable treatment and control groups.

Random allocation can be used with matching; for example, the researcher may match for race and sex. For a matched pair of white females, the researcher would randomly assign one subject to the treatment group and one subject to the control group. After each matched pair had been assigned, the two groups would then have the same sex and race distribution. The groups should also have about the same distribution for other variables because of the random allocation of subjects. Because random allocation is used frequently, the term "randomized clinical trial" or "randomized therapeutic trial" describes this experimental epidemiologic method.

Clinical and Community Epidemiology

Clinical epidemiology encompasses the study or knowledge of health states of groups or aggregates but is usually applied only to available, chosen clinical patients and is therefore selective. Clinical epidemiology includes the application of all research design strategies—cross-sectional, retrospective, prospective—in the trial of treatments, description of the natural history of illness, or tests of preventive care.

Clinical epidemiology is closely related to community epidemiology. For example, antihypertensive drugs (those that lower blood pressure) have been proven effective in therapeutic tests with selected hypertensive patients in randomized clinical trials. A community-oriented epidemiologist (or other professional) might decide to test effective antihypertensive agents on all, or a representative sample of, hypertensives in a community—aiming to lower blood pressure and thereby reduce complications (strokes, deaths). The community-oriented epidemiologist hopes for a reduction in the incidence rates of strokes or heart disease or death in all hypertensives in the whole community, and not merely in selected cases who came to the hospital or who volunteered for the experiment.

Such community intervention trials are currently in progress with control patients being assigned to the usual form of treatment, with evaluation being aimed at reduction of complications of hypertension. The community-oriented epidemiologist considers other health and social changes in the community produced concomitantly by the program (e.g., the possible increase in undesirable drug side effects, sickness absences, neuroses, or suicides) as conceptually related to a lifelong implication of being regarded as sick.

EXAMPLE

Experimental Trial: Lipid Research Clinics Coronary Primary Prevention Trial

This study tested the efficacy of cholestyramine in reducing the risk of coronary heart disease in asymptomatic middle-aged men with high serum cholesterol levels. In this randomized, multicenter, double-blinded trial, 3806 men were assigned to a treatment or a control group. For 7 to 10 years, the control group received a placebo and the treatment group received cholestyramine; both groups followed a moderate cholesterol-lowering diet. Serum cholesterol and LDL-cholesterol reductions averaged 13.4% and 20.3% in the treatment groups. These reductions were 8.5% and 12.6% greater than those in the control (placebo) group. A 24% reduction in CHD mortality and 19% reduction in nonfatal heart attacks in the treatment was also observed (Lipid Research Clinics Program, 1984).

Summary of Experimental Epidemiology

The main points covered in our discussion of experimental epidemiology include:

1. The elements of experiments
2. Ethical considerations in carrying out experiments
3. Random allocation procedures for establishing treatment and control groups
4. The relationship between clinical and community epidemiology
5. The sequence of applications and studies in developing innovations in clinical medicine and in community/public health practice

CHAPTER SUMMARY

We can see a logical progression to expansion of knowledge by the application of epidemiological methods. An idea or hunch develops, often from a series of cases or from cross-sectional studies. Then a case-control study may be done. Later, a cohort study may be done, which may lead to the implementation of a clinical trial—if the antecedent can be applied or reduced by the researcher to subjects. This may lead to changes in clinical practice, and may possibly be followed by a community intervention trial study on all (or a sample of) cases. If the cumulative sets of findings document the benefits of the intervention at the community level, the intervention may be implemented as part of community or public health practice with ongoing evaluation of its impact. To this end, we envisage the applications of epidemiology and the interface of clinical medicine, experimental epidemiology, and community epidemiology practice.

In this chapter we discussed the advantages and limitations of four general epidemiologic research methods—cross-sectional, case-control, cohort, and experimental. The Behavioral Risk Factor Survey and the Youth Risk Survey were presented as examples of cross-sectional studies. Examples of case-control, cohort, and experimental studies were also presented. In addition we explained the calculation of incidence rates, incidence density, cumulative incidence, attributable risk, population attributable risk, and odds ratios.

KEY TERMS

population at risk (PAR)
prevalence rates
point prevalence
period prevalence
association
positive association
dependent variable
independent variable
variance
standard error
confidence interval
absolute difference
z-statistic
prevalence ratio
case-control method
retrospective
matching
relative risk
odds ratio
confidence interval
Berkson's fallacy
prospective method
cohort
population at risk
cumulative incidence
person-years
incidence density
relative risk
attributable risk
population attributable risk proportion
historical cohort study
experiment
natural experiment
experimental epidemiology
clinical trials
internal validity
quasi-experimental
placebo
random allocation
clinical epidemiology

REFERENCES

Baer JT: Improved plasma cholesterol levels in men after a nutrition education program at the worksite. *Journal of the American Dietetic Association* 1993; 93:658-663.

Ballard JE, Koepsell TD, and Rivara F: Association of smoking and alcohol drinking with residential fire injuries. *American Journal of Epidemiology*, 1992;135:26-34.

Blair SN, Kohl HW, Paffenbarger RS, Clark DG, Cooper KH, Gibbons LW: Physical fitness and all-cause mortality: A prospective study of healthy men and women. *Journal of the American Medical Association*, 1989;262:2395-2401.

Centers for Disease Control and Prevention: Selected behaviors that increase risk for HIV infection among high school students—United States, 1990. *Morbidity and Mortality Weekly Report*, 1992;41(14):231, 237-240.

Centers for Disease Control and Prevention: *Principles of epidemiology: An introduction to applied epidemiology and biostatistics, 2d ed.* Atlanta, GA: CDC, 1992.

Danielson C, Lyon JL, Egger M, Goodenough GK: Hip fractures and fluoridation in Utah's elderly population. *Journal of the American Medical Association*, 1992;268:746-748.

Folsom AR, Kaye SA, Sellers TA, Ching-Pong H, Cerhan JR, Potter JD, Prineas RJ: Body fat distribution and 5-year risk of death in older women. *Journal of the American Medical Association*, 1993;269:483-487.

Frazier EL, Franks AL, Sanderson LM: Behavioral risk factor data. In Centers for Disease Control and Prevention, *Using chronic disease data: A handbook for public health practitioners*. Atlanta, GA: CDC, 1992.

Giovannucci E, Ascherio A, Rimm EB, Colditz GA, Stampfer MJ, Willett WC: A prospective study of vasectomy and prostate cancer in U.S. men. *Journal of the American Medical Association*, 1993;269:873-877.

Giovannucci E, Tosteson TD, Speizer FE, Ascherio A, Vessey MP, Colditz GA: A retrospective cohort study of vasectomy and prostate cancer in U.S. men. *Journal of the American Medical Association*, 1993;269:878-882.

Griffin MR, Ray WA, Fought RL, Melton III J: Black-white differences in fracture rates. *American Journal of Epidemiology*, 1992;136:1378-1385.

Johnson CL, Rifkind BM, Sempos CT, Carroll MD, Bachorik PS, Briefel RR, Gordon DJ, Burt VL, Brown CD, Lippel K, Cleeman JI: Declining serum total cholesterol levels among U.S. adults: The National Health and Nutrition Examination Surveys. *Journal of the American Medical Association*, 1993; 269:3002-3008.

Lesko SM, Rosenberg L, Shapiro S: A case-control study of baldness in relation to myocardial infarction in men. *Journal of the American Medical Association*, 1993;269:998-1003.

Lipid Research Clinics Program: The Lipid Research Clinics Coronary Primary Prevention Trial results I: Reduction in the incidence of coronary heart disease to cholesterol lowering. *Journal of the American Medical Association*, 1984; 251:351-363.

Paffenbarger RS: Conditions of epidemiology to exercise science and cardiovascular health. *Medicine and Science in Sports and Exercise*, 1988;20:426-438.

Sempos CT, Cleeman JI, Carroll MD, Johnson CL, Bachorik PS, Gordon DJ, Burt VL, Briefel RR, Brown CD, Lippel K, Rifkind BM: Prevalence of high blood cholesterol among U.S. adults: An update based on guidelines from the Second Report of the National Cholesterol Education Program Adult Treatment Panel. *Journal of the American Medical Association*, 1993;269:3009-3014.

Slome C, Brogan D, Eyres S, Lednar W: *Basic epidemiological methods and biostatistics: A workbook*. Boston: Jones and Bartlett, 1986. Figures and tables used with permission.

The Trials of Hypertension Collaborative Research Group: The effects of nonpharmacologic interventions on blood pressure of persons with high normal levels: Results of the Trials of Hypertension Prevention, phase I. *Journal of the American Medical Association*, 1992;267:1213-1220.

Trump DH, Hyams KC, Cross ER, Strewing JP: Tuberculosis infection among young adults entering the U.S. Navy in 1990. *Archives of Internal Medicine* 1993;153:211-216.

PROBLEMS

1. A study published in *Archives of Internal Medicine* (Trump, Hyams, Cross, and Struewing, 1993) determined the current prevalence of tuberculin reactors among young adults entering the U.S. Navy. 2,212 male recruits were tested in January and February 1990; 55 had tuberculin reactions. What was the overall prevalence rate of the male Navy recruit population (per 100 recruits)? Calculate the prevalence rate for the recruits according to the three age groups in the table below and according to race/ethnic group. Which age group and race/ethnic group had the highest prevalence rate of tuberculin reactors?

	Number of Reactors	*Number Tested*	*Prevalence Rate per 100*
Age group (yr)			
17-19	24	1,225	____________
20-24	22	855	____________
25+	9	134	____________
Race/Ethnic group			
White	12	1,588	____________
Black	20	386	____________
Hispanic	9	167	____________
Asian/Pacific Islanders	14	53	
Other	0	20	____________

2. In a survey of patients at a sexually transmitted disease clinic in San Francisco, 180 of 300 patients interviewed reported using a condom at least once during the 2 months before the interview. What is the period prevalence of condom use in this population during the last 2 months (per 100)?

3. Two surveys were done of the same community 12 months apart. Of 5,000 people surveyed the first time, 25 had antibodies to histoplasmosis. Twelve months later, 35 had antibodies, including the original 25. Calculate the prevalence of people with histoplasmosis antibodies at the second survey, and compare the prevalence with the 1-year incidence. (Calculate rates per 1,000 persons.)

4. Bakersville* is a village of 500 elves with two major ethnic groups—the Anorexies, who comprise 60% of the population, and the Pigouts, who constitute the remaining 40%. The folks of Bakersville suffered from a variety of maladies, especially donutitis. In 1980, the prevalence rate for this painful disease was 50 per 1,000 people. Unfortunately, there was a

*This problem was developed by Larry A. Tucker and is used with his permission.

severe outbreak of donutitis in 1981 with the people developing 125 new cases. Just when the problem was under control (only 50 new cases of donutitis in 1982), the townspeople hit a streak of bad luck and were overcome by an epidemic of cookienemia. Although 100 cases of this dreadful condition were reported during 1983, citizens who had previously contracted donutitis were totally resistant and not at risk (lucky for them). Responding rapidly to the emergency, the local health department commenced an intense immunization program which had a tremendously positive impact—only 5 new cases of cookienemia developed during 1984 (3 in Anorexies and 2 in Pigouts). The whole town celebrated, especially the Pigouts, who soon thereafter showed an increased risk to cola colic, developing 50 cases during 1985. Fortunately for the Anorexies, cola colic is confined to Pigouts. Unfortunately for the Pigouts, other diseases afford no protection against cola colic. Assuming there were no deaths, births, cures, or migration in Bakersville from 1980-1985:

a. What was the prevalence rate (per 100) of donutitis for 1980-81?
b. What was the incidence rate of donutitis in 1982 (per 100)?
c. What was the probability (risk) of cookienemia development among the citizens of Bakersville in 1983 (per 100)?
d. What was the prevalence rate of cookienemia in 1984 (per 100)?
e. What was the incidence rate of cookienemia in 1984 (per 100)?
f. What was the prevalence rate of cola colic for 1985 (per 100)?
g. What was the incidence rate of cola colic for 1985 (per 100)?
h. (For this question only) Ignoring the fact that donutitis provides resistance against cookienemia and assuming that 60 Anorexies and 40 Pigouts developed cookienemia during 1983, who was at greater risk of developing cookienemia during 1984, the Anorexies or the Pigouts?

5. Identify the following studies as either a cross-sectional, a cohort, a case-control, or an experimental study.

_______ a. Vietnamese Experience Study: Subjects were several thousand soldiers stationed in Vietnam from 1969-1971 and several thousand soldiers stationed in Europe from 1969-1971. In the mid-1980s, investigators determined and compared the death rate and prevalence of illness in both groups.

_______ b. Subjects were persons with laboratory-confirmed trichinosis, and one healthy friend of each. All subjects were asked about their consumption of pork and other meat products.

_______ c. Subjects were children enrolled in a health maintenance organization. At 18 months of age, each child was randomly given one of two types of vaccine against *Haemophilus influenzae*. Parents were asked to record any side effects on a card, and mail it back after 2 weeks.

6. In a case-control study, researchers wanted to determine whether females had a greater risk of developing pellagra than males. In this study involving 1,484 female subjects and 1,419 male subjects, it was observed

that 46 females had pellagra compared to only 18 males. What is the odds ratio showing the relationship between pellagra and gender?

7. In a prospective/cohort study, you have determined that graduate students have an incidence rate of 25 per 100 (25%) of carpal tunnel syndrome compared to only 5 per 100 (5%) of people employed in professional, white-collar occupations. This was a 2-year follow-up study that began when the cohort of interest received their undergraduate degrees (May 1991 through May 1993). What is a graduate student's relative risk of developing carpal tunnel syndrome (using the non-graduate student cohort as the reference group)? What percent of cases of carpal tunnel syndrome can be attributed to being a graduate student? (All subjects in the study were free from carpal tunnel syndrome at the beginning of the study.)

8. In a recent survey, investigators found that the prevalence of Disease A was higher than the prevalence of Disease B. The incidence and seasonal pattern of both diseases are similar. Explanations consistent with this observation include: (Circle ALL that apply.)

   a. patients recover more quickly from Disease A than from Disease B
   b. patients recover more quickly from Disease B than from Disease A
   c. patients die quickly from Disease A but not from Disease B
   d. patients die quickly from Disease B but not from Disease A

9. To investigate the association between Kawasaki syndrome (KS) and carpet shampoo, investigators conducted a case-control study with 100 cases (100 children *with* KS) and 100 controls (100 children *without* KS). Among children with KS, 50 gave a history of recent exposure to carpet shampoo. Among those without KS, 25 gave a history of recent exposure to carpet shampoo. For this study, the odds ratio is:

   a. 1.0
   b. 1.5
   c. 2.0
   d. 3.0
   e. cannot be calculated from the information given

10. A group of 1,000 female college seniors from a large university were "followed" for 20 years to investigate whether the use of oral contraceptives increases women's risk of developing blood clots (thrombo-embolism). Of these females, 550 were oral contraceptive users and at the end of 20 years, 48 had developed blood clots. Among those not using oral contraceptives, 17 developed clots. None of the females had clots when the study began. What type of study is this? Calculate the appropriate statistics to show how much greater the risk of blood clots was for women who used oral contraceptives.

ANSWERS

1. The overall prevalence rate for Navy recruits was 55/2,212 × 100 = 2.5 per 100 Navy recruits. Prevalence rates according to age and race/ethnic groups are listed in the table below. The prevalence rate (6.7 per 100) was highest in those 25 years of age and higher and in Asian/Pacific Islanders.

	Number of Reactors	*Number Tested*	*Prevalence Rate per 100*
Age group (yr)			
17-19	24	1,225	2.0
20-24	22	855	2.6
25+	9	134	6.7
Race/Ethnic group			
White	12	1,588	0.8
Black	20	386	5.2
Hispanic	9	167	5.4
Asian/Pacific Islanders	14	53	26.4
Other	0	20	0.0

2. 180/300 × 100 = 60 per 100, or 60%. Thus, the period prevalence of condom use for the 2 months was 60% in this population of patients.
3. The prevalence of antibodies at the second survey was 35/5,000 × 1,000 = 7 per 1,000 persons. The number of new positives during the 12-month period (35 − 25) is 10. The population at risk (5,000 − 25) is 4,975. Therefore, the incidence rate during the 12-month period is 10/4,975 × 1,000 = 2 per 1,000.
4. a. The prevalence rate in 1980 was 50 per 1,000. Because Bakersville included 500 elves, we can determine that there were 25 cases of donutitis in 1980. In addition, there were 125 new cases in 1981. Thus, there were 150 cases (25 + 125) in a total population of 500. So, the prevalence rate (per 100) in 1980-81 is 150/500 × 100 = 30 per 100 elves.
   b. The number of new cases in 1982 was 50. The population at risk was 350 (500 − the 150 who had donutitis in 1980 and 1981). Because elves could not be cured from donutitis, people with donutitis must be excluded from the population at risk. The incidence rate (per 100) in 1982 was 50/350 × 100 = 14.3 per 100 elves.
   c. Incidence rates reflect the probability or risk of developing a new disease. In 1983, there were 100 new cases of cookienemia (numerator). Because elves who have donutitis are resistant to cookienemia, they are not at risk. The number of these elves (25 in 1980 + 125 in 1981 + 50 in 1982 = 200), subtracted from the whole population (500) gives the population at risk (500 − 200), 300. The incidence rate for cookienemia in 1983 (per 100) is 100/300 = 33.3 per 100 elves.

d. There were 100 cases of cookienemia in 1983 and 5 cases in 1984, a total prevalence of 105. Since the total population of elves is 500, the prevalence rate in 1984 (per 100) is 105/500 × 100 = 21 per 100 elves.
e. The number of new cases of cookienemia in 1984 was 5. To determine the population at risk we exclude the 200 with donutitis and 100 with cookienemia (300) from the total population of 500 elves, leaving a population at risk of 200. The incidence rate of cookienemia in 1984 (per 100) is 5/200 × 100 = 2.5 per 100 elves.
f. There were 50 cases of cola colic in 1985 among a population of 500. The prevalence rate (per 100) in 1985 is 50/500 × 100 = 10 per 100 elves.
g. The number of new cases of cola colic in 1985 was 50. Because cola colic is confined only to Pigouts, the population at risk is the 200 Pigouts in Bakersville. The incidence rate (per 100) of cola colic in 1985 is 50/200 × 100 = 25 per 100 elves.
h. The risk of elves' developing cookienemia in 1984 can be determined by calculating 1984 incidence rates for the Anorexies and Pigouts. The population at risk for the Anorexies is the total number of Anorexies (300) minus those who had cola colic in 1983 (60), or 300 − 60 = 240. The number of new cases in 1984 among Anorexies was 3. The incidence rate for Anorexies in 1984 (per 100) is 3/240 × 100 = 1.25 per 100 elves.

   The population at risk for the Pigouts would be the total number of Pigouts (200) minus those who had cola colic in 1983 (40), or 240 − 40 = 160. The number of new cases in 1984 among Pigouts was 2. The incidence rate for Pigouts in 1984 (per 100) is 2/160 × 100 = 1.25 per 100 elves. So, the risk is the same between the Anorexies (1.25/100) and the Pigouts (1.25/100).

5.
$$\text{Odds ratio} = \frac{46 \times 1{,}401}{1{,}438 \times 18} = \frac{64{,}446}{25{,}884} = 2.5$$

6. a. cohort study, because subjects were enrolled on the basis of their exposure (Vietnam or Europe)
   b. case-control study, because subjects were enrolled on the basis of whether they had trichinosis (cases) or not (controls)
   c. experimental study, because the investigators rather than the subjects themselves controlled the exposure

7. Relative risk of carpal tunnel syndrome among graduate students is 25/5 = 5. Relative risk is calculated by dividing the incidence rate in the exposed group by the incidence rate in the nonexposed (reference) group. Thus, graduate students were 5 times more likely to develop carpal tunnel syndrome than those who did not go on to graduate school. Attributable risk is 25 (cases per 100) − 5 (cases per 100) = 20 cases per 100. This means that 20 cases of carpal tunnel syndrome per 100 were attributable to the exposure (being a graduate student).

8. The correct answers are b and d. Prevalence is based on both incidence and duration. If the incidence of the two diseases is similar, the difference in prevalence must reflect a difference in duration. Since Disease A is more prevalent than Disease B, the duration of Disease A must be longer and the duration of Disease B must be shorter. Two possible explanations for Disease B's shorter duration are rapid recovery or rapid mortality.

9. The correct answer is d.

$$\frac{50 \times 75}{25 \times 50} = \frac{3{,}750}{1{,}250} = 3.0$$

10. This study is a cohort or prospective study. The risk (incidence rate) of blood clots in oral contraceptive users was 48/550 × 1,000 = 87.3 per 1,000 females. The incidence rate in those who did not use oral contraceptives was 17/450 × 1,000 = 37.8 per 1,000. Relative risk = 87.3/37.8 = 2.3. Thus, oral contraceptive users were 2.3 times more likely than non-oral contraceptive users to develop blood clots. Attributable risk was 87.3 − 37.8 = 49.5 cases per 1,000. Thus, 49.5 cases of blood clots (per 1,000) were attributable to using oral contraceptives.

REVIEW QUESTIONS

1. What is the value of cross-sectional epidemiologic studies?
2. Why are cross-sectional studies described as "snapshot" studies?
3. Why does data derived from health facilities or providers of health services often yield incorrect or incomplete information about community health?
4. What are prevalence rates? How do point prevalence rates differ from period prevalence rates?
5. What are some factors that could raise or lower point prevalence rates?
6. In what ways can prevalence rates assist health care planners?
7. What is meant by the terms "association" and "positive association"?
8. What is an independent variable? a dependent variable?
9. Why do cross-sectional studies not permit cause-effect interpretation?
10. What are the limitations of cross-sectional studies?
11. What data are collected in the Behavior Risk Factor Survey and how are the data collected?
12. What are the advantages of telephone surveys? limitations?
13. What is prevalence ratio?
14. Why are case-control studies often referred to as retrospective?
15. Who are the cases and the controls in case-control studies?
16. What are some guidelines for selecting cases and controls?
17. What is matching? Why is matching often difficult?
18. List things that can potentially bias a study or lead to invalid findings in case-control studies.
19. Why is it not possible to establish antecedent-consequence relationships for case-control studies?
20. Why is it not possible to calculate relative risk in case-control studies?
21. What technique is used to estimate relative risk in case-control studies?
22. What does an odds ratio of 2.4 mean?
23. What is a confidence interval?
24. Why are cohort studies referred to as "prospective" (looking forward) studies?
25. What is a cohort? What are examples of cohorts?
26. Why is it necessary for a cohort used in an incidence study to be free of the health outcome of interest at the start of the study?

27. What do incidence rates measure?
28. What constitutes the population at risk in the calculation of incidence rates?
29. What are some factors that can produce strong influences on incidence rates?
30. How do measures that produce a cure for a disease influence incidence rates for that disease?
31. Describe the concept of incidence density. How is incidence density calculated?
32. How is cumulative incidence calculated?
33. Describe how relative risk is calculated. What does relative risk describe?
34. What is attributable risk? population attributable risk?
35. Discuss how cohort studies infer more evidence to support casual hypotheses than do cross-sectional or case-control studies.
36. What is a historical cohort study? Give examples.
37. What is an experiment? What is a natural experiment?
38. What are clinical trials? Give examples.
39. Why are experiments called the "Supreme Court" of epidemiologic research?
40. What is internal validity in relation to experiments?
41. What is the key distinguishing factor between experimental studies and other study methods?
42. What are quasi-experimental situations?
43. What are important ethical issues in human experimentation?
44. Describe the necessary conditions of control groups.
45. What are placebos and why are they sometimes used in experimental research?
46. How is random allocation performed?
47. What is clinical epidemiology? How does clinical epidemiology relate to community epidemiology?

4 Avoiding Common Pitfalls in Epidemiologic Research

OBJECTIVES

On completion of this chapter, you will be able to:

- List several sources of bias in epidemiological research studies
- Describe potentially erroneous conclusions that may result from incorrect labeling of cases and noncases and understand problems that are associated with categorization of data
- List ways of increasing the reliability and validity of studies
- Describe the concepts of ecological fallacy and cohort effect
- Describe how the use of ecologic indices can be potentially fallacious and list ways of controlling for ecological fallacy
- Discuss limitations of ecological indices
- Define sensitivity and specificity
- Discuss considerations in selecting data cutoff points and in classifying research subjects
- Provide examples of selection bias and potential selective forces on study populations
- Provide examples of cohort effects, events that can produce cohort effects, and steps that can be taken to confirm cohort effects

This chapter addresses certain aspects that must be considered in applying epidemiological methods if observations and their interpretations are to be meaningful. We will consider potential errors in:

- case labeling and the importance of reliability and validity in epidemiology
- classification of data
- forces of selection that may lead to spurious associations
- deriving relationships between indices that are based on group rather than individual characteristics
- failing to consider cohort effects

RELIABILITY AND VALIDITY: REDUCING INFORMATION BIAS

Potential problems in categorizing cases and/or characteristics are called information bias, or false labeling. Two important aspects of this bias are reliability (reproducibility, repeatability) and validity (accuracy, correctness).

What is bias?

The definition of bias depends on the frame of reference in which it is used. To a seamstress, bias is a line of direction across the weave of the cloth. To a bowler, it is a lopsided weight on the ball. To a racist, it is something often denied. To a statistician, bias is the difference between the average estimated value of a population parameter and the true (usually unknown) value of the population parameter.

In epidemiology, **information bias** is a conscious or unconscious tendency to mislabel observations in a nonrandom (systematic) manner so as to distort the estimate of effect. More simply, information bias is the tendency to misclassify variables in a consistent way that tips the scales in one particular direction.

In epidemiological studies, we are seeking information about differences in groups as shown by characteristics or by disease. Any differences produced artificially by labeling tendencies cloud the issue, give false answers to questions, and must be perpetually guarded against by checks built into the study design.

In every study, therefore, as part of the pretest or planning, an assessment of the intra- and/or inter-observer reliability should be obtained, and its dimensions assessed. Then we will know some of our errors, may be able to correct them, and thus be able to consider them as possible explanations for our findings.

Reliability of Observations

Consider bias from the standpoint of **reliability** or repeatability. In many epidemiological studies, for reasons of feasibility and time, more than one observer obtains data. For example, a variety of screening tests, questionnaires, or clinical examinations may be used to obtain information for classifying individuals (e.g., diseased or not diseased, smoker or nonsmoker, high cholesterol level or low cholesterol level). It is easy to imagine that the classification of results might differ when more than one observer interprets results or applies the instruments used in the study.

The following illustration is an example of erroneous conclusions that might result from nonrandom systematic mislabeling by one or more observers. A and B are observers studying disease distribution among men and women. If A examines only men and B examines only women, reproducibility is a potential hazard in comparing the two sexes. That is, differences between the sex-specific disease rates may be due only to the tendency of A and B to label certain symptoms differently for each gender group, rather than to "real" disease differences between the male and female populations. But if both A and B examine some men and some women, and the subjects are randomly assigned to A or B, any errors of A and B are spread throughout the two gender groups. Having both A and B examine men and women helps avoid spurious results obtained by a (potentially) high degree of nonreproducibility (low reliability) of a nonrandom nature.

However, even a single observer may vary over time in his/her precision of data collection. The measurement of this particular variability is called **intra-observer reliability** (within one observer). Consistency between two or more observers is called **inter-observer reliability** (between observers).

How is intra-observer reliability calculated?

Tests of reliability or reproducibility are valuable only if each labeling or examination result for a given test is independent of the knowledge of previous examination results on that specimen or person. Prior knowledge of earlier results can influence labeling and bias the results of the two examinations. It is important that we have no prior knowledge of previous results in testing for reliability.

The following hypothetical example illustrates the calculations of a test of reliability. To investigate intra-observer reliability a nurse was twice given the same 30 specimens of urine to test for the presence or absence of sugar. The nurse was not allowed to know her/his first findings when doing each repeat examination.

Table 4.1 shows the results of the two independent examinations for the presence or absence of sugar done by one observer on the same 30 specimens of urine. Results of the urine sugar tests were scored as negative (0), positive (+), or strongly positive (++). These data can be summarized by a frequency distribution for each examination, as shown in Table 4.2.

Looking at the results in Table 4.2, were the examinations 100% reproducible?

The answer to this question is no. The identical frequencies in Table 4.2 for 0, +, and ++ on the two examinations are misleading. The same totals were obtained even though different results were obtained for some individual specimens on the two examinations. Totals (or table marginals)

TABLE 4.1 Amount of sugar in urine specimen on two examinations

Urine Specimen Number	*Exam 1*	*Exam 2*	*Urine Specimen Number*	*Exam 1*	*Exam 2*
1	+	0	16	+	+
2	0	0	17	+	+
3	++	+	18	0	++
4	0	+	19	0	0
5	++	++	20	++	0
6	+	0	21	0	++
7	0	0	22	0	0
8	++	+	23	++	0
9	+	+	24	+	0
10	+	++	25	0	0
11	0	0	26	+	++
12	+	+	27	++	+
13	0	0	28	0	++
14	0	0	29	0	0
15	0	++	30	0	0

SOURCE: From Slome et al., 1986 (p. 150).

TABLE 4.2 Frequency distribution of amount of sugar in urine as shown by examination

Amount of Sugar	*Exam 1*	*Exam 2*
0	15	15
+	8	8
++	7	7
Total	30	30

SOURCE: From Slome et al., 1986 (p. 150).

never provide adequate information from which to judge reliability. We must compare the results of the two examinations *for each specimen*; that is, we need to know how many specimens had the same result on both examinations. Although the comparison of two independent examinations may look very good, unless it compares results for individual cases or specimens, it is not accurately assessing reliability.

We can put the results of the two examinations in a table (Table 4.3) to permit us to calculate the correct index of reliability. Number 3 in the first row of Table 4.3 represents that there were 3 specimens (out of 30) for which the nurse gave a result of + on the first examination and 0 on the second examination.

We can now determine how reproducible the nurse observer's examinations were. The reliability (repeatability) index for this observer is

$$\frac{10 + 3 + 2}{30} = \frac{15}{30} = 50\%$$

TABLE 4.3 Frequency distribution: Amount of sugar in 30 urine specimens, by results of two examinations

		Exam 1: Amount of Sugar			
		0	*+*	*++*	*Total*
Exam 2: Amount of sugar	0	10	3	2	15
	+	2	3	3	8
	++	3	2	2	7
Totals		15	8	7	30

SOURCE: From Slome et al., 1986 (p. 152).

Note that in the numerator the frequencies in the diagonal of the table were added. A reproducibility rate of 50% is not very good. It indicates that the observer arrives at a different result in one half of her/his reexaminations, a very inconsistent performance. Note that this index represents reliability as being 50% reproducible—not 50% correct. We do not know the correct results; in fact, every result may be incorrect. Reliability tests are *not* assessments of correctness.

Suppose that we care only whether the result of the urine examination is positive (+ or ++) or negative (0). The reproducibility is not necessarily the same as in our previous calculation. In fact, reproducibility is likely to be better than 50% because now the nurse needs only to distinguish between negative and positive (a dichotomous decision), as opposed to distinguishing between 0, +, and ++. Using the data from Table 4.3, Table 4.4 can be constructed.

In this case the reproducibility is (10 +10)/30, better than 50%. Although this index of reproducibility is better than the previous index, it is still not very good. This example shows that one observer may be so inconsistent that the findings are primarily an indication of the observer's inconsistency, rather than a true measure of the study group's health state.

What are the consequences of unreliability?

The unreliability of the nurse observer would have consequences in both treatment and epidemiological data-gathering situations. Any inconsistency is damaging in the clinical situation, where the inconsistent test results may influence clinical judgments and affect a patient's treatment.

When inconsistent information is gathered to indicate the status of groups of individuals (in the form of rates), the consequences may be less hazardous from the individual's point of view, but the resulting data may be useless in reflecting the comparative states of the groups—the data reflect only the observer's acumen (or lack of it) at that moment in time. Some unreliability in studies is expected, and if the population or sample

TABLE 4.4 Frequency distribution: Presence/absence of sugar in urine, by results of both examinations

		Sugar on Exam 1		
		Absent	*Present*	*Total*
Sugar on Exam 2	Absent	10	5	15
	Present	5	10	15
Totals		15	15	30

SOURCE: From Slome et al., 1986 (p. 153).

is large, a few "misses" cannot unduly exaggerate or depress rates, especially if the inconsistency involves data from only one particular group being compared. However, a few misses are important if the sample size is small. If reliability is poor, as with the nurse observer, there will be much uncertainty in defining cases. Any consistent direction of the unreliability can produce false rates. For example, if the unreliability on urine specimens is greater in female diabetics than in male diabetics, it will distort the effect measures and the conclusions drawn from them.

What are sources of unreliability?

Many clinical tests are not as reliable as we would like them to be. For example, readings of x-rays and laboratory tests vary from observer to observer and from test to test conducted by one observer. Characteristics that vary because of subjective perception on the part of an observer or subject run the risk of low reliability. Some examples are emotions, taste, smell, color, or attitude. Characteristics that are more quantifiable, such as age, gender, or marital status, have higher reliability. For example, if one sex consistently underreports age, there is high reliability even if the information is 100% invalid (incorrect).

There are several sources of unreliability. Sources attributable to the observer include inexperience, carelessness, poor sensory faculties needed to obtain information (e.g., ability to accurately hear telephone survey responses), previous knowledge or beliefs, inconsistencies in procedures of applying tests, coding errors, and human biases. Instrumentation problems such as leaking mercury from sphygmomanometers (for measuring blood pressure), unreliable measuring scales, and faulty laboratory equipment may be a source of unreliability.

Another source of unreliability is biological variability in research subjects. The nurse observer examined the *same* specimens twice. If the second examinations had been done on new specimens, even from the *same subjects,* the test of reproducibility would have been confounded by the biological variability expected to occur between urine samples from the same subject. The natural variability of any characteristic (e.g., sugar in urine) over time often presents a problem in checking intra- and inter-observer reliability. This is especially true for those characteristics which cannot be gathered and held for future observations (as many laboratory specimens can be) or for those that show a high degree of variability within short periods of time (i.e., blood pressure, pulse rate, emotions).

Training and providing opportunities for practice for observers can reduce unreliability, as does frequent checking and immediate repair (calibration) of any mechanical apparatus. Techniques used in data gathering should be as standardized as possible with a minimum of difference in method and style for individual observers.

How is inter-observer reliability calculated?

When more than one person gathers data, we are concerned with inter-observer reproducibility (reliability). This is measured by the amount of agreement between observers when they measure identical subjects or evidence.

In the following hypothetical example, data from a study of male cotton workers in No Where County, Alabama from 1988-1990 were used to determine cases of byssinosis, a chronic lung disorder due to the inhalation of cotton fibers. Two nurse practitioners gathered and classified the data. In order to investigate the amount of agreement between the two nurse practitioner observers, 183 male cotton farmers were examined independently and rated as "normal," having "Grade 1 byssinosis," or having "Grade 2 byssinosis." The results of the examinations are presented in Table 4.5.

Notice that there was agreement between the diagnosis of normal for 72 workers. Agreement was found in 47 diagnoses for Grade 1 byssinosis and in 20 diagnoses for Grade 2 byssinosis. Inter-observer reliability can be calculated by adding together the total number of diagnosis agreements (72 + 47 + 20) and dividing the total by the total number of workers

TABLE 4.5 Frequency distribution: Byssinosis ratings, by results of observers A and B, 183 male cotton workers, aged 40-59, Nowhere County, Alabama

		Observer A			
		Normal	*Grade 1*	*Grade 2*	*Total*
Observer B	Normal	72	6	0	78
	Grade 1	6	47	17	70
	Grade 2	1	14	20	35
Totals		79	67	37	183

SOURCE: From Slome et al., 1986 (p. 156).

observed (183). Therefore, inter-observer reliability for the three-way classification was (72 + 47 + 20)/183 = 139/183, or 76%.

Reliability on the presence (Grade 1 and Grade 2) or absence (normal) of byssinosis is (72 + 47 + 14 + 17 + 20)/183 = 170/183 = 93%. There were 14 workers whom observer A rated as Grade 1 and observer B rated as Grade 2. Similarly, 17 workers were rated as Grade 1 by observer B but Grade 2 by observer A.

Sometimes reliability is reported in the form of a correlation coefficient rather than as a proportion. A correlation coefficient is a statistical index showing the degree to which one variable changes as another variable changes. When correlation coefficients are used to measure degrees of reliability, they range in value from 0 (poor reliability) to 1 (superb reliability). What is "acceptable reliability" depends on the researcher and the situation; no absolute criteria govern acceptable values of reliability when a correlation coefficient (or a proportion) is used.

Validity of Observations

Another important part of information bias is **validity,** the correctness of labeling or measurement. In other words, validity is the ability of a criterion or tool to measure what it claims to measure, as well as the correctness of study participants' reports. Theoretically, observers can be 100% reproducible (reliable), yet be 100% incorrect (invalid). That is, observers can be very consistent in mislabeling or measuring in an invalid way. Inaccurate labeling is a potential bias in any epidemiologic study; study planners must take extreme care to avoid and reduce mislabeling of participants.

In categorizing participants in an epidemiologic study, there are four possible scenarios:

1. We can correctly categorize true cases (those with the disease or health condition of interest) as cases. We call these **true positives**; this is valid labeling.
2. We can correctly label the noncases (those without the disease or health condition of interest) as noncases. These are called **true negatives**; this categorization is also valid.
3. We can incorrectly label true cases as noncases. These are **false negatives.** Such labeling is incorrect, or not valid.
4. We can incorrectly label noncases as cases. These are **false positives.** This labeling is not valid.

What is sensitivity and specificity?

Let us return to the example testing sugar in the urine to illustrate validity. We ask a technician to test 100 specimens of urine, of which 50 are known to us to contain sugar; the remaining 50 are free of sugar. In the 100

TABLE 4.6 Frequency distribution: Technician's test results, by actual absence/presence of sugar in 100 urine specimens

		Actual Sugar Status		
		Present	*Absent*	*Total*
Technician's measure of sugar status	Present	(TP) 45	(FP) 20	65
	Absent	(FN) 5	(TN) 30	35
Totals		(Tot P) 50	(Tot N) 50	100

KEY: TP = True Positive FN = False Negative Tot P = Total Positive
FP = False Positive TN = True Negative Tot N = Total Negative

SOURCE: From Slome et al., 1986 (p. 163).

specimens, the technician labels 65 with sugar, 45 of which were known by us to contain sugar. This information is displayed in Table 4.6.

From this information, we can calculate sensitivity and specificity scores. **Sensitivity** is the percentage of all true cases correctly identified; in this example, a "case" is sugary urine. **Specificity** is the percentage of all true noncases (those with no sugary urine) correctly identified. The technician identified 45 of the 50 true cases (sugary urines) as cases. Therefore, the sensitivity is 45/50 = 90%. This technician correctly identified 30 of the 50 specimens with no sugar (noncases); therefore, his specificity is 30/50 = 60%.

Sensitivity measures an observer's ability to identify true positives, and specificity identifies an observer's ability to pick out the true negatives.

$$\text{Sensitivity} = \frac{TP}{TP + FN} \text{ or } \frac{\text{TRUE POSITIVES}}{\text{TOTAL POSITIVE}}$$

$$\text{Specificity} = \frac{TN}{TN + FP} \text{ or } \frac{\text{TRUE NEGATIVES}}{\text{TOTAL NEGATIVE}}$$

What are the consequences of invalid data for health services and research?

The technician's sensitivity rate (90%) indicates that he will probably not misidentify many true cases, but his low specificity rate (60%) suggests that he will mislabel as positive a large number of true negatives, and overestimate the number of cases. If the technician's test is the basis for patient referral, the number of false positives projected may overload a health service. In addition, the number of false positives is likely to create unnecessary alarm for patients and possibly needless treatment. On the other hand, false negatives mean that some cases will not be identified or treated. This is especially undesirable for conditions for which adequate treatment exists and is available.

In an epidemiological study, incorrectly labeled cases or characteristics may produce false etiologic associations or mask true causal findings. Unlike reliability, a determination of validity demands an objective standard of "truth" by which to judge. We may set up as "truth" a physician's diagnosis, or standards of growth, or biochemical levels. However, as knowledge increases, such standards may change or the decision based on the standard may change. For many characteristics, there is no consensus on standards among researchers. For characteristics which many researchers believe there are no standards, arbitrary standards are usually established.

It is difficult to find a standard for anything categorized on the basis of subjective or perceptive assessment. In addition to emotions and the sensations of color, smell, or pain, the diagnosis of neurosis and other psychiatric disorders can be very subjective. Self-esteem, self-efficacy, locus of control, and health attitudes are other examples. Behavioral scientists deal with variables of this type.

What are other types of validity used in behavioral sciences?

In the behavioral sciences, other types of validity are considered in establishing behavioral, cognitive, and affective measures. **Construct validity** is the degree to which a measure correlates with the characteristics one would expect. If a measure appears so logical to the study population that we can accept it at face value as valid, the measure has **face validity.** **Predictive validity** is the degree to which a measure forecasts the outcome of interest.

Predictive validity in epidemiology asks the following: Of the subjects that are labeled as cases, what percentage really are cases? This is essential information for health screening programs.

Applications of Reliability and Validity

The data in Table 4.7 are hypothetical results of two physicians' diagnoses of 30 cases and the correct diagnosis on those cases. From this data, we can calculate the inter-observer reliability of diagnoses of Dr. A and Dr. B, 8/30 = 26.7%. This suggests that similar physician training does not ensure high reliability. Note that all agreements between the two physicians were on coronary heart disease (CHD). On other disorders, the reproducibility was 0%.

As shown in Table 4.8, on "presence" or "absence" of CHD, they agreed 14/30 = 46.7%, as compared with 26.7% reproducibility on all other diagnoses. The reliability between these two observers is poor.

Table 4.9 shows the validity of the two physicians' diagnoses. We can calculate the validity (sensitivity and specificity) of Dr. A and Dr. B for their diagnoses of CHD, using the correct diagnosis as the standard (truth).

TABLE 4.7 Diagnosis, by phsyician, and correct diagnosis for 30 cases (hypothetical)

Case	*Dr. A's Diagnosis*	*Dr. B's Diagnosis*	*Correct Diagnosis*
1	Flu	CHD	Cancer
2	CHD	CHD	CHD
3	Suicide	CHD	CHD
4	Accident	Syphilis	Cancer
5	CHD	CHD	CHD
6	Homicide	Pneumonia	Cancer
7	Stroke	CHD	Flu
8	CHD	Flu	CHD
9	Cancer	CHD	Syphilis
10	CHD	CHD	CHD
11	CHD	CHD	Old Age
12	Cancer	CHD	CHD
13	Stroke	CHD	CHD
14	Homicide	Dysentery	Stroke
15	Old Age	CHD	Hysteria
16	CHD	CHD	CHD
17	CHD	CHD	CHD
18	Stroke	CHD	CHD
19	CHD	Sclerosis	Accident
20	Accident	Senility	Suicide
21	CHD	CHD	CHD
22	Cancer	Flu	Homicide
23	Drowning	CHD	Cancer
24	Stroke	CHD	CHD
25	Syphilis	Pneumonia	Accident
26	Pneumonia	CHD	CHD
27	Flu	CHD	CHD
28	CHD	CHD	Cancer
29	Pneumonia	CHD	CHD
30	CHD	Syphilis	Psychosis

SOURCE: From Slome et al., 1986 (p. 167).

TABLE 4.8 Frequency distribution: Presence/absence of CHD, by physician observer, for 30 cases

		CHD Status by Dr. A		
		CHD	*No CHD*	*Total*
CHD status by Dr. B	CHD	8	13	21
	No CHD	3	6	9
	Totals	11	19	30

SOURCE: From Slome et al., 1986 (p. 169).

TABLE 4.9 Frequency distribution: Presence/absence of CHD, by physician observer and by correct diagnosis, for 30 cases

		True Cases (CHD)	True Noncases (No CHD)	Total
CHD status by Dr. A	CHD	7	4	11
	No CHD	8	11	19
	Totals	15	15	30
CHD status by Dr. B	CHD	14	7	21
	No CHD	1	8	9
	Totals	15	15	30

SOURCE: From Slome et al., 1986 (p. 169).

Sensitivity is the ratio of true positives to all cases diagnosed as positive (true positives/all positives). Therefore, the **sensitivity** for Dr. A is 7/15 = 46.7%, and for Dr. B is 14/15 = 93.3%. **Specificity** is the ratio of true negatives to all cases diagnosed as negative (true negatives/all negatives). The specificity for Dr. A is 11/15 = 73.3%, and for Dr. B is 8/15 = 53.3%.

Which physician would be a better examiner for CHD in a screening program? Dr. A is likely to miss more than half the cases of CHD and is only fairly accurate in identifying noncases. Dr. B has a better record for identifying cases and thus would be the choice for a case-finding and treatment program.

Causes of Invalidity

The same types of factors that cause unreliable labeling also produce invalid or incorrect labeling. Observers' characteristics such as inexperience, poor sensory faculties, and previous knowledge and beliefs, as well as instrument shortcomings such as faulty equipment are some of these factors.

In addition, validity is influenced by the choice of the particular standard. Judgments about the best available standard change as knowledge and techniques of diagnosis advance. Thus, it is important in any study to reconsider the validity of all measurement techniques even though they may have been shown to be valid in the past. In practice, many researchers neglect this, a deficiency which may haunt them when they interpret their findings.

Can one always have confidence in a questionnaire that has been validated by other investigators? Not necessarily. Some studies have shown that validity is not constant across all groups. For example, the validity of the same test instrument can vary among different ethnic groups or age groups. This suggests that the degree of validity determined previously for a particular group of subjects may not hold true for similar groups at another point in time. Reestablishing validity for each subpopulation (cross-cultural validity) will produce confidence in the results.

POTENTIAL CAVEATS IN CLASSIFYING DATA

Classifying observations breeds potential hazards. In epidemiology, we classify persons into groups such as diseased or not diseased, or categories such as upper or lower social class. Criteria must be precisely defined for each group in an epidemiologic study. The criteria depend on current knowledge of the health outcome or other characteristics and on the type of data available. Data is either **quantitative** (e.g., blood pressure) or **categorical** (e.g., marital status, pregnancy status, gender).

Cutoff Points in Classifying Data

Table 4.10 shows hypothetical blood pressure recordings on 20 persons. We can use these data to examine the effects of cutoff points in classifying subjects as hypertensive. Let's look at four different cutoff points:

1. Hypertension defined as a systolic reading of 160 mm or higher. With this cutoff point, the rate of hypertension is 10/20 = 50%.
2. Hypertension defined as a diastolic reading of 90 mm or higher. With this cutoff as the criterion, the rate of hypertension is 8/20 = 40%.
3. Hypertension defined as a systolic reading of 160 mm or higher *or* a diastolic reading of 90 mm or higher. With these cutoff points, the rate is 14/20 = 70%. Although some patients may fit into both of the first two definitions, it is correct to count each hypertensive case only once.
4. Hypertensive cases defined as a systolic reading of 160 mm or higher *and* a diastolic of 90 mm or higher. With these criteria, the rate of hypertension is 4/20 = 20%.

As you can see, the rates of hypertension in this small sample of 20 subjects change from 20% to 70% as the cutoff classification criteria vary.

TABLE 4.10 Systolic and diastolic blood pressure (BP) readings on 20 individuals

Person	*Systolic BP (in mm Hg)*	*Diastolic BP (in mm Hg)*	*Person*	*Systolic BP (in mm Hg)*	*Diastolic BP (in mm Hg)*
1	160	90	11	120	80
2	212	74	12	164	92
3	110	54	13	156	92
4	162	86	14	200	88
5	146	94	15	120	64
6	184	64	16	150	96
7	200	110	17	148	84
8	158	94	18	210	110
9	140	60	19	140	86
10	210	86	20	160	88

SOURCE: From Slome et al., 1986 (p. 174).

The rates can be changed more by choosing different blood pressure levels as the cutoff points to define hypertension.

Thus, studies that use different criteria for defining the presence of any health state are not comparable with respect to reported rates of that health state. The use of different criteria or definitions in classification is a problem that can be solved only by cooperative decision by researchers. For example, epidemiological committees have urged general usage of agreed-on cutoff points for blood pressure. Because of this, hypertension studies using these criteria can be compared to each other with more confidence.

This does not imply, however, that epidemiological results are always comparable if identical diagnostic criteria were used. Investigations may differ on other important methodological points.

All study reports should state clearly criteria used for classifying variables. When we decide on classification criteria for investigations, using criteria of other researchers (even if it means reporting results in more than one way) improves comparability.

Quantitative and Categorical Variables

Blood pressure measured in mm of mercury is a quantitative variable because the number (e.g., 120 mm) indicates the amount of pressure in arteries. On the other hand, hypertension is a categorical variable (also called "nominal," from a Latin word that means "name"). In our hypertension example, subjects are classified as either hypertensive or not hypertensive. The quantitative blood pressure measurement (mm of mercury) was used to create two categories based on the concept that high blood pressure (hypertension) is a disease entity.

What are the ramifications of collapsing quantitative data into categories?

Some information on variability between persons is lost when quantitative data are categorized. For example, all those persons classified as hypertensive because their systolic blood pressure was 160 mm or higher are regarded as identical to each other, even though these persons do not have identical blood pressure measurements.

Collapsing a quantitative variable into a categorical variable with two or more categories may also obscure the fact that the underlying variable has a much larger range in one category than in another category. For example, at the cutoff point of 90 mm or more diastolic blood pressure, the range for hypertensives is 20 (90 to 110), whereas the range for non-hypertensives is 34 (54 to 88). (Note: the **range** of a collection of observations is the largest observation minus the smallest observation.) We must be careful in comparing ranges because a larger sample will generally have a larger range. One reason the range may be larger in the non-

Table 4.11 Classification of 100 consecutive patients in an outpatient clinic

Category	*Patients*
Bacterial infection	40
Anxiety	53
Cancer	10
Localized infection	15
Old age	8
Tiredness	3

SOURCE: From Slome et al., 1986 (p. 179).

hypertensive group is that (in our example) there are 12 subjects in that group compared with only 8 in the hypertensive group.

Collapsing quantitative variables into categories also limits the choices of appropriate statistical tests of significance.

Without categorization, however, we would never be able to calculate rates and make comparisons for some health conditions. Further, some categories have ecological meaning or social meaning. For example, we often use age 65 as "old" because so many legislative, health, and other services use this cutoff point. Commonly used categories such as five- or ten-year age bands in available data encourage our use of those same ranges. With adults, five-year age groups, such as 20-24 and 25-29, are frequent. But in studying infants, because they are very different in respect to likelihood of death, causes of death, and diseases in the first few days of life, as compared with the first four weeks and later weeks, we often categorize ages as perinatal (first week of life), neonatal (first 28 days of life), and postneonatal, or 29 days to one year.

In general, it is advisable not to start with wide ranges such as 20-year age groups, but with smaller components of the large category, such as five-year groups. If adjacent smaller categories do not differ on the health condition, and are not important in the test of the hypothesis or for other purposes, small categories may be combined into a larger category since differences are not masked any in so doing.

Application in Classifying Data

The classification scheme used in Table 4.11 might be a useful classification scheme for some specialists within a clinic. However, other specialists, such as psychiatrists, may want to know how many people have anxiety, no matter what additional afflictions they have.

Some modification of the classification scheme would be more generally useful for epidemiological purposes. Some patients have double (or more) pathology and thus appear in more than one category; this is indicated by the sum of the diagnostic frequencies (patient columns) which is greater than 100%. The problem of nonexclusive categories can be solved by creating separate categories or separate combinations of disorders, such as anxiety and cancer. Persons with double or triple pathology, along with patients with pathologies not mentioned in the list, can be categorized as "other." (This "catch-all" category may be detrimental if it includes many people.)

Mutually exclusive categories allow a subject to appear in only one category. **Exhaustive categories** include all classifiable subjects once in some category. Thus, the category of "other" may be necessary when all possible expected categories are not known, or included in case an unanticipated entity occurs.

Must all persons in an epidemiologic study be classifiable?

All persons in an epidemiologic study must be classifiable. This may require additional categories such as "refused to answer," "missing data," "unknown," and "other." Criteria for each classification category should be clearly established and strictly applied. The classification system must have conceptual meaning as related to the purpose of the study.

SELECTION BIAS

In the previous sections, we discussed potential pitfalls associated with information bias—errors in incorrect labeling of cases and noncases, and problems associated with categorization of data. This section is concerned with who gets into an epidemiological study—as participants, not as investigators. It addresses the population at risk and the forces of selection that can produce incorrect findings if the findings are not based on correct samples. Selection bias is an important area of potential error. **Selection bias** refers to the distortion of effect resulting from the way participants are accepted into studies.

Suppose the results of a study showed that the prevalence rate of patients with heart transplants was higher in Stanford, California, in 1993 than in any other city in the world. Why would this be likely? The Stanford University surgical expertise attracts those in need of heart transplants. This is a simple example of the effect of selective use of health services in producing a finding. We would be drawing a false conclusion if we decided that something about Stanford other than the surgeons' presence was associated with the high rate of heart transplants at Stanford.

A classic example of this type of selection is the initial description of the occurrence of thromboangeitis obliterans (Buerger's disease—a disease affecting peripheral blood vessels). In 1908 when Leo Buerger described the syndrome, he observed that the disease occurs frequently, although not exclusively, among Polish and Russian Jews. He also suggested that the dispensaries and hospitals of New York City provided a good opportunity for studying this condition. We realize now that any disorder described by Buerger might have appeared to be common among Polish and Russian Jews because he practiced at Mt. Sinai Hospital in New York, which at that time was used almost exclusively by Jews of Polish and Russian extraction.

Therefore, the sort of clientele (the characteristics of the population) using a health service may well determine an association that is not really epidemiologically significant. Such an association is artifactual and hence "noncausal," as a result of selection bias.

Hollingshead and Redlich (1958) studied psychiatric cases diagnosed and reported by psychiatrists and mental health agencies in a Connecticut community. The associations they found between mental illness and social class are shown in Table 4.12.

The prevalence rates in this table are derived from cross-sectional (point prevalence) studies, and the rates are adjusted for gender and age. Gender adjustment is a statistical manipulation used to prevent erroneous conclusions when data contain an unequal distribution of genders among social classes. Gender adjustment is used because mental illness and the characteristic of gender are associated. If genders are equally distributed in the classes, no adjustment for gender is necessary.

An inverse or negative association between social class and psychosis appears to exist (the higher the social class, the lower the psychosis rate), and also a direct or positive association between social class and neurosis (the higher the social class, the higher the neurosis rate). These associations were tested to be statistically significant.

Before accepting these associations at face value, we must consider alternative explanations to a "real" relationship or association. For example, could factors of information bias produce these results? If so, how?

Information bias could produce these results. One possibility relates to reproducibility. Since there are few agreed-on diagnostic criteria for the clinical syndromes of neurosis and psychosis, intra-observer and inter-observer reliability may be low. Either one of these aspects of reliability can produce artifactual differences in the rates of neuroses and psychoses among the social classes. One observer may apply different criteria for neurosis and psychosis in an artifactual difference in rates among social classes. Similarly, two observers may apply different criteria to different social classes or each may apply separate criteria consistently to all social classes but differ from each other on the criteria. If each observer sees subjects who are primarily from a particular social class, this type of inter-observer reliability could produce artificial differences in rates among social classes.

TABLE 4.12 Prevalence rates* per 100,000 of psychosis and neurosis by social class categories (sex- and age-adjusted), Connecticut, 1950

	Social Class	*Psychosis*	*Neurosis*
High	1 & 2	188	349
	3	291	250
	4	518	114
Low	5	1,505	97

*These rates were based upon people diagnosed by these practitioners. The data do not come from a population survey.

SOURCE: From Hollingshead AB, Redlich FC: Social class and mental illness. New York: John C. Wiley & Sons, 1958.

Another possibility for bias relates to the issue of validity. The people labeling cases were middle- and upper-class socially (psychiatrists and practitioners) who might prefer to label upper-class peers neurotic rather than psychotic, as less stigma is attached to neurosis. Because "neurosis" connotes a more promising prognosis, treatment might be sought more readily by the patient. Thus, the degree of validity might vary among different social classes. The same disorder might be labeled one way for upper-class people and another way for those in the lower class. These hypotheses do not exhaust the possibilities of bias as an alternative explanation, but they illustrate some ways in which social class bias can affect study findings.

Factors of selection bias could also produce these results. One factor of selection might be a belief that neurotics of low socioeconomic status do not have the ability, inclination, or money to seek diagnosis or treatment to the extent that neurotics in higher socioeconomic groups have. If so, neurotics of low status would not be available to the services or treatment net to become labeled and counted (an example of selective use of services). Such neurotic people may come to the attention of diagnosticians only when psychotic illness occurs.

We must also be alert to possibilities of selection out of the epidemiological net. Perhaps psychotic upper-class people are able to leave their geographic area when their behavior is at odds with the accepted behavior for their social group. If this happens, those who are seriously ill (psychotics) would not be available for labeling in the study (an example of "selective out-migration").

Because this was a cross-sectional or prevalence study, we should recognize that a disease (dependent variable) can place an individual in one or another category of the independent variable. Psychotics may drift down the social ladder because of their illness. Or there may be something about neurotics that produces "social climbers" ("selective interclass migration"). In cross-sectional studies, cause-and-effect considerations are not answerable—either characteristic may "cause" the other.

Thus, information bias and selection bias could have distorted the effect measures (the rates) producing the results in Table 4.12 and creating "noncausal," artifactual associations.

Because bias is a possible explanation for findings, it should always be considered before other hypothesized processes to explain associations.

A Classic Example of Selection Bias

The map in Figure 4.1, adapted from the classical study by Faris and Dunham (1939), depicts the prevalence rates of schizophrenia in Chicago in the 1930s. This map is famous in the annals of the epidemiology of schizophrenia. The rates are not age-adjusted, so we must consider whether age is a confounding variable producing an artifactual association. Rates are higher in the center city zone and generally decrease as the

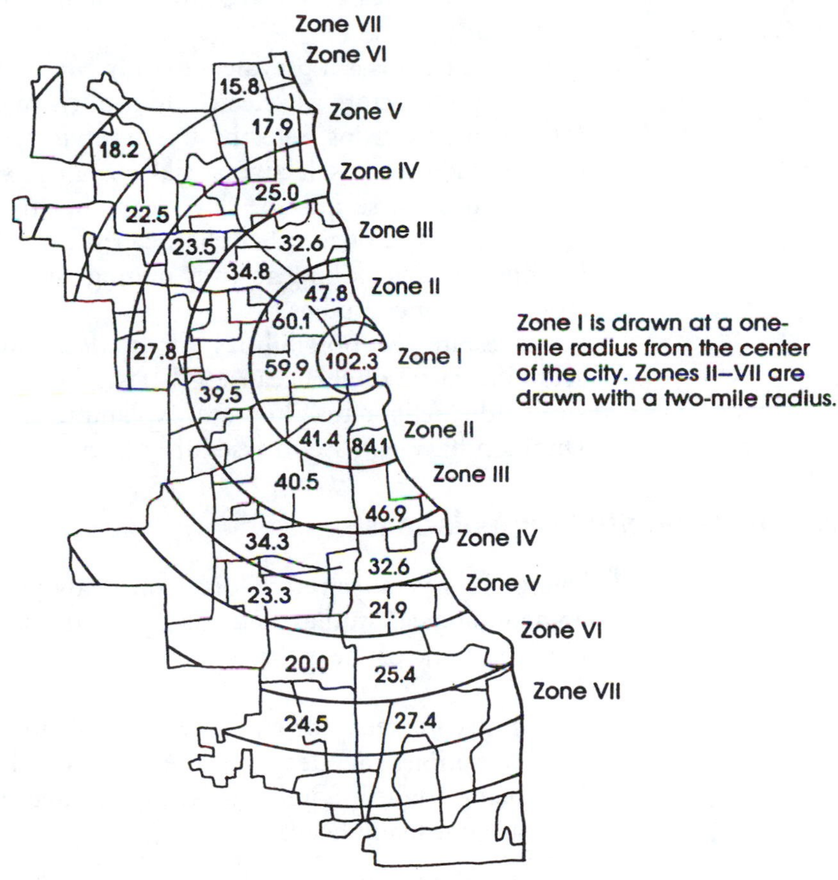

Rates per 100,000 population, aged 15-64, 1930. Subcommunities are based on census tracts of Chicago.

SOURCE: Adapted from Faris R, Dunham HW, *Mental Disorders in Urban Areas*. Chicago: University of Chicago Press, 1939.

FIGURE 4.1 *Average rates of schizophrenia, 1922-1934, by geographic zones and divisions of Chicago.*

concentric zones radiate. There are no great differences in the rates between the divisions within each zone.

The association between schizophrenia and geographic location may not be due to the locations in which the people were situated on the independent variable (distance from the center of the city in this case). Perhaps schizophrenics move to the center city for treatment. Or living in the center city may be easier for schizophrenics than living in the suburbs, and hence schizophrenics selectively migrate into the center city. Maybe there is a labeling bias against diagnosing schizophrenia among suburbanites. Perhaps suburbanites are more fortunate in their cure ratio. Or perhaps suburban schizophrenics are banished elsewhere (for example, to the center city) for cure or because of their socially "unacceptable" behavior. Perhaps there is an unknown risk factor that causes schizophrenics to die at a higher rate in the suburbs than in the center city (different case-fatality rates), so fewer cases survived to be counted in the suburbs in this prevalence study.

Because this is a prevalence study, we are applying as possible explanations such factors as selective mortality, migration, and different case-fatality or cure ratios. Selective use of services, selective migration in or out of the study area, selective social mobility, selective mortality/survival/cure—all of these may be due to the health state in question, or some antecedent of it, or to other characteristics. All of these possibilities must be considered in looking at study findings, especially when they are derived from prevalence studies.

Despite the possibilities for confounding, many findings become scientific facts, often because other studies replicate findings or because sub-studies eliminate alternate explanations. The findings of Faris and Dunham have withstood tests of both time and replication.

Selective Forces on Study Populations

There are several selective forces on study populations that can occur in epidemiological studies and may produce spurious associations. Listed here are some of these forces.

1. Volunteers for studies are almost invariably selective. Sometimes they fear that they have (or do not have) the condition being studied. Sometimes they volunteer because they believe they are unusually healthy.

2. Paid participants may be selectively different from the general population, especially if they are informed about payment before they participate.

3. Hospital and clinic data are invariably based on a selective population. Inferences to entire communities or other populations may be fallacious when based on selective samples of people. The statistician Joseph Berkson demonstrated the fallacy (called

Berkson's fallacy) that such data produces. Associations based on hospital or clinic data are influenced by differential admission rates among groups of people. A similar source of bias has been shown to occur when associations are based on autopsy data.

Controversies have been created by the publication of erroneous associations established from hospital patient data that later have been refuted when compared with data from nonhospital populations. An example is the assertion of an association between reserpine (a drug used for lowering blood pressure) and breast cancer, established by studies using hospital data but subsequently refuted by data gathered from nonhospital patients.

4. Studies of illness in industrial working populations have shown that risk of certain illnesses for these populations is lower than that in the general population. This is probably not due to the health-promotive environment of industries but to the "healthy worker effect" that results from pre-employment examinations which usually preclude ill people from being employed. (This effect may decline with time if ill-health effects of industries create illnesses in initially healthy workers.)

ECOLOGICAL FALLACY

We have considered potential errors in labeling cases and the importance of reliability and validity of epidemiology, the classification of data, and the forces of selection that may lead to spurious associations. Another potential problem is associated with deriving relationships between indices based on group characteristics rather than individual ones. There are many instances in which group or ecologic indices are compared and conclusions are drawn. These conclusions may be fallacious and should be pursued by further analysis for confirmation.

Ecological fallacy is the error that occurs by assuming that because two or more characteristics expressed as group indices occur together, they are therefore associated. For example, because a majority of a population has a particular characteristic and a majority of the population also has the disease, it may be assumed that the characteristic is associated with the disease. This assumption is the ecologic fallacy, as it is equally possible that the members of the population *without* the characteristic are the ones who have the disease.

Table 4.13 presents data from ten people, some of whom are young and some of whom are sick.

The proportion of the sample who are young is 6/10. The proportion who are sick is 7/10. In view of the fact that youth and sickness are common, we might conclude that young people are sick and older people are not. However, when we reconsider the data on an individual basis, we know only 3/6, or 50%, of the young people are sick; whereas, 4/4 (all) of

TABLE 4.13 Sample of ten persons, classified by age and health status (hypothetical)

Person	*Age*	*Health*
A	Young	Sick
B	Young	Sick
C	Young	Sick
D	Old	Sick
E	Young	Well
F	Old	Sick
G	Young	Well
H	Old	Sick
I	Young	Well
J	Young and Old	Sick

SOURCE: From Slome et al., 1986 (p. 196).

TABLE 4.14 Suicide rates per million population per proportion of Catholics, 15+ years, in Bavarian provinces, 1867-1875

Provinces with <50% Catholic		*Provinces with 50-90% Catholic*		*Provinces with >90% Catholic*	
Province	*Rate*	*Province*	*Rate*	*Province*	*Rate*
RP	167	LF	157	UP	64
CF	207	SA	118	UB	114
UF	204			LB	19
Average	192		135		75

SOURCE: From Durkheim E: *Suicide: A study in sociology*. Spaulding, JA and Simpson G (trans.) Glencoe, IL: The Free Press, 1951.

the old people are sick. Thus, a larger percentage of old people are ill, which refutes the association of sickness with age concluded when group indices were compared.

In his study of suicide in the late 1800s, Durkheim associated suicide with religion, as shown in Table 4.14.

Durkheim wrote the following about his findings (1951, p. 21):

> On the other hand, if one compares the different provinces of Bavaria, suicides are found to be in direct proportion to that of Catholics. Not only the proportions of averages to one and the other confirm the law, but all the numbers of the first column are higher than those of the second, and those of the second higher than those of the third without exception.[1]

[1]Durkheim E: *Suicide: A study in sociology*. Spaulding, JA and Simpson G (trans.) Glencoe, IL: The Free Press, 1951.

Durkheim has compared two ecologic or group indices: the suicide rate and the proportion of Catholics. This is potentially fallacious. Perhaps in provinces with a Catholic population greater than 90%, the Protestant minority committed suicide at a high rate and the Catholic majority committed suicide at a low rate; in provinces with a Catholic minority, the Catholics may have had a high suicide rate and the Protestants a moderate suicide rate. Durkheim's general conclusion or suggestion is that *rates of suicide for all Catholics are low,* which cannot be proven by these data alone. To avoid the problem of an ecologic fallacy, Durkheim should have calculated, if possible, religion-specific rates of suicide for each province. Each religious group in each province should have its own suicide rate with only its membership in the numerator and denominator. Durkheim did calculate religion-specific rates for many countries and presented "directly determined" rates from information about suicide and religion on an individual basis.

Note in Table 4.14 that 192 is not the average of the three numbers 167, 207, 204. The numeral 192 is a **weighted** average of 167, 207, and 204. The province with the largest population receives the largest weight and the province with the smallest population receives the smallest weight. The weighted average 192 means that if the populations of the three provinces RP, CF, and UF were added together and one suicide rate were calculated for the combined provinces, the rate would be 192.

Taking the average of the three numbers 167, 207, and 204 yields an **unweighted** average of suicide rates, which would not be appropriate *unless* all three provinces were of the same size with respect to population.

Certain characteristics are well suited to ecologic (group) indices. For example, if a town has only one water supply, exposure to the amount of a mineral such as lead in the water may be fairly constant for all inhabitants. It may be useful to consider several such towns to compare the quantity of lead in each town's water source with the rate of some health characteristic. Although the amount of lead received by persons in a given town is fairly constant, it does depend on the amount of water each person drinks and how much of the intake does not come from the town source, be it from imported beer, rainwater, or another source. Indices of air pollution in a neighborhood are also good indicators of individual pollution exposure, even with air conditioning. Some individuals may be exposed to additional or different pollution, for example, in their jobs. By applying logic and common sense we can decide whether to use an ecologic index in a particular situation and confirm its applicability by testing it in a sample of individuals.

In a study in 1849, Dr. Snow (see Chapter 1), in associating cholera with a water source, presented the comparison of mortality shown in Table 4.15.

In this example Snow calculated a specific mortality rate for each water source, the rate of cholera deaths per 10,000 houses receiving water from one source only. Later he calculated a more specific rate of deaths per 10,000 population, which further supported his hypothesis.

TABLE 4.15 Number of deaths per 10,000 houses in population supplied by three water souces during a seven-week epidemic

Water Supply	*Houses*	*Deaths from Cholera*	*Deaths per 10,000 Houses*
Southwark and Vauxhall Co.	40,046	1,263	315
Lambeth Co.	26,107	98	37
Rest of London	256,423	1,422	59

SOURCE: From Richardson BW: *Snow on cholera*. New York: The Commonwealth Fund, 1936.

Table 4.16 Average water hardness and death rates of white men, aged 55-64, from coronary heart disease and cerebrovascular disease in regions of North Carolina from 1956-1964

		Average Annual Death Rate per 100,000	
Region	*Average Hardness*	*Coronary Heart*	*Cerebrovascular*
Highland	23	585	147
Piedmont	61	778	172
Coastal plain	51	877	247
Tidewater	163	713	218

SOURCE: From Tyroler HA: Epidemiologic studies of cardiovascular disease in three communities of the southeastern United States. In: Kessler II, Levin M, eds., *The community as an epidemiologic laboratory: A case book of community studies*. Baltimore: Johns Hopkins Press, 1970.

Table 4.16 presents data from another study in which case investigators examined the association of hardness of water and mortality from coronary heart disease and cerebrovascular disease. In contrast to the generally shown negative association of water hardness and CHD deaths, the findings in Table 4.16 failed to demonstrate a relationship of average water hardness to coronary heart disease mortality.

This use of ecologic indices is potentially fallacious. The researchers combined counties with different water supplies into a regional average for water hardness and associated that average with mortality from CHD and cerebrovascular disease. These indices cannot assess whether more men aged 55 to 64 drinking hard water in a county or region died from CHD or cerebrovascular disease than those drinking soft water. However, these findings merit further study individually because of their potential importance.

Correcting for Ecological Fallacy

How could the investigators in the previous study have corrected for the potential of ecological fallacy?

To correct for this potential fallacy the investigators could have measured the hardness of the water and associated the hardness with CHD death rates derived from individual death certificates. Or they could have carried out the investigation in each of the 100 counties of North Carolina in which residents have a more consistently uniform water supply. However, such studies are often difficult, especially in rural areas where water comes from rainwater storage or wells that have not been tested for water hardness.

Because of the availability of ecologic indices—whether they are disease rates or demographic, social, agricultural, or environmental indices—they are easily used to generate hypotheses and test hunches. Some of the greatest epidemiological discoveries were based upon the use of ecologic indices. These include the association of Burkitt's lymphoma with malaria, the sickling trait with malaria mortality, and yellow fever with the mosquito. One presumes in assessing these studies that the association of each pair was so strong that fallacy was overridden, or that the assumptions made in using the ecologic indices were correct.

Limitations of Ecological Indices

Unless ecologic studies can create specific rates for subpopulations, they are not proof of an association. Because ecologic indices can produce incorrect associations or fail to reveal existing ones, we must rely on logic to assess the extent of possible error when we judge articles that report using this technique or when we use the technique. Ecologic indices can be productive if accompanied by wariness, thought, and additional study. Such considerations should be included in the interpretation of associations found by ecologic (group-based) indices. Many studies in the field of environmental epidemiology (for example, of radiation, air pollution, pesticides, and lead) use ecologic indices.

COHORT EFFECT

When data suggest the possibility that they are demonstrating the experience of one *particular group* over time, such a group is called a *cohort.* Its effect is termed a "cohort effect," borrowed from the use of cohort in ancient Roman days to refer to a group of warriors. We used the same term to describe one of the strategies used in epidemiology, namely, the cohort or prospective method (see Chapter 3). In this section, we are considering a cohort as a particular or unique group that shares some common experience relevant to health.

Some examples of cohorts are persons born in the same year or decade (birth cohorts), cohorts exposed to a war, cohorts exposed to radiation from the atomic bomb explosions of 1945, or persons exposed to a drug that is subsequently taken off the market (such as the daughters of mothers who took diethylstilbestrol during pregnancy).

Figure 4.2 depicts the hypothetical association of a disease with age in 1990. We considered this sort of association in Chapter 3 in our discussion of cross-sectional studies. The data are from a cross-sectional design.

One explanation of finding an association of a disease with age in the year the cross-sectional study is conducted might be that the old people

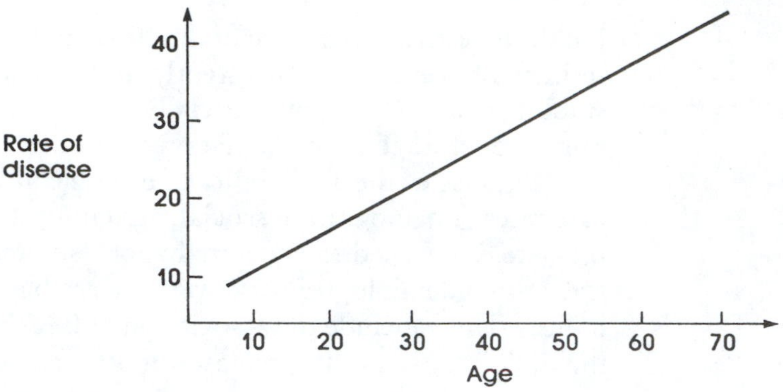

FIGURE 4.2 *Disease prevalence rate per 100,000, by age, 1990 (hypothetical)*

studied that year had *always* had a higher rate than any other age groups. They may have had the highest rate when they were 60 years old, when they were 50, 40, at any given age. If a birth cohort effect explains the association in Figure 4.2, then the particular group of old people studied in 1990 had always had higher rates throughout their lives.

Given this example, the highest rate in 1980 would be among the 60-year-old individuals. If this unique expression of disease began early in life, then the rate in 1920 would be the highest among infants.

A nonfatal persistent birth disorder can show an age cohort effect; that is, it can be highly prevalent at birth and persist in that birth cohort through time. An example is the cohort of "thalidomide babies" in Europe in the early 1960s (if they were common enough to be seen in a large population) or a cohort of blind babies exposed to excess administration of oxygen at birth (the retrolental fibroplasia syndrome of the 1960s). Thus, in 1980 in Europe (the United States was spared the widespread use of thalidomide and its consequences) there should have been a relatively high rate of thalidomide-affected adults among those aged 20, compared with others younger or older.

Another similar nondisease birth cohort recognized by demographers is the baby-boom babies of the late 1940s. (The baby boom refers to the high birth rate that followed the Second World War.) This birth cohort created a great need for colleges in the 1960s and 1970s, a need that disappeared in the early 1980s.

Another age cohort that manifests a high rate of a disorder in one particular period of time, and carries the disorder with them into older age, is the disabled American veterans of war cohort. Draftees aged 18 to 19 in 1970-1973 who were crippled by the Vietnam War show a higher rate of amputation, crippling, and so forth at age 30 to 31 (in 1982-1985) as compared with people younger than themselves and 25 or less years older than themselves. Similarly, we are aware of a high rate of leukemia and radiation effects in people who were exposed to the atomic bombs in Hiroshima and Nagasaki in 1945. Those afflicted are now older, manifesting higher rates of radiation-related disease than persons born later or earlier. Mothers who were exposed to the bomb's radiation while pregnant may have produced a birth cohort of defective babies.

Confirming Cohort Effects

Figure 4.3 gives the distribution of the prevalence of dental caries among black men in North Carolina in 1960-1963, as measured by the DMF Index (decayed, missing, and filled teeth). Dental caries are not cured as age increases, nor are they fatal. An edentulous (toothless) person would have a DMF of 32, and an adult with all 32 teeth filled would have the same score.

The shape of the distribution of average DMF is a bimodal distribution with two peaks (modes), at ages 25 to 29 and 70 or over, and two dips at ages 30 to 34, and 35 to 39. In this study of dental caries, a cohort effect among those 30 to 39 years old in 1960 seems likely. The 30-to-39 age cohort has an unusually low rate, lower than older persons but also lower than younger persons.

A note on bimodality: there are multiple modes in distributions of disease prevalence or death rates for several diseases. For example, leukemia has a peak (mode) in 2- to 5-year-olds and a later peak in persons over age 55. This suggests either two separate populations or diseases, or a cohort effect. Thus, with leukemia, young people may have a different disorder from those with the disease in older age. This has been confirmed clinically, for the disease is usually an acute type in youth and a more

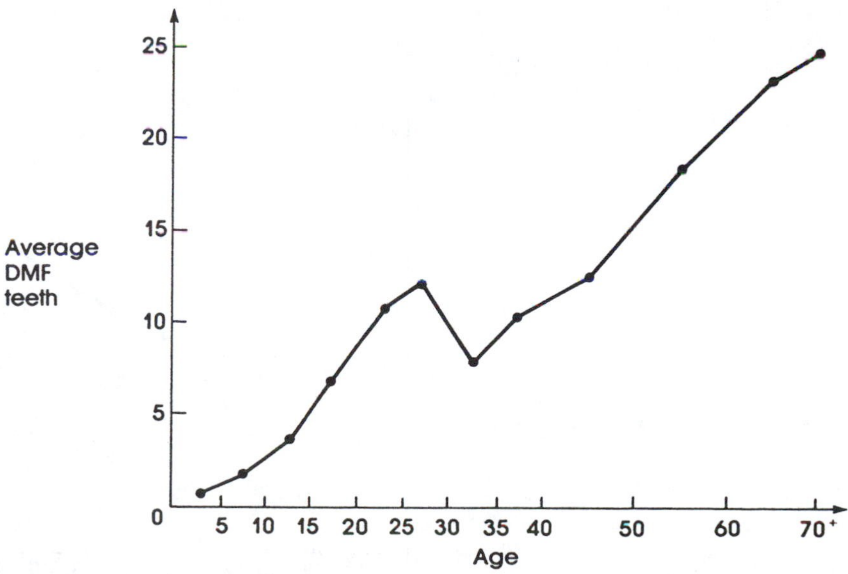

SOURCE: From Fulton JT and Hughes JT: *The natural history of dental diseases.* Chapel Hill: Department of Epidemiology, University of North Carolina, 1965.

FIGURE 4.3 *Average DMF for black men, by age, North Carolina, 1960-1963*

chronic type in older people. This also suggests different causation networks for each syndrome.

Similar evidence of two different syndromes and two different causations is seen in prevalence of diabetes by age, prevalence of deaths from automobile accidents by age, and prevalence of Down's syndrome by mother's age when pregnant.

Can additional steps be taken to confirm suggestions of a cohort phenomenon? If so, what steps?

Additional steps can be taken to confirm the suggestion of a cohort phenomenon. Using the example in Figure 4.3, we consider whether the unusually low rate of dental caries for ages 30 to 39 (in 1960-1963) is reflected in other gender-ethnic groups. In fact, it was found in men and women among both blacks and whites. The cohort effect could be confirmed if we repeated the prevalence study in another year, say 1980, and used exactly the same methods and criteria as in the first study. When the age-specific DMF rates for 1980 are plotted, the birth cohort with the low rate is 50- to 54-year-olds, as illustrated in Figure 4.4. Thus, the age cohort born in the period from 1926-1930 would show an unusually low DMF rate, indicating the possibility of exposure of this cohort to some protective effect early in life.

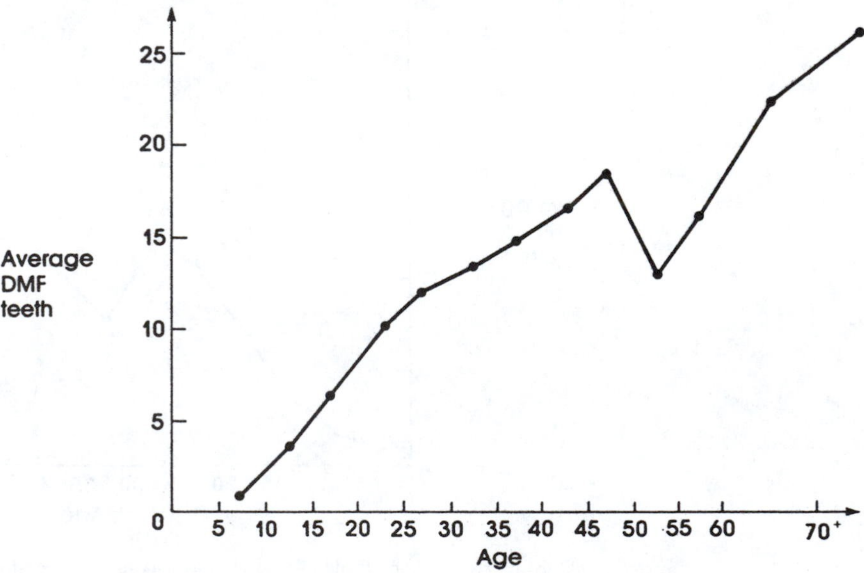

FIGURE 4.4 *Average DMF for black men, by age, North Carolina, 1980 (hypothetical)*

Factors Producing Cohort Effects

Let's consider possible events that could have produced such a cohort effect since a repeat of the study did *not* confirm the suspected cohort effect. If the cohort effect had been confirmed—in this instance an unusually low rate—something happened to those born around 1926-1930 that protected them from caries and may do so until their death. One possibility is that the Great Depression inculcated low candy-eating habits and other dietary practices promotive of good dental health. It is interesting to speculate about explanations as to why no cohort effect was confirmed. We would have to consider all the methods used as pitfalls and test the data for its potential contribution to non-confirmation of the cohort hypothesis.

When should a cohort effect be considered as a possibility?

A possible cohort effect should be considered in any cross-sectional studies or mortality data that show:

1. Any association of disease with age
2. An unexpected dip or increase in the distribution of a disease by age (this may be shown by a bimodal distribution)
3. An unexpected secular decline in a nontreatable disease (for example, the considerable decline in deaths from cancer of the stomach over time in the United States, for which there is as yet no satisfactory explanation)

In order to establish an age (birth) cohort phenomenon, we need data from several cross-sectional studies at different times, each one by age with similar methods used to gather data.

CHAPTER SUMMARY

The main points covered in this chapter include:

1. Information bias (incorrect labeling of cases, characteristics, or other variables) consists of two components: reproducibility and validity.
2. Reproducibility (reliability or repeatability) is assessed as the degree of agreement between two or more observers (inter-observer) or within one observer (intra-observer) on repeat tests.
3. Reliability varies with the skills of the observer, the variability of the characteristic being measured, and the consistency of instruments used.

4. Reliability can be improved by the training of observers and calibration of instruments or tests.
5. Validity is an indication of the correctness of labeling. It comprises sensitivity (percentage of true cases identified) and specificity (percentage of true noncases identified).
6. Both validity and reliability have important implications for health service and research.
7. The choice of categories for quantitative variables can affect the results.
8. Loss of information and analytical power in our statistical tests may follow such categorization.
9. For comparability with other studies, arbitrary cutoff points used in many studies are sometimes recommended for classification purposes.
10. In determining categories, the use of smaller ranges initially is indicated. Categories with large ranges may mask important differences if decided upon before examination of the data.
11. Classification systems should permit all persons in the study to be classified, and only once, including "refusal, unknown, or missing data" categories; that is, the categories should be exhaustive and exclusive.
12. Categories and cutoff points should be considered at the beginning of a study when variables and classification schemes are being considered for use in the study.
13. On occasion, the biological meaning of a cutoff point on a quantitative variable is confirmed, thereby providing support for clinical intervention. These categorical cutoff points, however, are frequently debated and change as knowledge advances.
14. Forces of selection can produce biased estimates of the effect. These include selective use of services, selective migration, and selective mortality or survival. They relate to people choosing various services or places, often because of illness, in order to be allowed to stay in an accepting area or to be employed. These forces must be considered in interpreting findings, for they may create associations that cannot be causal.
15. Consideration is given to the potential error (ecologic fallacy) that can arise in associating groups or ecologic indices with health outcomes.
16. Such an ecologic index assumes that the index reflecting a common characteristic in a group is applicable to all members of the group.
17. The fallacy is avoidable by using measurements derived from the individual's characteristics.
18. Ecologic indices are available and most useful in developing ideas for association or supporting hunches.
19. Logic should be used in assessing the extent of the fallacy.
20. Interpretation of association between ecologic indices should be reviewed carefully and warily.

21. Cohorts are groups of people that share a common experience.
22. Data are needed to determine whether a birth cohort effect exists.
23. There are specific steps that researchers can take to confirm a cohort effect.
24. The possibility of a cohort effect should be considered when interpreting data.

KEY TERMS

information bias
reproducibility
reliability
intra-observer reliability
inter-observer reliability
validity
true positive
true negative
false negative
false positive
sensitivity
specificity
construct validity
face validity
predictive validity
quantitative data
categorical data
range
mutually exclusive and exhaustive
selection bias
ecological fallacy
weighted
unweighted

REFERENCES

Faris R, Dunham HW: *Mental disorders in urban areas*. University of Chicago Press, Chicago, 1939.

Hollingshead AB, Redlich FC: *Social class and mental illness*. New York: John C. Wiley & Sons, 1958.

Slome C, Brogan D, Eyres S, Lednar W: *Basic epidemiological methods and biostatistics: A workbook*. Boston: Jones and Bartlett, 1986. Figures and tables used with permission.

EXERCISE APPLICATION 4.1

Locate three fairly recent epidemiologic studies in the library. In a 3- to 5-page paper describe what measures the authors/researchers took to avoid the pitfalls described in this chapter.

REVIEW QUESTIONS

1. What is information bias in epidemiology?
2. What is the reliability of observations?
3. What potentially erroneous conclusions may result from nonrandom systematic mislabeling by one or more observer?
4. What is intra-observer reliability? inter-observer reliability?
5. Describe how to calculate intra-observer reliability.
6. Describe how to calculate inter-observer reliability.
7. What are the consequences of unreliability?
8. What are several sources of unreliability?
9. What is validity?
10. What are the four possible scenarios in categorizing participants in an epidemiologic study?
11. Define sensitivity and specificity.
12. What is construct validity? face validity? predictive validity?
13. Identify potential causes of invalidity.
14. How is information on variability between research subjects lost when quantitative data are categorized?
15. What are some of the positive aspects of categorization of data?
16. What are mutually exclusive categories? exhaustive categories?
17. Discuss considerations in selecting cutoff points.
18. What is the range of a set of observations?
19. What are general recommendations for establishing age bands in classifying research subjects?
20. What is meant by the term "selection bias"?
21. Provide some examples of selection bias.
22. What is selective migration?
23. What are some potential selective forces on study populations?
24. Explain the concept of ecological fallacy.

25. Describe how the use of ecologic indices can be potentially fallacious.
26. What are ways of controlling for ecological fallacy?
27. Discuss limitations of ecological indices.
28. Describe the concept of cohort effect.
29. What are examples of cohort effects?
30. What steps can be taken to confirm cohort effects?
31. List possible events that can produce cohort effects.

5 Biostatistics

OBJECTIVES

Upon completion of this chapter, you will be able to:

- Mitigate fears about the use of statistical terminology
- Define biostatistics
- Differentiate between descriptive and inferential statistics
- Present fundamental points to consider when selecting a statistical test
- Describe concepts of populations and samples
- Introduce different types of inferences
- Describe probability sampling, random sampling, and nonprobability sampling
- Cite the basic assumptions underlying parametric and nonparametric statistical tests
- Describe and give examples of nominal, ordinal, interval, and ratio data
- List considerations in selecting appropriate statistical tests, particularly the chi-square test
- Describe the concept of degrees of freedom in statistical testing
- Explain under which conditions a two-tailed test of significance is appropriate
- Describe what sampling variability is
- Give examples of null and alternate hypotheses
- Explain the meaning of p-values in statistical testing
- Define Type I and Type II errors and list factors influencing the magnitude of these errors
- Describe computer resources for analyzing epidemiologic data

BIOSTATISTICS: AN INTRODUCTION

Biostatistics (a branch of applied mathematics) are procedures for condensing, describing, analyzing, and interpreting large sets of health-relevant information. These statistical procedures are analogous to "tools" in a toolbox as they are useful for doing a statistical job, for making sense of seemingly diverse information. We select the statistic (the tool) according to the information generated and the questions to be answered (the job to be done).[1]

What are descriptive and inferential statistics?

Biostatistical (statistical) methods are often classified as either **descriptive** or **inferential statistics. Descriptive statistics** are methods used to organize and produce quantitative summaries of numerical information, primarily by means of tables, charts, graphs, or diagrams (see Chapter 8). In epidemiology, the most commonly used descriptive statistic is a rate, a mathematical expression between a numerator and a denominator. Other descriptive statistics include frequencies, indices, ratios, proportions, and measures of central tendency and dispersion. Many of these descriptive statistic methods are discussed and illustrated in other chapters. The focus of this chapter is inferential statistical methods. **Inferential statistics** are used to make generalizations or "inferences" about a larger group or population on the basis of information derived from a representative subset or sample of the same group. The z, t, F, chi-square, Wilcoxon, and Mann-Whitney U tests are some of the most common inferential statistical methods.

POINTS TO CONSIDER WHEN CHOOSING A STATISTICAL TEST

To select the most appropriate inferential statistical test it is important to consider, at a minimum, the population objects (target population) and variables to study, the inferences to make about the target population, how the data are selected from the target population, how data on the variables of interest are distributed within the target population, and the level or type of data to analyze. Although these points of consideration are discussed separately because they are necessary but not always sufficient factors in determining which test or "tool" is appropriate for the statistical job at hand, they should be considered together when making a decision about which statistical test is best to use.

---

[1]An important caveat is that the terminology of statistics varies considerably. For example, quantitative data are also called measurement, variate, discrete and/or continuous data; qualitative data are often referred to as nominal or categorical data. If you persist in learning the concepts underlying statistical principles, you should be able to make a correct decision about which statistical method to apply to the data you intend to describe or analyze systematically.

Populations and Samples

Why do we study samples instead of populations?

Because it is often not feasible or even necessary to collect information on all objects in a **population** targeted for an epidemiologic investigation, statistics are intentionally limited to a group of objects called a **sample.** A sample is a subset of population objects selected in a way that they represent a well-defined population.

How are populations characterized?

When characterizing a population or a sample it is useful to differentiate between population **objects** and population **variables.** The objects within a population of interest to an epidemiologist are, in most instances, human beings. However, population objects can also include schools, churches, clinics, hospitals, dogs, or widgets (see Figure 5.1). Objects can have a number of different variables. **Variables** are the observable characteristics

Object	Variables (Traits or Characteristics)
Persons	Diastolic blood pressure
Persons	Height or weight
Persons	Race
Persons	Cholesterol value
Persons	Income
Persons	HLA type
Persons	An isolated clincial outcome like blood pressure
Persons	Single answer to a question
Persons	Patient status
Persons	Rating based on an observation of a behavior
Persons	Stress
Persons	Number of hospital days for stroke
Persons	Number of outpatient visits
Cars	Velocity
Light bulbs	Duration
Dogs	Breed
Corn fields	Bushels per acre
Coins	Number of tails

FIGURE 5.1 *Examples of population objects and corresponding characteristics within a statistical population*

of an object of interest in a sample selected for study. They are the constructs that epidemiologists enumerate (count) or measure. Some examples of population objects and their corresponding variables are provided in Figure 5.1.

Types of Inferences

What types of inferences do inferential statistics make?

There are four major types of inferences or generalizations that inferential statistics make. These are inferences relative to the *difference* between two magnitudes (e.g., Is there a difference in the mean serum cholesterol between men and women aged 25 to 35 years?); the *relationship* between two variables (e.g., Is there a relationship between mental health and stress?); the *appraisal* of two or more interventions, methods, devices or treatments (e.g., Is a sodium restriction diet more effective than a caloric restriction diet in preventing the development of hypertension?); and the *trend* of a variable of interest (e.g., Is there a pattern of change in asthma mortality in Maricopa County from 1979 to 1989?).

How Subjects Are Selected from a Population

What is nonprobability sampling and when is its use justified?

There are two alternatives for selecting a sample: **probability** and **nonprobability.** From a scientific perspective, a probability sample is preferred because it is the only type of sample that allows the epidemiologist to treat the sample as technically *representative* of the larger population about which she/he wishes to make inferences.

What is a random sample?

A probability, or **random,** sample is selected from the **target** or **study** population that the epidemiologist hopes to study. Selecting a random (probability) sample requires choosing a *representative* group of the members of a population in a way that ensures each member is independently chosen and has a known non-zero probability of being selected.

Sometimes it is not possible to obtain a probability sample because a list enumerating all objects of interest in the population is not available or because resources are restricted. In such situations, the decision must be between no sample at all or a nonprobability sample (i.e., purposive sample) obtained on a nonrandomly selected group of individuals in the population. A nonprobability sample may be justified if particular limitations are considered.

Data Distribution: Parametric and Nonparametric Statistics

Inferential statistical tests can be further classified as either **parametric** or **nonparametric** on the basis of how the data to be analyzed are distributed on a measurement scale. If data on the variable of interest in a study is proven or assumed to be distributed normally in the population from which a *representative* sample is chosen, then it is appropriate to use **parametric** statistics, e.g., the z-, t-, or F-test. Conversely, if the data on the variable of interest are not normally distributed in the target population, or are "distribution-free," **nonparametric** statistical tests should be applied; e.g., the chi-square, Wilcoxon, or Mann-Whitney U test. The following is offered as a guide for choosing between **parametric** and **nonparametric statistics.**

- If the data are taken from a normally distributed population, use a parametric procedure.
- If the distribution from which the data came is unknown, or if there is reason to suspect that the data are not normally distributed, use a nonparametric procedure.
- If the data are nominal (categorical), use a nonparametric procedure.
- If the data are quantitative (interval and ratio), use parametric procedures; if the data are qualitative (nominal and ordinal), do not use parametric procedures for most statistical testing.

What is a normal distribution?

The symmetrical clustering of values around a central location, typical of the distribution of many data distributions, is called the **normal distribution.** The bell-shaped curve that results when a normal distribution is graphed is called the **normal curve.** This common bell-shaped distribution is the basis of many tests of statistical inference that we use to draw conclusions or make generalizations from data (Centers for Disease Control and Prevention, 1992). To use parametric tests, data should be normally distributed; that is, it should show a normal curve if graphed. This distribution is also called the Gaussian distribution—named after Karl Friedrich Gauss who first applied the normal distribution to medicine (Kuzma, 1984).

What are other important distributions in the study of biostatistics?

One important distribution is the binomial distribution, a distribution of proportions (the absence or presence of a characteristic of interest) rather than quantitative values. While the normal distribution deals with the mean value of some characteristic of interest for a group of individuals, the binomial distribution is the distribution of the statistical estimate of the proportion of individuals who possess a certain characteristic. When the number of cases exceeds 30, the binomial distribution approximates the normal distribution. The Poisson distribution applies to discrete events (presence or absence of a characteristic) in cases when a sample is very large and the proportion of interest is very small.

The chi-square statistic is approximated by the chi-square distribution. Later in this chapter, we discuss the chi-square test and show a statistical application that provides experience with this distribution to determine whether a calculated chi-square test statistic is significant.

Types of Data and Levels of Measurement

Information (reports of observations) collected on variables identified with the objects of interest in a sample or population are called **data.** Because not all numerical values (data) share the same properties, it is important to distinguish between different types of data because the statistical "tool" selected must be appropriate for the type of data generated by the study. There are two types of numerical data basic to biostatistics: qualitative and quantitative. These data types are further subdivided, on the basis of the scale used to measure the data, into **nominal, ordinal, interval,** and **ratio data.**

Qualitative Data and Scales

Qualitative data are "all-or-none" information measured with **nominal** or **ordinal scales.** These data are sometimes labeled **nominal** or **ordinal data.** Variables measured on nominal or ordinal (qualitative) scales are appropriately referred to as qualitative, nominal, or ordinal variables.

Nominal Data

Nominal data include information on object characteristics that can be classified into mutually exclusive categories. Each response must fall into one, and only one, category and there is no natural order to the variables. For example, demographic data such as race, gender, and marital status are usually measured this way. If the variable of interest in a study is marital status, a study subject could be classified as "married," "unmarried," "divorced," or "widowed." If there are only two mutually exclusive categories (e.g., if seropositivity is the characteristic of interest, an individual is either "HIV positive" or "HIV negative"), the nominal data is referred to as **dichotomous** data.

The attribute gender also has no number associated with it but is simply labeled male or female; there is no attempt to measure "how much" of the variable a research subject has. Gender, therefore, is a variable measured on a nominal scale producing nominal data. Qualitative variables are also called **categorical variables** because different values of the variable indicate categories into which persons can be classified.

Ordinal Data

Data measured on an **ordinal scale** (**ordinal data**) are information on variables that may be counted, but these counts may also represent gradations of the variables. Ordinal data can be "ordered" in ranked categories with respect to the degree to which they possess a certain characteristic; this does not necessarily mean that one can tell how much difference there is between categories. It allows us only to recognize that an order to the responses may be legitimate. For example, a patient may be classified as "much improved," "slightly improved," or "not improved." We generally know that in health matters "much improved" is more desirable than "no improvement." However, we can not distinguish precisely how much difference there may be between these two responses.

Quantitative Data and Scales

Quantitative data are derived from a count or a standard measurement and have a frequency distribution. These data include information on variables that can be measured on **interval** or **ratio** scales and can be labeled as **interval** or **ratio data.** Variables measured on these scales can be classified as quantitative, interval, or ratio data.

What are interval and ratio data?

Interval Data

Interval data are measured in standard units. Any given difference between two numerical values has the same meaning, whatever the level of values; the difference between the values reflects the magnitude of the difference in the variable. With this scale it is possible for the researcher to report not only that one classification represents "more" or "less" of the variable being measured than another classification, but precisely how much "more" or "less" it represents.

Ratio Data

Ratio data are measured in standard units. The scale they are measured on has a true zero point that represents total absence of the variable. Examples of ratio data include age, length, time, volume, and mass.

What is the value of understanding types of data or level of measurement?

The scale and type of data are important to consider when selecting a statistical test. Understanding that age is measured on a ratio scale, and that gender is measured on a nominal scale producing nominal data, has implications for the types of statistical techniques to use when we describe or analyze data. For example, because age is measured on a ratio scale, one can calculate the average age (arithmetic mean) of a group of people.

Because gender is measured on a nominal scale, one can report the proportion (or rate) of persons that is female and the proportion that is male.

Sometimes in coding data for research studies, different values of the qualitative data are coded with numbers because most software used to analyze data are designed to input and analyze numbers rather than words. For example, marital status is a qualitative variable: "never married" may be coded as 1, "currently married" as 2, "divorced" as 3.

Consider the variable "self-perceived health status" measured on a four-point rating scale from excellent to poor. At first glance, self-perceived health status may appear to be a nominal variable (because its values are named excellent, good, fair, and poor), but it differs from marital status in that the different values of health status are ordered. Excellent health is better than good health, fair health better than poor health, and so forth. There is no implicit ordering among the different values for marital status or among different values for *any* nominal variable. Variables that have an order to them are called **ordinal variables.**

Although self-perceived health status does have an "order" about it, there is no way to measure exactly the "quantity" of health as we measure age (or weight or height or number of teeth). Some researchers apply numbers to the values on the ordinal scale (4 = excellent, 3 = good, 2 = fair, and 1 = poor) and then calculate a mean (average) self-perceived health status. Calculating a mean from these numbers is valid only if the difference between the numbers reflects actual differences between the levels of health. For example, the difference between excellent and good is 1 (4 − 3) and the difference between good and fair is 1 (3 − 2). Hence, the numbers applied to this scale assume that the difference between excellent and good is the same as the difference between good and fair.

Some researchers do not assume that the ordered values of the ordinal variable correspond to some numerical quantity of the variable. Instead, they use parametric statistical techniques for ordered or ranked data.

A quantitative variable, such as age, is often used as an ordinal variable (for example, age categories such as 20-29, 30-39, 40-49) or as a nominal variable (old versus young). If age is used as a nominal variable, it should be treated as a nominal variable for that study.

Consider the following two quantitative variables: "number of children ever born" and "weight." "Number of children ever born" can assume a value such as 0, 2, 5, or 13. It cannot assume a value like 3.02 or 3.27. However, "weight" can assume the value 105 pounds or 105.2 pounds or 105.23 pounds, depending on the accuracy of the scale in measuring weight.

These two kinds of quantitative variables are called *discrete* and *continuous* variables. This type of data is scaled on ratio or interval scales. A **discrete quantitative variable,** like "number of children ever born," can assume only a limited number of values. A **continuous quantitative variable,** like "weight," can assume an infinite number of possible values.

Averages or means are obtained for both discrete and continuous variables, but they have somewhat different interpretations. When an average weight of 105.37 pounds is reported, it is certainly possible for someone in that group to weigh exactly 105.37 pounds. However, when the average number of children ever born is reported to be 2.1, it is not possible for anyone in that group to have had 2.1 children. Although it is appropriate to obtain averages of both discrete and continuous variables, one needs to be careful of interpretation.

PUTTING IT ALL TOGETHER: A GUIDE FOR SELECTING THE RIGHT STATISTICAL TEST

Certain statistical tests are frequently used in epidemiology. The guide provided in Figure 5.2 shows statistical tests often used in epidemiology and the social sciences.

The guide is intended to help one select from many statistical techniques the most appropriate "tool" (i.e., a particular statistic) for a particular analysis, given certain data and sample constraints. The guide is designed for health science students and practicing social and behavioral scientists who have a basic knowledge of statistics and who want a condensed, systematic chart of currently used statistical techniques. The chart is not comprehensive. There are other statistics a researcher may elect to

		Nonparametric / Not Normally Distributed		*Parametric / Approximately Normally Distributed*	
	Data	*Nominal*	*Ordinal*	*Interval*	*Ratio*
		DISCRETE			*CONTINUOUS*
One Sample		Binominal Test χ^2 1-variable Test		Kolmogorov- Smirnov Goodness of Fit	*t* Test *z* Normal curve
Two Samples	Inde-pendent	Fisher Test χ^2 Test of Independ-ence Mantel-Haenszel Log Linear Analysis	Tukey Test Mann Whitney Median Test	Kolmogorov- Smirnov 2-sample Test	*F* Test *t* Test
	Correlated	Sign Test McNemar Test	Wilcoxon Matched Pairs Spearman Rank		*t* Test Pearson's R Linear Regression
>2 Samples	Inde-pendent	χ^2 Test Contingency Co-efficients	Median Test Kruskal Wallis 1-way ANOVA		ANOVA Multivariate Methods
	Correlated	Cochran's Q	Friedman 2-way ANOVA Wilcoxon Multiple Comparisons		ANOVA Multivariate Methods

SOURCE: From Seigel S: *Nonparametric statistics for the behavioral sciences*. New York: McGraw-Hill, 1956; Daniel WW: *Applied nonparametric statistics*. Boston: Houghton Mifflin, 1978; and Andrews FM, Klem L, Davidson TN, O'Malley PM, Rodgers WL: *A guide for selecting statistical techniques for analyzing social science data*, 2d ed. Ann Arbor, MI: Institute for Social Science Research, 1981.

FIGURE 5.2 *Selecting a statistical test*

use. Additionally, the researcher is strongly urged to examine the requirements and assumptions that may correspond with each technique.

In Figure 5.2, each row lists, cumulatively across, those tests applicable to the sample and the given level of measurement for the data. For example, if one had two correlated samples, with ratio data, one might choose a statistical technique such as the t-test, Pearson's R, or linear regression. If one had a single sample and nominal data, one might use the binomial test or the chi-square one-variable test. The following are some specific references for selecting appropriate statistical tests.

Andrews FM, Klem L, Davidson TN, O'Malley PM, Rodgers WL: *A guide for selecting statistical techniques for analyzing social science data*, 2d ed. Ann Arbor: Institute for Social Research, 1981.

Blalock HM: *Social statistics*, 2d ed. New York: McGraw-Hill, 1979.

Daniel WW: *Applied nonparametric statistics*. Boston: Houghton Mifflin, 1978.

Duncan RC, Knapp RG, Miller MC: *Introductory biostatistics for the health sciences*, 2d ed. New York: John Wiley & Sons, 1983.

Ingelfinger JA, Mosteller F, Thibodeau LA, Ware JH: *Biostatistics in clinical medicine*. New York: Macmillan, 1983

Kahn HA: *An introduction to epidemiologic methods*. New York: Oxford University Press, 1983.

Kahn HA, Sempos CT: *Statistical methods in epidemiology*. New York: Oxford University Press, 1989.

Kuzma JW: *Basic statistics for the health sciences*. Palo Alto, Calif.: Mayfield, 1984.

Rosner B: *Fundamentals of biostatistics*, 3d ed. Boston: PWS-Kent, 1990.

Siegel S: *Nonparametric statistics for the behavioral sciences*. New York: McGraw-Hill, 1956.

Wassertheil-Smoller S: *Biostatistics and epidemiology: A primer for health professionals*. New York: Springer-Verlag, 1990.

Some Commonly Used Statistical Tests

As Figure 5.2 displays, there are a variety of statistical tests available; the choice of a particular test depends on the type of data to be analyzed and the research question to be answered. In this section, we briefly review the purposes of some common statistical tests.

t-Test

The t-test is suitable to determine whether two means are significantly different at a selected probability level. For example, if a researcher were interested in whether the cholesterol level of men differs from that of women in a particular sample, a t-test would be an appropriate statistical test. The *t*-test is also appropriate to test for mean differences in cholesterol levels between subjects (those who underwent a low-fat diet and control subjects who did not consume the diet).

Analysis of Variance

When a researcher wishes to know whether two or more means differ at a selected probability level, one-way analysis of variance can be used. This test tells whether there is a significant difference between groups, but does not tell which specific groups differ. As a result, a researcher must use one of many multiple comparison techniques to determine which groups differ. Examples of multiple comparison tests are the Scheffe test and the Duncan multiple range test.

Researchers who are interested in determining the effect of two or more independent variables and the interactions between them on the means of two or more groups can rely on factorial analysis of variance or analysis of covariance, a technique for controlling extraneous variables and means of increasing statistical power.

Multivariate Tests

A variety of multivariate tests are available for the statistical analysis of variance—multiple regression, multivariate analysis of variance, discriminant analysis, factor analysis, logistic regression, and canonical correlation. These sophisticated tests allow for more than one independent or dependent variable and are called multivariate tests to distinguish them from univariate tests such as the *t*-test and one-way analysis of variance. Powerful computers are necessary for running these increasingly used tests.

Nonparametric Tests

Nonparametric tests are often used in epidemiologic studies because they have fewer restrictions than parametric tests and computation is easier. Nonparametric tests are referred to as distribution-free tests because a researcher does not have to assume that the data distribution he/she is working with is normally distributed (follows a "bell-shaped" curve). However, nonparametric tests are less efficient than parametric tests. Examples of nonparametric tests are the chi-square test, Mann-Whitney test, sign test, median test, Wilcoxon matched-pairs signed rank test, and the Kruskal-Wallis test.

HYPOTHESES AND RESEARCH QUESTIONS

Epidemiologic studies often include descriptive studies that give the researcher a profile of the sample group being studied. For example, one can speak of the elements in the sample as having an average age, as being divided into a specific number of males and females, as being mostly from one area or another area, and so forth. However, the researcher sometimes needs to know more. Particularly in biostatistical research, the researcher often wants to know whether one group is different from another group. These types of questions lead to the formation of **hypotheses.** Most analytical studies involve testing hypotheses about population parameters; a **hypothesis** is essentially a testable statement about the world.

In clinical research, hypotheses are usually statistical statements about the difference between two groups on a variable of interest (e.g., the relative effectiveness of drug A versus drug B). Statistical hypotheses are usually concerned with the differences in population parameters (i.e., the population variables that can be estimated and are measurable) and are usually expressed numerically. For example, one might want to know whether the population mean for cholesterol levels is the same for two groups when one group received medication and one group did not.

In behavioral research, hypotheses are often written statements about the question of concern (research questions), not mathematical expressions. For example, one might be interested in whether or not an intervening technique, such as teaching 6th grade students the advantages of postponing sexual activity until marriage or how to resist peer pressure to engage in sex, will delay the mean or median age of onset of sexual activity within a target population and, in turn, reduce the incidence of STDs or HIV among adolescents.

In both instances, the researcher is primarily concerned with procedures that allow evaluation as to whether the data gathered provide evidence against a hypothesis about a population parameter. No method, short of examining an entire population, provides absolute certainty regarding whether a hypothesis about a population parameter is true. If the data provide evidence against a hypothesis, we can reject the hypothesis; if the data do not provide evidence against a hypothesis, we cannot reject the hypothesis.

How do we decide whether data provide evidence against a hypothesis?

We begin by temporarily assuming that the hypothesis is true. Then we can determine how likely the newly generated data set is true, relative to the questions of interest, assuming the hypothesis is true. If data like those generated are extremely unlikely, assuming the hypothesis is true, the data provide evidence against the hypothesis. If data like ours are not unlikely, assuming the hypothesis is true, the data do not provide evidence against the hypothesis. This process is the same regardless of whether the hypotheses are expressed as research questions alone or as statistical hypotheses. Most of the time, hypotheses are expressed as research questions.

TABLE 5.1 Male subjects, aged 40-49, by stress status at beginning of study and stroke status at end of study

	Stress Status		
Stroke Status	*Stressed*	*Nonstressed*	*Total*
Developed stroke	300	100	400
Did not develop stroke	700	900	1,600
Totals	1,000	1,000	2,000

SOURCE: From Slome et al., 1986 (p. 218).

STATISTICAL TESTING

In previous chapters, we compared groups' rates of diseases or the means of health attributes, such as blood pressure. Comparisons such as these are the basics of epidemiology. We found differences, one group being higher or lower than the others, and noted the need to exclude any effects due to sampling variability in interpreting these differences. Such exclusion requires tests of significance. Statistical tests are based on statistical concepts and do not by themselves determine the biological, social, or "real life" meaning or importance of differences.

In this chapter, we look more closely at differences between groups in health status and consider in more detail "statistical tests of significance."

Determining Statistical Significance

The data presented in Table 5.1 were obtained from a hypothetical ten-year cohort study of a random sample of 2,000 men aged 40 to 49 to test the association of stroke and stress. Our random sample of 2,000 men resulted in 1,000 "nonstressed" men. Because it is a cohort study, all subjects were free from stroke at the start. Because we have a random sample of men free of stroke, the prevalence of stress in this population can be estimated from Table 5.1 as 1,000/2,000 = 0.50.

Gender and age are controlled for by subject selection because all of the subjects are men 40 to 49 years old at the beginning of the study. The incidence rate of stroke among stressed men is 300/1,000 = 0.30. The incidence rate of stroke among nonstressed men is 100/1,000 = 0.10. The relative risk is 0.30/0.10 = 3.0. Attributable risk (simple attributable risk) is 0.30 − 0.10 = 0.20. The population attributable risk percent (PARP) can be calculated from the formula:

$$\frac{P(RR - 1)}{P(RR - 1)} \times 100$$

where P is the prevalence of the risk factor (in this instance, stress) in the population and RR is the relative risk for stressed men. Therefore, in this study,

$$\text{PARP} = \frac{0.50(3-1)}{0.50(3-1)+1} = \frac{1}{2} = 0.50 = 50\%$$

Because this is a cohort study, we are able to estimate the attributable risk and use it in the alternate formula: PARP = P(AR)/RT, where AR is the attributable risk, RT is the disease rate in the total sample, and P is the prevalence of the risk factor. Applying the data, we get PARP = (0.50)(0.20) = 0.50, as before. The PARP calculation is the same by either formula.

Keep in mind that we are using hypothetical data for illustration. Therefore, any conclusions about the real association of stress with stroke are also hypothetical.

The two calculated incidence rates differ from each other, since 0.30 and 0.10 differ from each other. From an epidemiological and practical viewpoint, the difference is meaningful, in that a difference of 20% is large, particularly where the risk factor (stress) is common.

What "pitfalls" discussed in Chapter 4 could potentially produce artifacts in this hypothetical study and should be avoided?

We need to consider whether the difference found may be an artifact due to any pitfall of methods before we try to interpret the process by which stress produces strokes in men. Entities such as the validity of the diagnosis of stroke and the classification of stress are not indicated in the table. Sex and age are not confounders, but we know that other potential confounders are not controlled for in this table. In particular, we know that blood pressure is associated with stress and with stroke, so blood pressure may create an artifactual association between stroke and stress.

When all confounding effects are eliminated, we should consider the possibility that sampling variability produces the difference. Only when we have studied a *sample* can its variability be relevant.

Sampling Variability

If the 2,000 men in the example were the entire population, the difference in stroke incidence would be real because the incidence rates are the actual population parameters and are not derived from samples. In reality, therefore, if the total population is included in a study, tests of significance are not necessary because no sampling variability is involved. In that instance, such findings are not *estimates* of the truth (of real parameters of the population) but the truth itself.

Since entire populations of interest are not often included for research studies because they are usually too large, and it is too costly and too time-consuming to include everybody, a sample of the members of the population is generally used.

The idea that "total" populations, even those such as the world population, are samples of larger populations or samples of future populations from the same place, and that, therefore, even total populations should be regarded as samples, is a debatable notion. Believers in the idea that all populations are samples claim that they wish to apply the results of their current research to all current or future populations similar to the one under study. A believer of this idea would consider sampling variability for every study, even when the entire population is used. Opponents regard the idea as a way to provide employment for statisticians.

In the study under consideration, we know that the 2,000 men constituted a random sample of stressed and nonstressed men; thus, the sample estimates reflect the population parameters. We cannot yet conclude that the population parameters differ from each other. What *is* clear is that the incidence rates *in the two samples* differ (0.10 and 0.30 are different). However, it is not known whether the incidence rates in the two populations differ because all members of these two populations were not measured. From the samples, we can estimate the parameters and therefore the difference, but the estimates will vary with each sample drawn. If another sample of 1,000 stressed men and 1,000 nonstressed men had been selected, the two incidence rates might have resulted in 0.15 for nonstressed and 0.28 for stressed men. If yet another sample had been selected, the sample incidence rates might have been 0.09 and 0.31. Variability is produced by different samples.

If, in fact, the parameters (the two population incidence rates) are exactly the same, and if samples of 1,000 stressed and 1,000 nonstressed men are followed for ten years, we must consider whether the sample incidence rates would be the same. They *might,* but in general the answer is *no,* because both sample incidence rates are subject to sampling variability. That is, each sample incidence rate may differ somewhat from the population parameter because a sample was measured rather than the entire population.

Thus, when two (or more) observed sample rates are compared with each other, they may differ only because of sampling variability *or* because of sampling variability *and* a difference between the population parameters. All statistical tests of significance address that issue, and that is their correct place in our epidemiological pursuits. In this study, the researcher tests the working hypothesis that the incidence rate for stroke is greater among stressed men than among nonstressed men.

Stating Hypotheses

Statisticians prefer to express hypotheses as if no differences were there; that is, in the null fashion, and then to disprove the null hypothesis by using a test of significance. (The word "null" is derived from the Latin *nullus,* which means "none.") In a sense, statisticians are saying that if we can disprove the nonexistence of an association, we prove the existence of that association.

Suppose that a court case followed our hypothetical stress/stroke study and the defending lawyer for the stress industry pleaded "not guilty" to a damage suit brought by the stroke victims. The no-guilt plea presumes that there is no association of stress with stroke in the population (the null hypothesis). In rejecting this plea, the jury accepts the opposite and rules that an association does exist.

In statistical shorthand the null hypothesis H_0 is that the incidence rate of stroke in stressed men (one true parameter) is the same as the incidence rate of stroke in nonstressed men (the other true parameter). IR_s and IR_{ns} are the population parameters, the incidence rates for stressed and nonstressed men, respectively. Thus, the null hypothesis is written

$$H_0{:}IR_s = IR_{ns} \quad \text{or} \quad H_0{:}IR_s - IR_{ns} = 0$$

(which is why it is called "null").

What is an alternate hypothesis?

Many studies, particularly descriptive epidemiological ones, do not specifically indicate any null hypotheses. However, the researchers reflect their null hypotheses implicitly in the comparisons they make. Most researchers state explicitly the hypotheses they wish to substantiate with their study data; for example, that stress and stroke are related. This kind of hypothesis, expressing some sort of inequality, statisticians call the *alternate hypothesis*. Any null hypothesis and its corresponding alternate hypothesis should cover all possible situations in reality. Thus, if the null hypothesis is not true, the alternate hypothesis must be true, and vice versa.

What are some common symbols used in statistics?

Statisticians use symbols to distinguish between population parameters and estimates of these parameters from sample data. A common practice in biostatistics and scientific writing is to make a distinction between the population parameter and a sample estimate of the population parameter. If the population parameter is represented by IR, for instance, a "hat" (^) written over IR is used to represent symbolically the sample estimate. It is read aloud as "IR hat."

If the null hypothesis is true, we expect the difference between IR_s and IR_{ns} to be close to zero or very small. Sampling variability is likely to keep the difference from being equal to zero.

If the null hypothesis is not true, we expect the difference to be quite different from zero. The difference is produced by sampling variability *and* by the differences in the population parameters.

If the observed difference between IR_s and IR_{ns} is close to zero or very small, we do not reject the null hypothesis. If the difference is close to zero, it seems likely that this difference is due only to sampling variability, indicating that the hypothesis is not false (it is true).

When the observed difference between IR_s and IR_{ns} is large, we reject the null hypothesis. If the difference is large, it seems likely that the difference is not caused *only* by sampling variability, indicating that the null hypothesis is false.

Probability and Hypothesis Testing

There must be a rational basis for determining what is "very small" and what is "large" in regard to differences. An appropriately chosen test of significance allows us to calculate the probability of obtaining a difference between sample estimates as large as the observed difference, given that the null hypothesis is true. If the calculated probability is large, it means that the difference between these estimates was unlikely to occur if the null hypothesis were true. If, however, the probability turns out to be small, it means that the difference between the sample estimates was unlikely to occur under the assumption that the null hypothesis is true; that is, because of sampling variability *only*. Hence, we would probably reject the null hypothesis with that degree of probability.

What is the "p-value" of a statistical test?

The calculated probability is often called a "p-value" and is denoted by "p" (because p is the first letter of the word probability).

Recall that the two incidence rates for the stress/stroke example are 0.30 and 0.10. Suppose a p-value of 0.50 is calculated by the test of significance. We would not reject the null hypothesis because the chances are 50-50 that a difference as large as 0.20 could occur due only to sampling variability when the null hypothesis is true. Thus, we would conclude that the population parameters IR_s and IR_{ns} do not differ.

If the p-value were 0.002 instead of 0.50, we would come to a different conclusion. Chances are only 2 out of 1,000 that a difference as large as 0.20 would be found due only to sampling variability if the null hypothesis were true. Thus, we would reject the null hypothesis and conclude that the population parameters IR_s and IR_{ns} do differ.

Avoiding Type I and Type II Errors

When we use a test of significance to decide whether to reject a null hypothesis, it is possible to err in either of two directions. We can (a) disagree with something that is true or (b) fail to disagree (agree) with something that is false.

One error is that we reject the null hypothesis when it is really true. Researchers call this a **Type I error.** Another possible error is that we fail to reject a null hypothesis that is false. This is called a **Type II error.**

Returning to the hypothetical "stress industry" trial illustrates these two types of errors. On one hand, if stress is not associated with stroke (the null hypothesis is true) and the jury finds the stress industry guilty (it rejects the null hypothesis), then the jury has made a Type I error. On the other hand, if stress is associated with stroke (the null hypothesis is false) and the jury finds the stress industry not guilty (it does not reject the null hypothesis), then the jury has made a Type II error.

It is also possible to make *correct* decisions, using tests of significance. We can be correct in our decisions when we reject a null hypothesis when it is false and fail to reject a null hypothesis when it is true.

Table 5.2 helps distinguish between Type I and Type II errors. In reality, the null hypothesis is either true or not true. As a result of doing a test of significance we decide whether to reject the null hypothesis. The table illustrates four possible outcomes. The two cells marked "OK" illustrate a decision that corresponds to reality. The other two cells show the two types of errors.

If we reject the null hypothesis, we do not know for certain that the null hypothesis is false. The null hypothesis could be false, but it is also possible that we could be making a Type I error. When doing a test of significance, researchers decide the maximum probability that they are willing to tolerate in making a Type I error. This is called the "size" of the Type I error and is denoted by the Greek symbol α ("**alpha**").

Choosing α or the α-level to be equal to zero does not prevent making a Type I error. A test of significance will *never* reject the null hypothesis—that is how the test of significance avoids making any Type I error. When the size of the Type I error equals zero, doing the study is unnecessary because, no matter what data are gathered, the test of significance will never reject the null hypothesis.

Because most researchers *want* to reject the null hypothesis to prove their point, they choose some non-zero value, usually a low one, for α and accept that degree of error. A common choice for the size of a Type I error is 0.05, but there is nothing special about that number. We could choose 0.10, 0.08, 0.03 or any value for the α-level.

If we do not reject the null hypothesis, we do not know for certain that the null hypothesis is true because we could be making a Type II error. Unlike the size of the Type I error, which researchers choose rather arbitrarily, the size of the Type II error is influenced by three components of the

TABLE 5.2 Distinguishing between Type I and Type II errors

Your Decision as a Rssult of a Test of Significance	Reality	
	H_0 True	*H_0 Not True*
Reject H_0	Type I error	Correct decision
Accept H_0	Correct decision	Type II error

SOURCE: From Slome et al., 1986 (p. 231).

study: (1) the sample size, (2) the chosen level of Type I error, and (3) the size of the difference between the population parameters.

The size of the Type II error is often denoted by β (“**beta**”). The larger the sample size, the smaller the sampling variability and, thus, the smaller the Type II error (β). The smaller the size of the Type I error, the larger the Type II error (the smaller α is, the larger β is). The greater the difference between the population parameters, the smaller the size of Type II error.

In planning a good study, we first choose the size of the Type I error because it will influence the size of the Type II error. Then from other published studies or from a pretest we estimate the size of the expected difference between the population parameters being studied and specify a tolerable size for Type II error. With the help of a statistician or statistical tables, we determine how large the sample needs to be to meet our specifications. If the required sample size is larger than we can afford to include in the study, we have to accept either a larger size of Type I error or a larger size of Type II error.

How critical is the size of a sample?

The size of a sample does not determine whether we can relate our findings to a population; that is, make generalizations from the sample. In order to make such generalizations, the sample (whether small or large) must truly represent the population, which is why considerable care must be taken in the way we select our sample. There are many studies in which a researcher has not considered the interrelationships of size of Type I and Type II errors, size of sample, and expected differences between population parameters. All these choices require deliberation; in the process it is wise to include help from a statistician or a statistical textbook.

Statistical Testing Guidelines

If we have chosen our α- and β-level values, determined the necessary sample size for the expected difference in the population parameters, completed the study, and applied the appropriate test of significance to the data, we will have the p-value.

The p-value is the *probability* that, *if* the null hypothesis were true, we will obtain a difference in sample estimates as large as the difference we have. Alternately, the p-value is the probability that the sample estimates differ only because of sampling variability.

Suppose we have a p-value of 0.01 and a chosen α-level of 0.05. Because the p-value is less than the chosen size of Type I error, we reject the null hypothesis. That is, the probability is 1 in 100 that we would obtain the difference in sample estimates we have *if* the null hypothesis is true. Therefore, the probability that we will make a Type I error by rejecting the null hypothesis is tolerable.

In another case, suppose an obtained p-value is 0.17 and our chosen α-level is 0.10. We will not reject the null hypothesis because our p-value is greater than our α-level.

Understanding these concepts and their place in epidemiology permits us when reading scientific articles to realize that these concepts are often used incorrectly and/or inappropriately. Many articles or scientific presentations do not elucidate these concepts. For example, the null hypothesis may never be stated, although it is always implied, and no concern about the size of Type II error may be evident. Also, the chosen α level may not be stated; only the p-value may be reported. Researchers do not always report exact p-values but indicate its size by writing $p < 0.01$, $p < 0.05$, $p < 0.001$, and so forth.

Some researchers attempt to rate the relative *importance* of their data in terms of the size of the p-value because they believe that a smaller p-value indicates more importance. That is why terms such as "highly significant," "very highly significant," "approaching significance," and "almost significant" are used. This practice should not be encouraged, we believe, because the size of the p-value has no relationship to the potential practical significance of the findings.

P-Values and Confidence Interval Estimation

Although the p-value had traditionally been the statistic of choice in hypothesis testing, it is limited in that it reveals nothing about the magnitude of effect (i.e., how much one group differs from another) or the precision of measurement (i.e., the amount of random error). Because of these limitations, it is not uncommon for researchers to reject a null hypothesis on the basis of a p-value when, in fact, the data indicate a strong treatment effect. The statistical procedure known as interval estimation (the calculation of confidence intervals) can remedy these flaws and provide added insight concerning whether a null hypothesis should be accepted or rejected. More important, this procedure uses the sample mean to construct an interval (range) of numbers to estimate the effect. This interval provides some indication of how probable it is (e.g., 68%, 90%, 95%), or how "confident" one can be, that the true mean lies within the range of numbers included in the interval estimate. Confidence intervals are not limited to means but are also used with sample proportions, rates, risk ratios, odds ratios, and other measures of epidemiologic interest. A 95% confidence interval, for example, indicates that there is a 95% probability that the parameter of interest lies within the confidence interval.

There are a variety of methods (formulas) for calculating confidence intervals for different epidemiologic parameters. These formulas and their interpretation relative to the different parameters of epidemiologic concern are readily included in nearly all statistics books.

An Application of Statistical Analysis and Testing

Knowing the type of variables we have in our study allows us to decide which statistical tests of significance may be appropriate for the study. Let us review the example of the possible relationship between stress and stroke, discussed earlier.

The independent variable is the presence or absence of stress, and it is a nominal variable. (It might also be considered an ordinal variable because people with stress have more of the variable than people without stress. However, when there are only two possible ordered values of the variable, as in this case, it is usually considered nominal rather than ordinal.)

The dependent variable is the presence or absence of a stroke over some defined time period. This is also a nominal variable.

This example illustrates a very common research design in epidemiology—the investigation of the relationship between two nominal variables. Often the independent variable is the presence or absence of the characteristic and the dependent variable is the presence or absence of a disease. The statistical test of significance that assesses whether the observed differences between rates in this study design are due only to sampling variability is called a **chi square (χ^2) test.** (The symbol χ is "chi," pronounced "kigh," which rhymes with "high.")

The data from the hypothetical cohort study of stress/stroke are shown in Table 5.3. Using the notation we used earlier in the chapter, the null hypothesis is H_0: $IR_s = IR_{ns}$. This is equivalent to stating that the incidence rate for stroke is "independent of" or "not associated with" or "not related to" the presence of stress. The sample proportions or incidence rates IR_s and IR_{ns}, which equal 0.30 and 0.10 respectively, are compared.

In order to find the p-value, it is necessary to calculate a test statistic that quantifies the difference between the observed outcome (the data in Table 5.3) and the outcome we expect if the null hypothesis is true. If the null hypothesis is true, the sample incidence rates will be relatively close to each other and will differ only because of sampling variability. What value would they be? If we know what the incidence of stroke is in 40- to 49-year-old men, that information could be used to specify the expected sample incidence rates. (Usually such information is not available.)

TABLE 5.3 Frequency of male subjects, aged 40-49, by stress status at beginning of study and stroke status at end of study

	Stress Status		
Stroke Status	*Stressed*	*Nonstressed*	*Total*
Developed stroke	300	100	400
Did not develop stroke	700	900	1,600
Totals	1,000	1,000	2,000

SOURCE: From Slome et al., 1986 (p. 245).

TABLE 5.4 Observed and expected subjects, by stress status and by stroke status

	Stress Status		
Stroke Status	*Stressed*	*Nonstressed*	*Total*
Developed stroke	O = 300 E = 200	O = 100 E = 200	400
Did not develop stroke	O = 700 E = 800	O = 900 E = 800	1,600
Totals	1,000	1,000	2,000

SOURCE: From Slome et al., 1986 (p. 248).

In most cases it is necessary to use the sample data itself to estimate what the sample incidence rates will be if the null hypothesis is true. Under this assumption, all 2,000 persons in the sample will be at the same risk of stroke. The data indicate that 400 of these persons developed a stroke. Hence, an estimate of the common incidence rate or overall rate, if the null hypothesis is true, is 400/2,000, or 0.20.

Using an overall incidence rate of 0.20, which assumes the null hypothesis is true, how many of the 1,000 stressed persons and how many of the 1,000 nonstressed persons will be expected to develop a stroke? The calculation is the same for each group: (1,000) × (0.20) = 200. Therefore, one expects 200 of the stressed men and 200 of the nonstressed men to develop a stroke, if the null hypothesis is true.

How many of the 1,000 subjects in each group will be expected *not* to develop a stroke, assuming the null hypothesis is true? If 200 per group are expected to suffer a stroke, then 800 per group (1,000 − 200) will be expected not to suffer a stroke.

Consider now the four "cells" in Table 5.4, stressed with stroke, nonstressed with stroke, stressed without stroke, and nonstressed with stroke. Compare the expected number of subjects (abbreviated as E) with the observed number of subjects (abbreviated as O) in each of the four cells. The observed number of subjects is derived from Table 5.3.

If the null hypothesis is true, the observed number and the expected number of subjects per cell probably will be relatively close to each other. But, we also know they would differ somewhat due to sampling variability.

What does the χ^2 statistic quantify?

The χ^2 statistic quantifies the amount of discrepancy between the observed and the expected number of subjects per cell. For each cell, we calculate the difference between the observed number of subjects and the expected number of subjects. This is denoted by $(O_j - E_j)$, where the subscript j refers to a particular cell. Some of the values of $(O_j - E_j)$ will be positive and some will be negative. To have a measure of discrepancy that is never negative, the quantity $(O_j - E_j)$ is squared, or multiplied by itself $(O_j - E_j)^2$. Because a larger difference between O_j and E_j is likely to occur as the value of E_j grows, the squared difference is adjusted for the size of E_j by dividing by E_j; that is, $(O_j - E_j)^2/E_j$.

This quantity (ratio) is calculated for each of the four cells in Table 5.4. The sum of these four quantities is the χ^2 statistic, which quantifies the amount of discrepancy between the observed number of subjects and the expected number of subjects.

For each cell in Table 5.4, we can calculate $(O_j - E_j)^2/E_j$. To obtain the χ^2 statistic we add together the four quantities derived from each cell. For the stressed/stroke cell we have $(300 - 200)^2/200 = (100)^2/200 = 10{,}000/200 = 50.0$. For the nonstressed/stroke cell we have $(100 - 200)^2/200 = (-100)^2/200 = 10{,}000/200 = 50.0$. Recall that $(-100) \times (-100) = +10{,}000$.

For the stressed/nonstroke cell, we have $(700 - 800)^2/800 = 10{,}000/800 = 12.50$. For the nonstressed/nonstroke cell, we have the equation $(900 - 800)^2/800 = 10{,}000/800 = 12.50$. Adding these four quantities, we obtain $\chi^2 = 125.0$.

The smallest possible value for the χ^2 statistic is zero. This will occur only if the expected number equals the observed number of subjects in every single cell. The largest possible value approaches infinity.

What should we expect if the hypothesis is true? is not true?

If the null hypothesis is true, then the expected number and the observed number of subjects per cell should be fairly close, any variation resulting only from sampling variability. Hence, the resulting χ^2 statistic should be fairly small, but not equal to zero, although a χ^2 statistic summed over a large table with many cells would probably be larger than a χ^2 summed over a smaller table with fewer cells.

If the null hypothesis is false, then the value of the χ^2 statistic should be large, since a false null hypothesis results in larger discrepancies between the expected number and observed number of subjects per cell.

How can we determine the probability that the χ^2 statistic is significant?

Over the years, statisticians have studied the χ^2 distribution and have provided tables that allow us to make probability statements about the χ^2 statistic. Using these tables, we can figure out the probability that we would obtain a χ^2 statistic as large or larger than the one we obtained in our study, *if* the null hypothesis is true (if there is no association). Table 5.5 is an abbreviated table of the χ^2 distribution. This table is sufficient for most researchers' purposes.

Actually, there are several different χ^2 distributions, each depending on how many quantities were added together to obtain the χ^2 statistic. (In our stress/stroke example, four quantities were added to obtain our χ^2 statistic.)

What are "degrees of freedom"?

Each of the different χ^2 probability distributions is specified by a quantity called its "**degree of freedom**," abbreviated as df. Each line of Table 5.5 gives the probability distribution for a particular χ^2 distribution defined by its df.

Note that the column that denotes "degrees of freedom" is the right-hand column. There are 37 different χ^2 distributions in Table 5.5, and the degrees of freedom are 1, 2, 3, . . . 29, 30, 40, 50, 60, 70, 80, 90, 100. One way to figure out the df in tables such as Table 5.3 is to use a general formula:

$$\text{degrees of freedom} = (\text{number columns} - 1) \times (\text{number rows} - 1)$$

where the number of columns and numbers of rows refer to those in the table under consideration.

For the data presented in Table 5.3, the degree of freedom is one. The degree of freedom is one because the number of columns is two ("stressed" and "nonstressed") and the number of rows is two ("developed a stroke" and "did not develop a stroke"). Note that the product of the number of rows and columns ($2 \times 2 = 4$ in this example) is the number of cells added to obtain the χ^2 statistic. (We do *not* count the "total" column and "total" row as one of the rows or columns when we use this formula for df.)

TABLE 5.5 Upper percentage points of the χ^2 distribution

a = 0.10	a = 0.05	a = 0.025	a = 0.010	a = 0.005	df
2.70554	3.84146	5.02389	6.63490	7.87944	1
4.60517	5.99147	7.37776	9.21034	10.5966	2
6.25139	7.81473	9.34840	11.3449	12.8381	3
7.77944	9.48773	11.1433	13.2767	14.8602	4
9.23635	11.0705	12.8325	15.0863	16.7496	5
10.6446	12.5916	14.4494	16.8119	18.5476	6
12.0170	14.0671	16.0128	18.4753	20.2777	7
13.3616	15.5073	17.5346	20.0902	21.9550	8
14.6837	16.9190	19.0228	21.6660	23.5893	9
15.9871	18.3070	20.4831	23.2093	25.1882	10
17.2750	19.6751	21.9200	24.7250	26.7569	11
18.5494	21.0261	23.3367	26.2170	28.2995	12
19.8119	22.3621	24.7356	27.6883	29.8194	13
21.0642	23.6848	26.1190	29.1413	31.3193	14
22.3072	24.9958	27.4884	30.5779	32.8013	15
23.5418	26.2962	28.8454	31.9999	34.2672	16
24.7690	27.5871	30.1910	33.4087	35.7185	17
25.9894	28.8693	31.5264	34.8053	37.1564	18
27.2036	30.1435	32.8523	36.1908	38.5822	19
28.4120	31.4104	34.1696	37.5662	39.9968	20
29.6151	32.6705	35.4789	38.9321	41.4010	21
30.8133	33.9244	36.7807	40.2894	42.7956	22
32.0069	35.1725	38.0757	41.6384	44.1813	23
33.1963	36.4151	39.3641	42.9798	45.5585	24
34.3816	37.6525	40.6465	44.3141	46.9278	25
35.5631	38.8852	41.9232	45.6417	48.2899	26
36.7412	40.1133	43.1944	46.9630	49.6449	27
37.9159	41.3372	44.4607	48.2782	50.9933	28
39.0875	42.5569	45.7222	49.5879	52.3356	29
40.2560	43.7729	46.9792	50.8922	53.6720	30
51.8050	55.7585	59.3417	63.6907	66.7659	40
63.1671	67.5048	71.4202	76.1539	79.4900	50
74.3970	79.0819	83.2976	88.3794	91.9517	60
85.5271	90.5312	95.0231	100.425	104.215	70
96.5782	101.879	106.629	112.329	116.321	80
107.565	113.145	118.136	124.116	128.299	90
118.498	124.342	129.561	135.807	140.169	100

SOURCE: Thompson CM: Tables of the percentage points of the χ^2 distribution, *Biometrika* 32:188-189. Reproduced by permission of the *Biometrika* Trustees.

The concept "degrees of freedom" also has an intuitive interpretation; it is the number of cells whose expected number of subjects does not depend upon the expected number of subjects in other cells. For instance, in the cell "stressed and stroke" in Table 5.4, it was determined that 200 subjects would be expected in that cell if the null hypothesis were true. Given that, the expected number of subjects in the cell "stressed and no stroke" is 800, because there is a total number of 1,000 stressed persons in the study. Likewise, because 400 persons out of the total sample size of 2,000 developed a stroke, and it was calculated that 200 of these would be expected in the stressed group, then 200 subjects are expected in the "nonstressed and stroke" cell. Similarly, 800 subjects are expected in the "nonstressed and no stroke" cell, because there is a total of 1,000 nonstressed persons.

Thus, once one expected number is calculated for any cell in the table, the expected numbers in the remaining three cells are automatically determined due to the fixed marginal totals in the table (1,000 stressed, 1,000 nonstressed, 400 who developed a stroke, 1,600 who did not develop a stroke). Because there is only one cell whose expected value does not depend on expected values in other cells, the df = 1. It does not matter which one of four cells is selected to make the first calculation of expected number of subjects.

Consider the χ^2 distribution with df equal to one, the first line of Table 5.5. The columns of Table 5.5 are selected probability levels. For example, looking in the column marked 0.10 and the row labeled 1, we see the number 2.70554. This is interpreted in the following manner: If the null hypothesis is true, the probability is 0.10 that a χ^2 variable with 1 degree of freedom will be 2.70554 or larger. (A value of 2.70554 or larger for a χ^2 variable with one degree of freedom is somewhat unlikely if the null hypothesis is true.)

If the null hypothesis is true, the probability is 0.01 that a χ^2 variable with one degree of freedom will be 6.635 or larger. Hence, if a calculated χ^2 statistic with 1 df is equal to 6.635, the p-value corresponding to 6.635 is 0.01 (see the column labeled 0.010 and the row labeled 1 in Table 5.5).

If the calculated χ^2 statistic for the stress/stroke example is 125.0, and if it has one degree of freedom, what is the probability that the χ^2 statistic, with one degree of freedom, would be as large as 125.0, or larger, if the null hypothesis is true?

In Table 5.5, look along row 1 (df = 1) for a number in the table close to 125.0. The closest available is 7.879. Hence, the p-value being sought here is not in Table 5.5, but we know that the p-value is less than 0.005. Why? Because the probability is 0.005 that a χ^2 variable with df = 1 will be as large as or larger than 7.879 if the null hypothesis is true. Because larger values of the χ^2 variable are *more likely* under the null hypothesis, the p-value corresponding to a value of 125.0 must be smaller than 0.005 (sometimes written as $p < 0.005$).

If an alpha level (or size of Type I error) of 0.05 is used for this statistical test of significance, and the p-value is less than 0.005, the null hypothesis is rejected. Because the p-value, whatever it is, is less than 0.005, it must be less than 0.05. Therefore, the null hypothesis is rejected.

Rejection of the null hypothesis means that the incidence rates of stroke are not the same in the stressed and nonstressed populations. Because the sample incidence rate is higher in the stressed group, the conclusion can be drawn that the incidence of stroke is higher in that population.

The χ^2 test for tables with two rows and two columns (called 2 × 2 contingency tables) is appropriate *only* if all four cells have met their expected number of observations—equal to or larger than five. This condition was met in Table 5.4. If this condition is *not* met, another statistical test of significance, called Fisher's Exact Test for 2 × 2 tables, can be used. (This shows how knowing the assumptions of a statistical test allows us to use it in appropriate situations.)

What are two-tailed and one-tailed statistical tests?

Those with a biostatistical background may have noted that the χ^2 example we used was a *two-sided* or *two-tailed* χ^2 test of significance. This means that our alternate hypothesis allowed for the possibility that the null hypothesis could be false in one of *two* possible ways—$IR_s > IR_{ns}$ or $IR_s < IR_{ns}$. The data indicated that the null hypothesis was false in the direction $IR_s > IR_{ns}$. Some might argue a priori (before data are collected) that it is inconceivable or impossible that the null hypothesis would be false in the direction $IR_s < IR_{ns}$. These people would perform a *one-sided* or *one-tailed* χ^2 test of significance, assuming that the null hypothesis could only be false in the direction $IR_s > IR_{ns}$. The χ^2 statistic would be calculated the same way as in our example. However, the p-value would be calculated differently, resulting in a smaller p-value. Because the same empirical data yield a smaller p-value for a one-sided test than for a two-sided test, many researchers prefer to do a one-sided test. When comparing two groups, one needs to be absolutely certain, a priori, that the null hypothesis could be false in only one possible direction. Those who like to "play it safe" usually choose to do a two-sided test.

Can the chi-square test be used for variables with more than 2 classification categories?

Tests for association of two variables need not be performed only in 2 × 2 contingency tables. If appropriate, tables with more rows and columns can be used. Consider a modification of the stress and stroke study discussed in the chapter. Instead of classifying subjects as stressed or nonstressed, we expand the classification to three levels: nonstressed, mildly stressed, and highly stressed. Assume there is a random sample of 150 nonstressed, 100 mildly stressed, and 100 highly stressed—all males. The outcome of such a cohort study is given in Table 5.6. The null hypothesis is: $H_0: IR_{ns} = IR_{ms} = IR_{hs}$, where IR denotes incidence rate for stroke

TABLE 5.6 Male subjects, by stress status and stroke status

	Stress Status			
Stroke Status	*None*	*Mild*	*High*	*Total*
Developed a stroke	20	20	30	70
Did not develop a stroke	130	80	70	280
Totals	150	100	100	350

SOURCE: From Slome et al., 1986 (p. 258).

TABLE 5.7 Expected and observed subjects, by stress status and stroke status

	Stress Status			
Stroke Status	*None*	*Mild*	*High*	*Total*
Developed stroke	O = 20 E = 30	O = 20 E = 20	O = 30 E = 20	70
Did not develop stroke	O = 130 E = 120	O = 80 E = 80	O = 70 E = 80	280
Totals	150	100	100	350

SOURCE: From Slome et al., 1986 (p. 260).

over a period of time and ns, ms, and hs mean no stress, mild stress, and high stress, respectively.

What can we conclude from our calculated χ^2 statistic?

The table for the observed and the expected numbers of subjects per cell is presented in Table 5.7. The calculated value for the χ^2 statistic is 10.41. This was obtained by using the formula (rows − 1) × (columns − 1) yields (2 − 1) × (3 − 1) = (1) × (2) = 2. Recall from calculating the expected number of subjects per cell that there were two cells for which the expected number needed actually to be calculated; the expected number of subjects for the remaining four cells was then determined because the marginal totals were fixed. Hence, df = two.

If we look at row two of Table 5.5, for df = 2, a χ^2 value of 10.41 is not found. However, 10.41 is between 9.2 (which corresponds to a p-value of 0.01) and 10.6 (which corresponds to a p-value of 0.005). Hence, the p-value corresponding to χ^2 = 10.41 is somewhere between 0.005 and 0.01.

Because the p-value is less than 0.01, the null hypothesis is rejected. The inference is that the incidence rates for stroke are not the same in all three stress populations. However, they could be "unequal" in a variety of ways. For example, the nonstressed could have a low incidence rate, whereas both the mildly and the heavily stressed could have the same incidence rates higher than the nonstressed. Or all three incidence rates could differ from each other. The χ^2 statistic calculated does not indicate which of these various situations is the case; additional statistical techniques need to be used to address this issue.

Many researchers, obtaining a significant χ^2 statistic such as the 10.41 above, look at the different sample incidence rates and make a personal judgment about which ones appear to be different from each other. Although such a procedure is not desirable from a statistician's point of view, it is frequently used when it is "obvious" which incidence rates differ from each other. In Table 5.6, where the sample incidence rates or proportions are 0.13, 0.20, and 0.30, it is "obvious" that the sample rates 0.13 and 0.30 are significantly different from each other. Whether 0.13 and 0.20 are significantly different, and whether 0.20 and 0.30 are significantly different, is not quite so obvious. Techniques to address this issue can be found under the topic of "partitioning of the χ^2 statistic" in the statistics books listed as references earlier in this chapter.

As in the case for 2×2 tables, there are guidelines for larger contingency tables regarding how large the expected cell frequencies should be. One common guideline for tables larger than 2×2 is that no more than 20% of the expected cell frequencies can be less than five *and* no expected frequency can be less than one. Table 5.7 meets these conditions.

We have calculated and evaluated two χ^2 tests—one on a 2×2 table and one on a 2×3 table. The χ^2 statistical test of significance is of great use in research and in understanding others' use of the test.

There are many other tests of significance commonly used in epidemiology. For quantitative variables, t-tests and z-tests are often used, as are tests for analysis of variance and regression analysis. For nominal dependent variables, discriminant analysis sometimes is used. For ordinal variables, there are many nonparametric statistical techniques.

COMPUTER RESOURCES FOR EPIDEMIOLOGIC DATA ANALYSIS

We present a few guidelines for determining what capacity is needed for analyzing epidemiologic data. Several standard software packages that support epidemiologic analyses are cited as well as two of the Center for Disease Control and Prevention's information systems for public health research.[2]

---

[2]This section is adapted from Franks AL, Mendlein JM, Blount SB: *Using chronic disease data: A handbook for public health practitioners.* Atlanta, GA: Centers for Disease Control and Prevention, 1992.

Hardware

The computer resources required for analyzing health-relevant data depend on the complexity of the statistical analyses, the number of observations, and the number and type of variables in the data set. The amount of information recorded about each death, each hospitalization, or each population object (i.e., survey respondent) determines the length of the corresponding computerized record.

The number of observations, or records, involved in a calculation is usually the most important determinant of the computer capacity required. Analyses of a data set for a state with a large population (for example, California, which has more than 200,000 deaths and 2 million hospitalizations per year) require more computer capacity than do analyses for a state with a small population (such as Maine, which has about 11,000 deaths and 200,000 hospitalizations per year).

In California, most analyses are performed on a 386-series personal computer system, and in Maine, on a 286-series computer. For analyzing data from the Behavioral Risk Factor Surveillance System (see Chapter 3), the minimum equipment required is a 386-series computer. For analyses that require complex computations or have large data sets, you may need to upload/download data to/from a mainframe computer.

Software

Various software packages are available for different types of epidemiologic analyses. They are briefly described below with the address of the organization from which they are available. Users with a university affiliation may have access to these packages through the university's site licenses. The first three packages are multipurpose programs for data management and statistical analysis.

SAS System

SAS is a set of programs that control data access, management, computation and analysis, and reporting. Versions are available for both mainframe and personal computers.

SAS Institute, Inc.
SAS Campus Drive
Cary, NC 27513

SPSS Information Analysis System

This integrated data management, report writing, and statistical analysis system is available in versions for both mainframe and personal computers.

SPSS, Inc.
444 North Michigan Avenue
Chicago, IL 60611

BMDP Statistical Software

The BMDP program library of data analysis procedures, for mainframe and personal computers, can be used to manage data, test statistical significance, evaluate relationships between variables, and perform many other advanced statistical analyses.

Software: BMDP Statistical Software, Inc.
1440 Sepulveda Boulevard
Suite 316
Los Angeles, CA 90025

Documentation: University of California Press
2120 Berkeley Way
Berkeley, CA 94720

SUDAAN

SUDAAN software is available for mainframe and personal computer analysis of data from complex sample surveys. It can be used for analyzing responses from the Behavioral Risk Factor Surveillance System or other types of complex survey data. Its predecessor, SESUDAAN, is a mainframe package.

Research Triangle Institute
P.O. Box 12194
Research Triangle Park, NC 27709

SAMMEC II

Smoking-Attributable Mortality, Morbidity, and Economic Costs, Release II (SAMMEC II), is a spreadsheet software that estimates the disease impact of smoking.

Office on Smoking and Health
National Center for Chronic Disease Prevention and Health Promotion
Centers for Disease Control and Prevention
Mailstop K-50
1600 Clifton Road, NE
Atlanta, GA 30333

Epi Info

This is a program for data entry, word processing, and analysis of questionnaire data. Epi Info can be used to manage data obtained through epidemiologic investigations and disease surveillance.

USD Incorporated
2075A West Park Place
Stone Mountain, GA 30077

Information Systems

In addition to the packages described above, two Centers for Disease Control and Prevention products are particularly helpful to public health workers whose time is limited and to persons inexperienced with computer programming and data analysis. These two information systems, designed to simplify access to information, are described below.

WONDER

Wide-Ranging Online Data for Epidemiologic Research (WONDER) is a computerized information system designed by CDC to simplify online access to public health databases maintained at CDC. WONDER provides state and local health departments with rapid access to information, and its use requires neither programming skills nor expensive computer resources.

Data available through WONDER that support health and disease research include the following:

- Alcohol abuse and alcoholism data from the Alcohol, Drug Abuse, and Mental Health Administration
- Behavioral risk factor data from the Behavioral Risk Factor Surveillance System
- Surveillance, Epidemiology, and End Results (SEER) data from the National Cancer Institute
- Population data by age, race, sex, and county from the U.S. Bureau of Census and a private organization
- Disease codes from the International Classification of Diseases, Ninth Revision (ICD-9), and the ICD-9 Clinical Modification.
- National Hospital Discharge Survey results from the National Center for Health Statistics
- Underlying and multiple-cause-of-death files from the National Center for Health Statistics

Depending on the data set accessed, data can be displayed by year, state, demographic variables (such as age, race, and sex), or other variables. Results can be presented as tables, charts, or maps, and tables, graphics, and documentation from the computer screen can be created and printed. Because WONDER is a menu-driven system supported by extensive online documentation, no programming skills are required for its use.

In a single online session, you can access multiple data sets, tabulate data, view the results, and print them for later use. For example, to obtain lung cancer mortality data for specific counties, one might first search the ICD-9 listings for diagnostic codes appropriate for classifying lung cancer. Then, one might access the multiple-cause-of-death files and search for information by these codes. Results can be displayed by state, organized by county, and restricted to selected years. By pressing the "PrintScrn" key on the computer, the data could be immediately output to a printer at your site. To access WONDER, obtain an account on the CDC/Atlanta mainframe by calling (404) 332-4569 and asking for a registration form. A few days after you mail in the form, you will receive an account number, a password, a diskette that contains a communications package called MAINLINK, and a user manual. The basic equipment required is a DOS-based microcomputer, a modem, and the MAINLINK diskette. The only costs are telephone charges.)

HIRS

Health Information Retrieval System (HIRS), originated by one of the authors of this text and developed in conjunction with the CDC, is a PC-based information system that can simplify access to data sets maintained at a local site. With HIRS, you decide which data sets you need rapid access to, and you specify which information you want to be available from the data set. The data are pre-tabulated so that their subsequent use requires minimal computer time and no specialized computer skills. The only resource equipment is a 286-series personal computer (or more powerful machine with a larger disk drive). HIRS eliminates the need for programming skills, a mainframe computer for storing data, and lengthy processing each time information is needed.

Various combinations of variables, such as demographic variables, risk factors, diagnostic information, dates of health events, and other values, can be included in the pre-tabulated data file. HIRS permits immediate access to tabulations for any subset of your choice, stratified by any variable in the data set. Population data can also be included in a data set so that the system can calculate measures such as crude, adjusted, and cause-specific rates (see Chapter 2).

Data made available to HIRS could come from hospital and public health clinic databases, cancer registries, local vital records, and other sources. For example, information could be evaluated on outpatient clinic and emergency room visits made within a state during a given period. The record for each visit might include demographic data for the patient, date of visit, diagnosis, and location of clinic or hospital. By using HIRS, health department staff may determine, within seconds, the number of visits made for treatment of asthma, by month, as well as by age and race of patients. HIRS makes immediate and detailed analyses of local data possible.

The data sets and variables to include in HIRS are selected locally. The actual importation of data into HIRS takes from several minutes to several days, depending on the size of the data sets and the speed of the computer. The importation process requires some data management skills; however, technical assistance is made available by CDC whenever possible.

Once the system is set up, it can be used by persons with no computer experience. At each step in a data search, all allowable options are displayed, and a user need only select one from the list. Results can be printed directly to a local printer or output as an ASCII file. Selected information can also be copied into a text-processing area for further manipulation and incorporation into word-processed reports to spreadsheets.

For information on obtaining HIRS contact the Office of Surveillance and Analysis, National Center for Chronic Disease Prevention and Health Promotion, Centers for Disease Control and Prevention (telephone: (404) 488-5281). The system is provided free of charge.

CHAPTER SUMMARY

Some of the main points covered in this chapter are:

1. Descriptive statistics are methods used to organize and produce quantitative summaries of numerical information, primarily by means of tables, charts, graphs, or diagrams.
2. Inferential statistics are used to make generalizations or "inferences" about a larger group or population of objects on the basis on information derived from a representative subset or sample of the same group.
3. Inferential statistical tests can be further classified as either parametric or nonparametric on the basis of how the data to be analyzed are distributed on a measurement scale.
4. To select the most appropriate inferential statistical test it is important to consider the population objects and variables to study, the inferences to make about the target population, how the data are selected from the target population, how data on the variables of interest are distributed within the target population, and the level or type of data to analyze.
5. Variables can be classified as nominal, ordinal, or quantitative.
6. Quantitative variables are either discrete or continuous.
7. Arithmetic means can be calculated from quantitative data.
8. Proportions (rates) are applied to qualitative (categorical or nominal) data.
9. Some researchers may apply numbers to nominal or ordinal variables and pretend that these variables are quantitative.
10. A statistical test of significance tells whether sample estimates differ only because of sampling variability.
11. The format of a test of significance is to reject or not reject a null hypothesis.
12. One can make two possible kinds of errors in performing a test of significance—a Type I error and a Type II error.
13. The design of a study should include specification of the acceptable sizes for Type I and Type II errors, the expected difference between the population parameters, and the sample size necessary to attain these acceptable levels.

14. A decision to reject or keep the null hypothesis is made by comparing the α-level with the p-value obtained from the test of significance.
15. The nature of the sample, *not the p-value,* will determine whether inferences to the population of interest can be made. In order to make such inferences, the sample must be representative of the population.
16. A commonly used statistical test of significance is the chi square test, used to test whether two nominal variables are associated.
17. Many other statistical tests of significance are available for different combinations of nominal, ordinal, and quantitative variables.
18. A brief review of computer resources for epidemiologic data analysis was provided.

KEY TERMS

biostatistics
descriptive statistics
inferential statistics
sample
population
target or study population
population variable
probability
nonprobability
random sample
parametric statistics
nonparametric statistics
normal distribution
normal curve
nominal data
qualitative variable
categorical variable
ordinal data
interval data
ratio scale
quantitative variable
ordinal variable
discrete quantitative variable
hypothesis
Type I error
Type II error
alpha
beta
chi-square test
degrees of freedom

REFERENCES

Centers for Disease Control: *Principles of epidemiology: An introduction to applied epidemiology and biostatistics*, 2d ed. Atlanta, GA: Centers for Disease Control and Prevention, 1992.

Kuzma J: *Basics statistics for health sciences*. Palo Alto, CA: Mayfield Publishing, 1984.

Slome C, Brogan D, Eyres S, Lednar W: *Basic epidemiological methods and biostatistics: A workbook*. Boston: Jones and Bartlett, 1986. Figures and tables used with permission.

EXERCISE APPLICATION 5.1

Formulate 4 hypothetical studies—cross-sectional, case-control, cohort/prospective, and experimental. For each one list an appropriate null and alternative hypothesis, describe how research subjects would be selected and sampled, and how data would be collected.

REVIEW QUESTIONS

1. For what are descriptive statistics used?
2. For what are inferential statistics used?
3. What is the difference between parametric and nonparametric statistics?
4. List 5 things to consider when selecting a statistical test.
5. Distinguish between nominal, ordinal, interval, and ratio data.
6. What is sampling variability?
7. Give an example of a hypothesis that is stated in a null fashion.
8. What is an alternate hypothesis?
9. What is meant by the p-value of a statistical test?
10. What are Type I errors? Type II errors?
11. What factors influence the sizes of Type I and Type II errors?
12. What are biostatistics?
13. What is meant by the term "population?"
14. What is a probability sample? random sample? nonprobability sample?
15. What is meant by quantitative data?
16. What are hypotheses?
17. When is a chi-square test appropriate?
18. Discuss the concept of degrees of freedom in statistical testing.
19. What is meant by a two-tailed test of significance?
20. Provide examples of computer software available to analyze epidemiologic data.

6 Epidemiologic Inference

OBJECTIVES

On completion of this chapter, you will be able to:

- Discuss considerations in establishing association between an attribute and a health outcome
- List steps in establishing causality between an attribute and a health outcome
- Define practical significance
- State and explain Hill's nine rules of evidence
- Provide five explanations to consider as potential causes of artifactual associations

Previous chapters have dealt with various strategies and methods, potential errors and fallacies, tests of significance, and types of data used in epidemiology. These entities come together when we consider the meaning of findings and their possible implications. This chapter is a guide to thinking through some of the ramifications of epidemiological inferences in the search for causal factors.

ESTABLISHING ASSOCIATION

In a study that compares the occurrence of a health attribute in two or more populations, the first consideration is whether there is an association between the health attribute and the other characteristic (i.e., whether the null hypothesis is false). When there is a possible relation between two variables there is **association.** A statistical measure of an association is a **correlation.** Association and correlation do not necessarily imply causation, but they often provide an impetus for more study and confirmation (Cohn, 1989).

How can association be determined?

This can be done by testing whether there is a numerical difference between the health indices (rates, means, and so forth) that describe the populations. Although more sophisticated techniques exist to assess the presence of an association, such as correlation coefficients and other association coefficients, we shall not pursue them here.

If there were no numerical differences between the health indices for the various populations and if we expected a difference, we might consider potential errors (bias) in method, sampling, data collection, and so forth, which may have masked a true difference in the populations studied. If such errors are likely to have happened, the study needs to be redesigned and repeated.

However, the absence of a numerical difference may be a reality, and that in itself may be very useful information. Two examples illustrate this. First, certain populations in the world do not manifest the generally accepted association of increasing blood pressure with increasing age. Such absence of association may suggest a cultural or biological immunity to a disorder that afflicts the vast majority of all older people. Second, if we expected an improvement in health status among patients who received home visits but we did not observe the expected improvement, it may be true that home visits do not improve health status. The finding of "no difference" is important to health planners and administrators.

Another consideration, discussed earlier, may explain the absence of an expected difference in a study—a Type II error. That is, an association may exist in the population but, due to sampling variability, sample size, and the true differences in the parameters, the particular sample used may not reflect the true differences in the populations. Thus, in doing a statistical test of significance, we would not reject the null hypothesis (because there is no numerical difference) and we would be making a Type II error.

ESTABLISHING PRACTICAL SIGNIFICANCE

If there is a numerical difference, the next consideration is whether the difference is meaningful, or of **practical significance.** Some may disagree with the particular order in which we deal with all these considerations; there is no established order.

What is practical or meaningful difference?

By practical or meaningful difference, we mean a difference large enough to have important implications within the conceptual context of the study.

For example, if a preventive program reduces the incidence of a rare, nonfatal, mild disease by a small amount, perhaps 1 per 10,000, the difference may not be meaningful in terms of continuing the preventive program, especially if it is expensive. Similarly, if a study shows that a factor is independently associated with a disease with a relative risk slightly over 1, this may be very important in the search for causes of the disease. However, the population attributable risk percent (PARP) may be quite small and, thus, not useful in terms of launching a program to reduce this factor.

Making a decision about the meaning of a difference is up to the researcher who knows the purpose of the study, its context, and the practicality of the findings. Reviewing published articles and consulting with others who have made similar decisions is helpful in deciding what constitutes "meaningful difference."

RULING OUT ARTIFACTUAL ASSOCIATION

If there is a numerical difference, and if it is meaningful, several explanations may need to be considered before accepting the association as nonartifactual.

What are five explanations which may make an artifactual association between a factor and a health outcome?

We must consider at least five explanations, any or all of which may make your association artifactual (that is, spurious or secondary).

1. *Information bias.* In Chapter 4 we discussed potential hazards involved in labeling disease states and characteristics.

2. *Selection bias.* In Chapter 4 we also discussed how selective forces can produce artifactual associations.

3. *Failure to control for confounding variables.* This was presented in Chapter 2 and subsequently throughout the book. Knowledge about factors already known to be associated with the occurrence of the health state or outcome (dependent variable, effect variable) is necessary to discern whether these factors are potential confounders in a study.

4. *Ecologic fallacy.* Chapter 4 discussed how ecologic indices used in establishing an association may create an artifactual association.

5. *Sampling variability or chance.* In Chapter 5 we discussed using an appropriate statistical test of significance to find out whether difference is likely to be due *only* to sampling variability (corresponding

to a large p-value) or to sampling variability *plus* true differences between the parameters (corresponding to a small p-value). A large p-value would cause us not to reject the null hypothesis, and thus assume that the difference is artifactual and produced only by sampling variability. A small p-value would cause us to reject the null hypothesis, and assume that the association really exists in the population.

Friedman (1980, pp. 187-88) comments on a classic example which shows how researchers rule out potential artifactual associations:

> An interesting example of a search for other explanations comes from a case-control study showing an association between oral contraceptives and thromboembolic disease (Vessey and Doll, 1968). Since it is easy to overlook the diagnosis of deep-vein thrombosis or pulmonary embolism, the investigators considered the possibility that a history of oral contraceptive use would alert the physician to these conditions, resulting in a spurious association. They reasoned that a spurious association of this type would be strongest among patients with the least evident disease, since this group would contain women whose condition was diagnosed only because they were known to have taken oral contraceptives. Cases were therefore classified by degree of certainty as to the presence of thromboembolism. It was found that the association with oral contraceptive use was actually less marked among the less certain and milder cases than among the definite and severe cases. Thus, this alternative explanation could reasonably be rejected, lending greater credence to the idea that thromboembolism was actually caused by oral contraceptives.

ESTABLISHING CAUSALITY: THE GREATEST CHALLENGE IN EPIDEMIOLOGY

Morton, Hebel, and McCarter (1990, p. 158) say the following about causal association:

> Medicine is concerned with limiting or preventing disease. The search for etiology is pursued in the hope that, once the cause of a disease is found prevention will follow. Causality is assumed when one factor is shown to contribute to the development of disease and its removal is shown to reduce the frequency of disease. This concept of causality is different from that applied in law or philosophy. In prevention, it is sufficient to identify an exposure without necessarily identifying the ultimate cause of the disease. For example, cigarette smoke has been identified as the contaminated substance that is associated with increased rates of lung and other cancers as well as heart and respiratory diseases. It is unnecessary to identify precisely which component in the smoke is the prime offender before instituting preventive measures.

If our association "survives" the previous considerations described about artifactuality and is meaningful, the association is likely to be real.

Next, it is necessary to determine whether the association is causal and where it fits into the network of causes.

Establishing epidemiologic associations as causal is a difficult process and the greatest challenge to epidemiological (or other behavioral) sciences. We offer some rules of evidence to use when considering whether an association is causal.

What are the rules of evidence for considering an association as causal?

The following rules of evidence are adapted from an article by Sir Austin Bradford Hill (1965). We present Hill's titles for his nine rules, with a short explanation of each one.

1. *Strength.* A large relative risk for a factor associated with a disease increases the likelihood that the association is causal. The size of the attributable risk bears no relation to this likelihood, but is of importance to the program implications of the association.

2. *Consistency.* If the association has been confirmed by others in different situations, in different populations, at different times, and with different methods of inquiry, then this increases the likelihood that the association is causal.

3. *Specificity.* If the association is particular to one factor and to one disease, this increases the likelihood that the association is causal. Such specificity is a rare event, because most diseases have more than one cause, and suspected causes often are associated with more than one disease. As a result, Hill suggests that this rule of evidence not be overemphasized.

4. *Temporality.* Which came first, the disease or the characteristic? Obviously, in search of causality, we wish to show that the characteristic preceded the disease. Power is added to the inference that the association is causal if it is produced by a cohort or experimental study instead of a case-control or cross-sectional study.

5. *Biological gradient.* If the association demonstrates a dose-response relationship between the characteristic and the effect, the association is more likely to be causal.

6. *Plausibility.* The association should be acceptable in light of current biological knowledge. However, with the extremely rapid advance of this knowledge, the absence of such plausibility should not refute a causal inference.

7. *Coherence.* The association should be in accordance with other facts known about the disease, including its natural history.

8. *Experiment.* Association derived from experiments (animal experiments, health programs, clinical traits, or natural experiments) add considerable weight to the evidence supporting a causal nature of the association.

9. *Analogy.* If similar associations have been shown to be causal, then, by analogy, the association is more likely to be causal. For example, because rubella in pregnancy is accepted as a cause of congenital abnormalities in infants, credence is added to the assertion of the causal nature of any new association of another infection or drug during pregnancy and congenital abnormalities.

AN EXAMPLE OF ESTABLISHING A CAUSAL ASSOCIATION: SMOKING AND DISEASE

Tens of thousands of studies have documented the associations between cigarette smoking and a large number of serious diseases. It is safe to say that smoking represents the most extensively documented cause of disease ever investigated in the history of biomedical research.[1]

Previous Surgeon General's reports, in particular the landmark 1964 Report of the Surgeon General's Advisory Report on smoking and cancer, examined these associations with respect to the epidemiologic criteria for causality. These criteria include the consistency, strength, specificity, coherence, and temporal association of the relationship. Based on these criteria, previous reports have recognized a causal association between smoking and cancers of the lung, larynx, esophagus, and oral cavity; heart disease; stroke; peripheral artery occlusive disease; chronic obstructive pulmonary disease; and intrauterine growth retardation. The 1990 Surgeon General's Report is the first to conclude that the evidence is now sufficient to identify cigarette smoking as a cause of cancer of the urinary bladder; the 1982 Report concluded that cigarette smoking is a contributing factor in the development of bladder cancer.

The causal nature of most of these associations was well established long before publication of the 1990 Surgeon General's Report. Nevertheless, it is worth noting that the findings of this Report add even more weight to the evidence that these associations are causal. The criteria of coherence requires that descriptive epidemiologic findings on disease occurrence correlate with measures of exposure to the suspected agent. Coherence would predict that the increased risk of disease associated with an exposure would diminish or disappear after cessation of

---

[1]This section is from U.S. Department of Health and Human Services: *The health benefits of smoking cessation: A report of the Surgeon General, executive summary,* Washington, DC: U.S. Government Printing Office. DHHS Publication No. (CDC) 90-8416, 1990.

exposure. This report shows in great detail that the risks of most smoking-related diseases decrease after cessation and with increasing duration of abstinence.

Evidence of the risk of disease after smoking cessation is especially important for the understanding of smoking-and-disease associations of unclear causality. For example, cigarette smoking is associated with cancer of the uterine cervix, but this association is potentially confounded by unidentified factors (in particular by a sexually transmitted etiologic agent). The evidence reviewed in the 1990 Surgeon General's Report indicates that former smokers experience a lower risk of cervical cancer than current smokers, even after adjusting for the social correlates of smoking and risk of sexually acquired infections. This diminution of risk after smoking cessation supports the hypothesis that smoking is a contributing cause of cervical cancer.

CHAPTER SUMMARY

The main points covered in Chapter 6 include:

1. A series of considerations applied to association to arrive at possible causality.
2. Exclusion of artifactuality as a confounder.
3. Exclusion of bias and selection-method pitfalls.
4. Measurement of sampling variability effect by a statistical test of significance.
5. Consideration of possible causation, using rules of evidence for making a decision of causation.
6. Recognition that no definite decision is provided by any one study.

KEY TERMS

association
correlation
practical significance

REFERENCES

Cohn V: *News and numbers: A guide to reporting statistical claims and controversies in health and other fields.* Ames, Iowa: Iowa State University Press, 1989.

Friedman GD: *Primer of epidemiology,* 2d ed. New York: McGraw-Hill, 1980.

Hill AB.: The environment and disease: Association or causation? *Proceedings of the Royal Society of Medicine,* 1965;58:295-300.

Morton RF, Hebel JR, McCarter RJ: *A study guide to epidemiology and biostatistics,* 3d ed. Gaithersburg, MD: Aspen Publishing, 1990.

Vessey MP, Doll R: Investigation of relation between use of oral contraceptives and thromboembolic disease. *British Medical Journal,* 1968;2:199-205.

APPLICATION EXERCISE 6.1

In the library locate the following articles that review the epidemiology of a particular disease. For each article, write a one-page paper summarizing the "state of the art" (what is known and what is not known) in epidemiologic understanding of the etiology of the particular disease. Use the following articles:

Bretler MMB, Claus JJ, van Duijn CM, Launer LJ, Hoffman A: Epidemiology of Alzheimer's disease. *Epidemiologic Reviews,* 1992;14:59-82.

Guess HA: Benign prostatic hyperplasia: Antecedents and natural history. *Epidemiologic Reviews,* 1992;14:131, 131-153.

Kilbourne EM: Eosinophilia-myalgia syndrome: Coming to grips with a new illness. *Epidemiologic Reviews,* 1992;14:16-36.

REVIEW QUESTIONS

1. What is the first step in establishing causality between an attribute and a health outcome?
2. What is meant by practical significance?
3. What are five explanations to consider as potential causes of artifactual associations?
4. What are Hill's nine rules of evidence?

7 Thinking Through a Study: The Application of Basic Epidemiologic Research Methods

OBJECTIVES

On completion of this chapter, you will be able to:

- Describe the progressive steps in addressing a research problem or question
- Explain the importance of thoroughly reviewing relevant literature in the research process
- Describe how a research question (hypothesis) guides the research process
- Design research specifications and protocol that meet the purposes of a study, including sample selection, pretesting or piloting methods, and instruments
- Recognize the need to modify research protocols based on pretest results and conduct a study according to modified protocol
- Draw conclusions and recommendations from tested hypotheses
- Control for potential confounding variables

In the previous chapters, we have considered many aspects of the epidemiological method. In this chapter, we combine these elements to consider how they are related in the course of a epidemiologic research study.

Because epidemiology is an observational science that addresses the health of humans, many compromises in scientific rigor, practicality, and ethics have to be made in conducting a study. A researcher or investigator makes such compromises knowingly and uses them to interpret data and draw conclusions.

Each time we seek answers about health status and disease, health behaviors, or health care a step-by-step process can be followed beneficially. Some steps proceed sequentially; others occur concurrently. We present a general outline of factors that should be considered in carrying out a sound epidemiologic research study. A pilot could hop in an airplane and take off, trusting to the instruments and the winds to arrive at a desired destination. Or a pilot (with whom we would prefer to ride) could prepare a flight plan, check equipment lists, and navigate the flight. Planning, checking, and thinking increase the probability of the pilot's arriving safely at the correct destination. We, too, can structure a study to reach "the correct destination" by relying on logic, and not serendipity. The following exercise is designed to apply the skills presented thus far in this book.

Suppose that the manager of a large manufacturing firm tells you that routine company statistics indicate more cases of peptic ulcer are occurring in the company than in past years and that the increase is related somehow to job dissatisfaction among workers. She suspects this may explain a recent decline in worker productivity and a concomitant decrease in company profits. If a study confirms her hunches, she intends to institute a program to improve worker satisfaction. Because of your epidemiological skills, she asks for your help.

1. How would you begin?

Begin by asking to see the data that caused her concern. These data might include subjective or anecdotal histories of workers with ulcers and company statistics on sickness, absences, or medical reimbursement claims. You might also talk with a group of workers and administrative people about the problem.

In addition, request a description of the total population of company workers categorized by as many social and demographic characteristics as are available, such as sex, age, race, and so forth. This will help you decide whether to study the entire work population in the company or a portion of it. For example, if only a small percentage of the work force is male, you may choose to study just females.

Confirm whether preemployment examinations identify applicants with an ulcer and whether these applicants are excluded from employment. If they are not excluded from working at the company, job dissatisfaction at *this* company will not have caused their ulcers. (However, you will omit them from the population used in your study since it concerns workers who developed ulcers at *this* company.)

2. The manager shows you Table 7.1, which she prepared for the last board meeting. What do you conclude from this table?

There is a yearly increase in the number of workers reported to have an ulcer. But these are numerator (case) data. You need rates because the number of employees may have increased over the years. These data may also reflect increased *reporting* rather than an actual increase in the number of persons with an ulcer.

TABLE 7.1 Employees reported to have an ulcer, 1986-1990

Year	*Employees*
1986	46
1987	123
1988	135
1989	124
1990	180

SOURCE: From Slome C, Brogan D, Eyres S, Lednar W: *Basic epidemiological methods and biostatistics: A workbook*. Boston: Jones and Bartlett, 1986. Figures and tables used with permission.

3. What other data do you need to continue your explorations?

You need (1) the number of employees, which would provide the PAR for each year, and (2) information about whether the numbers reported are for individual employees with ulcers or for episodes of ulcer problems. (If they are the latter, the same employees could be counted more than once.)

The apparent increase in ulcers may be artifactual because of bias, such as changes in diagnostic custom or reporting, or from selective migration of workers with an ulcer in or out of the company. Request data about these issues from the manager.

With the data provided, we can construct Table 7.2

4. Does Table 7.2 confirm the likelihood that there has been an annual increase in the prevalence rate of ulcers?

Since we have a common base of comparison (per 100 workers), Table 7.2 does show an increase in the prevalence rate.

5. The manager reiterates that she believes the problem is caused by job dissatisfaction among workers and she wants her hunch tested in a scientific manner. What is your next step?

The first step is to outline the purpose of the study. At this stage, the make the study questions specific; it is more difficult, if not impossible, to answer unclear questions.

TABLE 7.2 Prevalence rate per 100 of workers with an ulcer, 1986-1990

Year	*Rate*
1986	2.3
1987	4.1
1988	5.4
1989	6.2
1990	10.0

SOURCE: From Slome C, Brogan D, Eyres S, Lednar W: *Basic epidemiological methods and biostatistics: A workbook*. Boston: Jones and Bartlett, 1986. Figures and tables used with permission.

Studies need not be restricted to one question; usually several questions are involved. Multiple hypotheses are recommended to avoid overzealousness or attachment to one hypothesis. Although it is not necessary to limit a study to answering only one question, it is necessary to limit the questions to a manageable number. Otherwise the study becomes overburdened by too many questions and too many data.

Having confirmed the annual increase in the rate of workers with an ulcer, you must now state the question(s) or hypothesis(es) to be addressed by the study.

6a. How would you state the question of the association between dissatisfaction and occurrence of an ulcer?

Your question might be: Is there a positive association between job dissatisfaction and occurrence of an ulcer? (If you want to state the question in null hypothesis form, you say: There is no association between job dissatisfaction and occurrence of an ulcer.)

6b. What other questions might you add?

You might consider whether the association is stronger among certain subgroups, for example among smokers as compared with nonsmokers, or among those exposed to noisy working conditions as compared with those not so exposed. These additional questions may not only enhance scientific knowledge, but may be important to the company if it implements a program to reduce job dissatisfaction among workers.

6c. What is the next step in planning your study?

At this point you should search published material to help in the study design:

1. Find out what is known about the topic under study. In this case, the topic is occurrence of ulcers, particularly in industrial populations. It is important to know the experiences, options, findings, and methods of others who have given attention to your study topic. Personally contacting investigators can provide information beyond that included in publications, as well as information too recent to have been published.

2. Researching the topic may lead you into other disciplines. In this particular study, you may need to read material from the areas of occupational medicine, epidemiology, industrial psychology, sociology, and so forth. Experts in these fields may be useful sources to contact. Be careful in applying the findings or methods from other studies to your population because populations studied by others will differ from yours. In other words, use information from other studies with care.

3. A review of published material helps to identify potential confounding variables. You will need to account for these variables by (a) definition of the study population, (b) method of sampling (if a sample is studied rather than the entire study population), or (c) analysis of data. In part, the review identifies necessary information to collect.

For example, you might find that the type of work hazard exposure, level of responsibility, presence of a chronic disease, socioeconomic status, or length of employment are important to consider. The number of variables that must be considered as potentially confounding is usually a function of how much research has been done on the subject; that is, how many associations have already been discovered to be potential confounders in your study. Potential confounders must be associated with the exposure variable (dissatisfaction) and with the effect or outcome (occurrence of an ulcer).

4. It is also helpful to examine the research designs others have used to answer similar questions, and to analyze the designs for their strengths and weaknesses in interpreting their findings.

5. Research may also show what rates of occurrence of job dissatisfaction and ulcers are reported, especially in similar occupational settings. These will guide you in estimating the number of reported ulcer cases and of dissatisfied workers, and may also help you determine the size of the sample(s) you need for your study.

6. The review may provide an indication of various statistical and analytical techniques that other researchers have used in dealing with a similar problem.

7. The review may provide indices and instruments others have used to measure variables, including the reliability and validity as used in those studies. These may include criteria for ascertaining and diagnosing ulcers and ways of measuring worker satisfaction. By providing information about the usefulness of these instruments, the research may increase your confidence about using the instruments in your study. In addition, using similar instruments or indices may enable you to compare the findings of your study with those of other investigators.

8. Research may provide names of others whom you could contact for information on their work on similar problems.

For many of us, scientific writing is not easy; for all of us, it is essential. As you review published information, elaborate on the conceptual framework addressing your study, and develop ideas on methods of ascertaining cases, measuring satisfaction, analyzing your findings, and so forth, and *write these things down.* However good your memory, make sure to record the bases of the decisions you make for your study, the reasons for compromises that you make, and the reasons you choose one method or another.

These and other issues will arise as you read relevant publications and discuss your study with others; not to record your ideas and decisions invites later regret. After the study is completed, you will include your considerations and justifications in any report you write or present; only on-going recording of the development of your considerations and decisions will allow rational explanation of them later. There is no perfect study; you must make compromises knowingly and substantiate your choices.

7. In choosing a study design, you may prefer a cohort or historical cohort study. Are these options feasible?

The prevalence rate of ulcer in this firm has ranged from 2.3 to 10.0 per 100 from 1976 to 1980. The incidence rate is probably less than this, although the data may give no indication of what the incidence rate actually is. Although you may wish to do a cohort study, the possibility of a fairly low incidence rate and a relatively small population of workers discourages this option. Also, a cohort study takes a fairly long period of time, and the manager would have to wait—something she is not willing to do.

Perhaps there is sufficient data to conduct a historical cohort study since the manager has past data on job dissatisfaction in the form of complaints, nonsickness absences, and poor relationships with other workers. But with the anticipated small incidence rate for an ulcer (learned from other studies) and the small population at risk in this study, a historical cohort study is not feasible.

8. You rapidly discard any notions of an experimental study; it would be unethical and inhumane in this situation because it would involve manipulating job dissatisfaction among workers and then assessing the effect on the incidence of ulcer. What study designs are left to consider?

There are two other possibilities:

1. One is a cross-sectional study in which you associate job dissatisfaction with the concurrent presence of an ulcer at one point in time. However, this does not allow a time relationship between job dissatisfaction and the occurrence of an ulcer to be established; that is, you cannot determine which happened first.

2. Another possibility is a case-control study in which you compare the job dissatisfaction histories of workers with an ulcer (the cases) with similar histories of workers without an ulcer (controls).

A case-control study is indicated when the condition (ulcer) is rare or when you are looking for a time relationship between a presumed cause and effect. In addition, it quantifies the relative risk and, under certain assumptions, permits you to estimate the etiologic fraction, the population attributable risk percent that will give the company a reasonable estimate of the number of cases of ulcer that would be preventable if job dissatisfaction is removed.

Hence, under these circumstances, your best choice would be a case-control study.

9. Pursuing a case-control study, how would you identify workers with an ulcer (cases)?

The best method is a clinical examination of all workers, but that may not be feasible, ethical, or acceptable to the workers. In your research readings, you may have noticed an instrument used by other investigators to measure the presence of an ulcer. This instrument was a questionnaire with four to five questions about symptoms that suggest the presence of an ulcer. Such an instrument seems inexpensive, quick, and reasonably satisfactory for identifying cases.

10. What else would you want to know about this instrument before deciding to use it?

Using instruments available from other studies is a common issue in epidemiology. Generally, if possible, we prefer to repeat the tests of reliability and validity of the instrument with our own study population or one similar to it, especially if the instrument was devised in another cultural setting. To check validity, you apply the instrument to known ulcer cases (perhaps obtained from clinical settings), and to non-ulcer cases. For reproducibility or reliability, you must apply the same instrument on more than one occasion to a number of persons. If the sensitivity, specificity, and reliability of the instrument are high enough, you may elect to use it.

Just as there is no perfect study, there is no perfect instrument or set of diagnostic criteria to determine a case. The instruments or diagnostic criteria are selected because they are the best available, although we know that there is a possibility of making errors in so doing.

11. On behalf of the company, the manager accepts the proposed case-control study. What is the first step in implementing your study?

To implement your study, draw up an initial study protocol, including a definition of the study population, which variables (any characteristics or attributes that can be measured) you need to collect, how you will collect the variables, how you will code the variables, how cases and controls will be identified, what matching of cases and controls will be done, and any other relevant details. At this stage you may need to consult experts for additional advice.

At this point, you should ask a series of questions about each piece of information to be gathered. Such questions include: (1) Why is this information being gathered? (2) Is this variable to be used in the identification of cases and controls? (3) Is it a variable to be used in measuring the presumed cause (job dissatisfaction)? (4) Is it a potential confounding variable? (5) Is this variable to be used only for administrative purposes? (6) Is it ethical to ask people for this information? (7) How does this variable fit into the overall analytical scheme for this study?

Any variable or piece of information that does not help answer the hypotheses or questions raised, or any which contribute solely to the administration of the study, should not be collected. Do not collect data "because they may show something" or "because you may want them later." Collect only what you need to answer your study questions.

12. Would you obtain the name, age, sex, race, and address of all cases and all controls? If so, why?

Names generally have relevance only for administrative purposes; for example, to check the medical history or to identify the workers in the company. However, if names beginning with a particular letter or names having five letters prove to be associated with job dissatisfaction and the presence of an ulcer, then names would be collected and dealt with as a potentially confounding variable. (Such an event is unlikely, given the current state of knowledge.)

Age is nearly always collected because it is associated with almost all health outcomes and factors associated with these outcomes. Age is a universal variable (effect modifier). In your review of published material, you may find that the presence of an ulcer is related to age and that age may be associated with job dissatisfaction. Hence, age is a potential confounder in your study, as it is in most epidemiological studies. You should confirm its confounding nature when you analyze your data.

Similar reasoning applies to the collection of data on sex and race. Collecting an address is often used for administrative purposes to check the identity of the worker or to locate subjects if follow-up data will be collected. Sometimes an address is used as an indicator of socio-economic status.

Each variable *must* have a reason for data to be collected; if in doubt, leave it out.

13. When the manager asks how many workers you need for the study, what considerations do you have in replying to this question?

The size of the sample is always a difficult problem because cost, feasibility, and other factors may require compromising the ideal sample size. There is no easy answer to the manager's question.

The first thing to determine is the number of cases you would like to have in your study. This is influenced by the difference in job dissatisfaction between the two groups that the manager considers meaningful, or, alternatively, the magnitude of the relative risk that is meaningful to the manager. It is also influenced by what levels of data you recommend and the range of scores for job dissatisfaction you expect to obtain. Another factor is the number of cases and controls you will use—an equal number of cases and controls, or two, three, four, or more controls per case. If matching cases and controls is your choice for dealing with some confounding variables, multiple controls per case is often recommended; however, it is not easy to find multiple controls that match given cases. Hence, you may need to settle for less than the ideal number of controls per case. In fact, many case-control studies are conducted with an equal number of controls and cases. Consulting with experts may be of use in making your decision.

Once you determine the desired number of cases for the study, it is easy to determine from known rates of occurrence of ulcer how many workers need to be examined to obtain the desired number of cases and controls. For example, if 80 cases are needed and the rate of ulcer is 20 per 1,000, you need to examine 4,000 workers to obtain 80 cases. But you would need 3,920 others from which to select the controls for your study. This may not be possible, either because the company personnel is not large enough or the process is too time-consuming or too expensive. You may need to settle for fewer cases.

14. The sample size you determine as necessary is too large to be feasible, according to the manager. What do you do now?

First, explain that this sample size is necessary for all the specifications you and the manager discussed. If the sample size is still not feasible, either compromise on some of your specifications or conduct the study on the largest possible sample size you can obtain. Use appropriate sampling procedures, and make sure the sample is as representative of the study population as possible. *Conduct the study,* knowing that your compromise of a smaller sample size will reduce the chances of statistical significance at your preset levels; that is, it will increase the chance of Type II error.

All too frequently we are confronted by logistic, financial, and situational realities and must conduct studies on available or convenient samples. But we do this knowingly, and are then more circumspect about conclusions we draw from that sample.

15. You have revised the protocol, including the sampling plan to select cases and controls, and you show it to the manager and representatives of the workers. Do you need to do a pretest?

The pretest of a study protocol will be very helpful for the final study. With your pretest you carry out the study, as if it were the final study, on a sample as similar to your study population as possible. It is not advisable to do a pretest on a sample of the workers who will actually be in the study, but on a sample of workers from another similar industry. The pretest will indicate whether the questions are understandable, the persons questioned are at ease and comfortable, how long each interview takes, and the number of interviews that can be done in one day. On that basis, the number of staff required to carry out the study can be estimated. The experience of the pretest will suggest training needs and any changes that may be required in the final version of the protocol. A pretest can confirm the expected number of cases in the study population and the distribution of variables you can expect in your study population.

If your pretest sample is large enough, you may be able to decide on categories for the variables you wish to categorize. You may be able to test your analytic models on the pretest data to see how well the data meet the assumptions of the planned statistical tests. When a pretest is feasible, it is advisable.

16. The pretest has been completed. What do you do before conducting the actual study?

Modify the protocol in the light of the administrative and substantive findings of your pretest. The protocol must include an approved, informed consent form signed by each participant in the study. Obtain approval of the revised protocol from the manager, representatives of the workers, and all consultants. Then recruit and train staff.

17. Are there any more preparatory steps before implementing the actual study?

No. Go ahead with the first stage of the study, collecting information to identify cases and controls (noncases). You will collect these data on the entire study population if it is small and does not contain many cases, or on a random sample from the study population if it is large and contains many more cases than you need for your study.

Ensure throughout that the interviewers who administer questionnaires or who carry out any required examinations have been trained to apply the protocol in a consistent, objective manner. All data received should be scrutinized for errors, omissions, and possible biases.

18. The data have been collected. What is the next step to identify cases and controls?

After you code the data, apply your pretest criteria for a case (a person with an ulcer). This will give you a listing of cases for your study. The controls are chosen from the list of noncases.

19. You may want to consider matching cases and controls on some variables. How would you proceed to match them?

In most studies, investigators decide which variables to match after they have reviewed other studies. Many times they match universal variables such as age, sex, and race, in addition to specific variables relevant to the outcome and antecedent of the particular study. If you decide to match universal variables, you will now match the cases to controls.

There is an alternative approach. Given the cases and controls you have identified, and assuming that you have measured the antecedent variable on these subjects, you may use these data to identify which variables are confounding variables *in the data you have*. When you identify the confounding variables, you may wish to match to control for some or all of the confounding variables. In this approach, the variables to be matched are *not* decided on before you collect the data, but *after* you collect the data. This procedure may not be feasible if it is expensive for your study to collect information on the antecedent variable.

A confounding variable should not be part of the causative network. If it is, you must quantify its association with the outcome variable. If you make cases and controls similar on this variable by matching, you will not be able to measure the strength of the association between cause and outcome. Second, the association between the confounding variable and the outcome variable should be predictive; that is, the confounding variable must precede the outcome variable. Third, the confounding variable or the association found cannot confound if they are not found *in your data*. Fourth, the confounding variable should be shown to be associated with the outcome variable in the unexposed group; it should change the outcome (effect) measure without the exposure variable.

20. If you cannot find the ideal number of controls for each case, what do you do?

Use as many controls per case as you can. Sometimes it is better to have the *same* number of controls per case so that statistical analysis does not become unduly complicated.

21. What is the first thing to look for in the data?

If you matched controls with cases, compare the matching characteristics of the cases and their controls to assess your success in matching. You need to see that the two groups are similar on matched criteria. By comparing cases and controls on a "dummy" variable that was not relevant to the study, you can tell whether the "dummy" variable is similarly distributed among cases and controls. If so, chances are good that your cases and controls are well matched.

Be cautious about using the median or mean alone in making these comparisons because these are not good indicators of whether the characteristic has the same distribution in both groups. For example, the distribution of age can be very different in two groups although the mean age of each group is the same.

22. You find good matching, and no significant differences between cases and controls on the matched variables. What is the next step?

Look for more confounding variables among unmatched variables. If you find no more confounding variables, test your hypothesis. If you find other confounding variables, adjust by using a control table or other statistical adjustment techniques to test your hypothesis. Such adjustments include stratification of confounder scores, regression techniques, and others. Seek guidance from references on the subject or from experts if you are uncertain about how to make adjustments.

23. Are you now ready to test your hypothesis?

Yes. You have confirmed good matching on the cases and controls and identified other variables that need to be adjusted since they are confounders. Now answer your initial question by calculating the relative risk (risk ratios) for dissatisfied workers.

If there are no other confounding variables to be controlled for in the analysis, proceed as discussed in Chapter 3 in the section on case-control studies.

24. Assume that you find the risk for ulcers among dissatisfied workers to be 3.7 times that of satisfied workers (a relative risk is 3.7). This is statistically significant at your preset value of Type I error. What is the next step?

Present your results to the manager, orally and in a full written report. The writing of the report should be as succinct and scientific as possible, with conclusions drawn strictly in light of the findings. The field of epidemiology is one of relative uncertainty because of its observational nature, so all conclusions may be guarded, but conclusions must be drawn. The conclusion you draw from the study must encompass the compromises you made and any other problems that arose in the study. Honestly presented explanations of findings are expected of scientists; such explanations indicate your awareness of compromises and show that you have no interest other than a scientific one in reaching your conclusions, and that you recognize there is no perfect study.

25. The manager accepts the report and asks you what needs to be done. What suggestions do you have?

First, you calculate the population attributable risk from the risk ratio and explain how much reduction of ulcers should be anticipated, theoretically, if dissatisfaction is removed. However, before recommending a company-wide program to remove or reduce job dissatisfaction, suggest an experiment to confirm whether dissatisfaction *can* be removed or reduced to achieve the anticipated effect of reduction in ulcers. (Such an experiment is a randomized clinical trial.)

26. If the randomized clinical trial is effective in removing job dissatisfaction, with the consequent reduction of ulcers, what would you then recommend to the company?

Recommend that the intervention (treatment) for removal of dissatisfaction be implemented for the whole company, with monitoring over subsequent years to confirm the anticipated reduction in ulcer occurrence.

Then complete your report and publish it.

Addendum

We have used a case-control strategy as an example. Similar steps and considerations apply to cross-sectional, cohort, or experimental studies. In each of these, you would pose specific questions; seek help from published material and other researchers; estimate necessary sample size, given specifications; test for reliability and validity; do a pretest; redesign your protocol based on pretest results; conduct the study; analyze the data; reach conclusions; and produce a written report.

CHAPTER SUMMARY

Chapter 7 outlines the main considerations in carrying out a study:

1. There is no perfect study.
2. The progressive steps in addressing a problem or question are sequential and concurrent.

3. A review of published material and opinions of other researchers is helpful.
4. The statement of the problem, question, or hypothesis is based on specifications that include what a meaningful difference or degree of association is as well as the statistical inferential requirements.
5. Compromises are likely in the size of the sample to be studied.
6. A study protocol is drawn up.
7. Tests of reliability and validity are carried out, where indicated.
8. If possible, the protocol is pretested to provide information regarding the administrative cost and feasibility of the method.
9. The protocol is modified, based on pretest results.
10. The study is carried out according to the modified protocol.
11. The data are analyzed, confounding variables are considered and controlled for, and the hypothesis is tested.
12. Conclusions and recommendations are formulated, however tentative they may be.
13. The study is described in written form, including the reasons for any compromises made and their implications for the conclusions. A written report is necessary so that interested persons can learn from your study.

8 Organizing Epidemiologic Data

OBJECTIVES

On completion of this chapter, you will be able to:

- Correctly prepare tables with one, two, or three variables
- Correctly prepare the following types of graphs: arithmetic-scale line graphs, semilogarithmic-scale line graphs, histograms, frequency polygons, and scatter diagrams
- Correctly prepare the following types of charts: bar charts, pie charts, spot maps, area maps, and box plots
- Describe when to use each type of table, graph, and chart

When we collect more records than we can review individually, we can use tables, graphs, and charts to organize, summarize, and display the data clearly and effectively. With tables, graphs, and charts we can analyze data sets of a few dozen or a few million. These tools allow us to identify, explore, understand, and present distributions, trends, and relationships in the data. Thus tables, graphs, and charts are critical tools not only when we perform descriptive and analytic epidemiology, but also when we need to communicate our epidemiologic findings to others.

INTRODUCTION TO TABLES, GRAPHS, AND CHARTS

Data analysis is an important component of epidemiologic practice. To analyze data effectively, an epidemiologist must first become familiar with the data before applying analytic techniques. The epidemiologist may begin by examining individual records such as those contained in a line listing, but will quickly progress to summarizing the data with tables.

Note: This chapter is adapted from *Principles of Epidemiology: An Introduction to Applied Epidemiology and Biostatistics*. Atlanta: Centers for Disease Control and Prevention, 1992.

Sometimes, the resulting tables are the only analysis that is needed, particularly when the amount of data is small and relationships are straightforward. When the data are more complex, graphs and charts can help the epidemiologist visualize broader patterns and trends and identify variations from those trends. Variations may represent important new findings or only errors in typing or coding which need to be corrected. Thus, tables, graphs, and charts are essential to the verification and analysis of the data.

Once an analysis is complete, tables, graphs, and charts further serve as useful visual aids for describing the data to others. In preparing tables, graphs, and charts for others, you must keep in mind that their primary purpose is to *communicate* information about the data.

TABLES

A table is a set of data arranged in rows and columns. Almost any quantitative information can be organized into a table. Tables are useful for demonstrating patterns, exceptions, differences, and other relationships. In addition, tables usually serve as the basis for preparing more visual displays of data, such as graphs and charts, where some of the detail may be lost.

Tables designed to present data to others should be as simple as possible. Two or three small tables, each focusing on a different aspect of the data, are easier to understand than a single large table that contains many details or variables.

A table should be self-explanatory. If a table is taken out of its original context, it should still convey all the information necessary for the reader to understand the data. To create a table that is self-explanatory, follow the guidelines below:

- Use a clear and concise title that describes the what, where, and when of the data in the table. Precede the title with a table number (for example, Table 8.1a).
- Label each row and each column clearly and concisely and include the units of measurement for the data (for example, years, mm Hg, mg/dl, rate per 100,000).
- Show totals for rows and columns. If you show percents (%), also give their total (always 100).
- Explain any codes, abbreviations, or symbols in a footnote (for example, *Syphilis P&S = primary and secondary syphilis*).
- Note any exclusions in a footnote (*1 case and 2 controls with unknown family history were excluded from this analysis*).
- Note the source of the data in a footnote if the data are not original.

TABLE 8.1a Primary and secondary syphilis morbidity by age, United States, 1989

Age Group (years)	*Number of Cases*
≤14	230
15-19	4,378
20-24	10,405
25-29	9,610
30-34	8,648
35-44	6,901
45-54	2,631
≥55	1,278
Total	44,081

SOURCE: CDC, 1989c.

TABLE 8.1b Primary and secondary syphilis morbidity by age, United States, 1989

	Cases	
Age Group (years)	*Number*	*Percent*
≤14	230	0.5
15-19	4,378	10.0
20-24	10,405	23.6
25-29	9,610	21.8
30-34	8,648	19.6
35-44	6,901	15.7
45-54	2,631	6.0
≥55	1,278	2.9
Total	44,081	100.0*

*Percentages do not add to 100.0% due to rounding.
SOURCE: CDC, 1989c.

One-Variable Table

In descriptive epidemiology, the most basic table is a simple frequency distribution with only one variable, such as Table 8.1a. In such a frequency distribution table, the first column shows the values or categories of the variable represented by the data, such as age or sex. The second column shows the number of persons or events that fall into each category.

Often, a third column lists the percentage of persons or events in each category, as in Table 8.1b. Note that the percentages in Table 8.1b add up to 100.1% rather than 100.0% due to rounding to one decimal place. This is common in tables that show percentages. Nonetheless, the total percent should be given as 100.0%, and a footnote explaining that the difference is due to rounding should be included.

TABLE 8.1c Primary and secondary syphilis morbidity by age, United States, 1989

	Cases		
Age Group (years)	*Number*	*Percent*	*Cumulative %*
≤14	230	0.5	0.5
15-19	4,378	10.0	10.5
20-24	10,405	23.6	34.1
25-29	9,610	21.8	55.9
30-34	8,648	19.6	75.5
35-44	6,901	15.7	91.2
45-54	2,631	6.0	97.2
≥55	1,278	2.9	100.0
Total	44,081	100.0*	100.0%

*Percentages do not add to 100.0% due to rounding.

SOURCE: CDC, 1989c.

The one-variable table can be further modified to show either cumulative frequency or cumulative percent, as in Table 8.1c. We now see that 75.5% of the primary and secondary syphilis cases occurred in persons less than 35 years old.

Two- and Three-variable Tables

Tables 8.1a, 8.1b, and 8.1c show case counts (frequency) by only one variable: age. Data can also be cross-tabulated to show counts by a second variable. Table 8.2 shows the number of syphilis cases by both age and gender of the patient.

A two-variable table with cross-tabulated data is also known as a **contingency table.** Table 8.3 is an example of a common type of contingency table, which is called a **two-by-two table** because each of the two variables has two categories. Epidemiologists frequently use contingency tables to display the data used in calculating measures of association and tests of statistical significance.

Epidemiologists also use two-by-two tables to study the association between an exposure and disease. These tables are convenient for comparing persons with and without the exposure, and those with and without the disease. Table 8.4 shows the generic format of such a table. As shown there, disease status (e.g., ill versus well) is usually designated along the top of the table, and exposure status (e.g., exposed versus not exposed) is designated along the side. The letters a, b, c, and d within the 4 cells of the two-by-two table refer to the number of persons with the disease status indicated above and the exposure status indicated to its left. For example,

TABLE 8.2 Newly reported cases of primary and secondary syphilis by age and sex, United States, 1989

	Number of Cases by Sex		
Age Group (years)	*Male*	*Female*	*Total*
≤14	40	190	230
15-19	1,710	2,668	4,378
20-24	5,120	5,285	10,405
25-29	5,304	4,306	9,610
30-34	5,537	3,111	8,648
35-44	5,004	1,897	6,901
45-54	2,144	487	2,631
≥55	1,147	131	1,278
Total	26,006	18,075	44,081

SOURCE: CDC, 1989c.

TABLE 8.3 Follow-up status among diabetic and nondiabetic white men, NHANES follow-up study, 1982-1984

	Dead	*Alive*	*Total*	*Percent Dead*
Diabetic	100	89	189	52.9
Nondiabetic	811	2,340	3,151	25.7
Total	911	2,429	3,340	

SOURCE: Kleinman, et al., 1988.

in Table 8.4, c is the number of persons in the study who have the disease, but who did not have the exposure being studied. Note that the "H" in the row totals H1 and H2 stands for horizontal; the "V" in the column total V1 and V2 stands for vertical. The total number of subjects included in the two-by-two table is represented by the letter T (or N).

When displaying data to others, it is best to use one- or two-variable tables, like those on the preceding pages. Sometimes, however, you may want to include a third variable to show a set of data more completely. Table 8.5 shows such a three-variable table for the variables of age, race, and sex. As you can see, a three-variable table is rather busy. It is the maximum amount of complexity you should ever include in a single table.

Tables of Other Statistical Measures

Tables 8.1 through 8.3 show case counts (frequency). The cells of a table can just as easily contain means, rates, years of potential life lost, relative risks, and other statistical measures. As with any table, the title

TABLE 8.4 General format for 2 × 2 table

	Ill	Well	Total
Exposed	a	b	H1
Unexposed	c	d	H2
Total	V1	V2	T

TABLE 8.5 Primary and secondary syphilis morbidity by age, race, and sex, United States, 1989

		Race			
Age (years)	*Sex*	*White*	*Black*	*Other*	*Total*
≤14	Male	2	31	7	40
	Female	14	165	11	190
	Total	16	196	18	230
15-19	Male	88	1,412	210	1,710
	Female	253	2,257	158	2,668
	Total	341	3,669	368	4,378
20-24	Male	407	4,059	654	5,120
	Female	475	4,503	307	5,285
	Total	882	8,562	961	10,405
25-29	Male	550	4,121	633	5,304
	Female	433	3,590	283	4,306
	Total	983	7,711	916	9,610
30-34	Male	564	4,453	520	5,537
	Female	316	2,628	167	3,111
	Total	880	7,081	687	8,648
35-44	Male	654	3,858	492	5,004
	Female	243	1,505	149	1,897
	Total	897	5,363	641	6,901
45-54	Male	323	1,619	202	2,144
	Female	55	392	40	487
	Total	378	2,011	242	2,631
≥55	Male	216	823	108	1,147
	Female	24	92	15	131
	Total	240	915	123	1,278
Total for all ages	Male	2,804	20,376	2,826	26,006
	Female	1,813	15,132	1,130	18,075
Total		4,617	35,508	3,956	44,081

SOURCE: CDC, 1989c.

TABLE 8.6 Newly reported cases of primary and secondary syphilis, age- and race-specific rates per 100,000 (civilian) population, United States, 1989

	Rate (per 100,000) by Race			
Age Group (years)	*White*	*Black*	*Other*	*Total*
≤14	0.0	2.4	0.8	0.4
15-19	2.4	131.5	51.0	24.3
20-24	5.8	323.0	139.2	55.9
25-29	5.4	270.9	117.9	44.1
30-34	4.7	256.6	83.2	38.8
35-44	2.9	135.0	47.8	19.0
45-54	1.7	76.7	29.6	10.5
≥55	0.5	19.4	10.4	2.4
Total	2.2	115.8	45.8	17.7

SOURCE: CDC, 1989c.

and headings must clearly identify what data are presented. For example, both the title and the top heading of Table 8.6 indicate that rates are presented.

Table Shells

Although we cannot analyze data before we have collected them, we should design our analyses in advance to expedite the analysis once the data are collected. In fact, most protocols, which are written before a study can be conducted, require a description of how the data will be analyzed. As part of the analysis plan, we develop **table shells** which show how the data will be organized and displayed. Table shells are tables that are complete except for the data. They show titles, headings, and categories. In developing table shells that include continuous variables such as age, we create more categories than we may later use, in order to disclose any interesting patterns and quirks in the data.

The following sequence of table shells was designed before conducting a case-control study of Kawasaki syndrome. Kawasaki syndrome is a pediatric disease of unknown etiology which occasionally occurs in clusters. Two hypotheses to be tested by the case-control study were the syndrome's association with antecedent viral illness and with recent exposure to carpet shampoo. A previously reported association with increasing household income was also to be evaluated.

TABLE SHELL 1 Clinical features of Kawasaki syndrome cases with onset October-December, 1984

Clinical Feature	# with Feature	Percent
1. Fever ≥ 5 days	___	( )
2. Bilateral conjunctival injection	___	( )
3. Oral changes		
• injected lips	___	( )
• injected pharynx	___	( )
• dry, fissured lips	___	( )
• strawberry tongue	___	( )
4. Peripheral extremity changes		
• edema	___	( )
• erythema	___	( )
• periungual desquamation	___	( )
5. Rash	___	
6. Cervical lymphadenopathy <1.5 cm	___	( )
Total	___	(100)

TABLE SHELL 2 Demographic characteristics of Kawasaki syndrome cases with onset October-December, 1984

Demographic characteristic		Number	Percent
Age	<1 yr	___	( )
	1 yr	___	( )
	2 yr	___	( )
	3 yr	___	( )
	4 yr	___	( )
	5 yr	___	( )
	≥6 yr	___	( )
Sex	Male	___	( )
	Female	___	( )
Race	White	___	( )
	Black	___	( )
	Asian	___	( )
	Other	___	( )
Total		___	(100)

Table Shell 3

County of Residence	Number	%
	___	( )
	___	( )

Table Shell 4

Household Income ($)	Number	%
≤10,000	___	( )
10,001 - 15,000	___	( )
15,001 - 20,000	___	( )
20,001 - 25,000	___	( )
25,001 - 30,000	___	( )
30,001 - 35,000	___	( )
≥ 35,001	___	( )

Table Shell 5

Number of Days in Hospital	Number	%
0	___	( )
1	___	( )
2	___	( )
3	___	( )
4	___	( )
5	___	( )
	Mean = ___	
	Median = ___	

Table Shell 6

Serious Complication	Number	%
cardiac	___	( )
arthritis	___	( )
death	___	( )
	___	( )

Table Shell 7

Demographic Characteristic		Cases		Controls	
		Number	%	Number	%
AGE	< 1 yr	___	( )	___	( )
	1 yr	___	( )	___	( )
	2 yr	___	( )	___	( )
	3 yr	___	( )	___	( )
	4 yr	___	( )	___	( )
	5 yr	___	( )	___	( )
	≥ 6 yr	___	( )	___	( )
SEX	Male	___	( )	___	( )
	Female	___	( )	___	( )
RACE	White	___	( )	___	( )
	Black	___	( )	___	( )
	Asian	___	( )	___	( )
	Other	___	( )	___	( )
Total		___	(100)	___	(100)

Table Shell 8

Household Income ($)	Cases		Controls	
	Number	%	Number	%
≤10,000	___	( )	___	( )
10,001 - 15,000	___	( )	___	( )
15,001 - 20,000	___	( )	___	( )
20,001 - 25,000	___	( )	___	( )
25,001 - 30,000	___	( )	___	( )
30,001 - 35,000	___	( )	___	( )
≥ 35,001	___	( )	___	( )

Table Shell 3: Distribution by county of residence; Table Shell 4: Distribution by household income; Table Shell 5: Number of days of hospitalization; Table Shell 6: Distribution by serious complications; Table Shell 7: Demographic characteristics; and Table Shell 8: Household income.

FIGURE 8.1 *Illustration of table shells designed before conducting a case-control study of Kawasaki syndrome*

Alternatively, Table Shell 2 could have been drawn as a 3-variable table of number of cases by age by sex by race.

The sequence of table shells shown in Figure 8.1 and in Table Shell 9 on page 250 provides a systematic, logical approach to the analysis. Of course, once the data are available and plugged into these tables, additional analyses will come to mind and should be pursued.

TABLE SHELL 9 Epidemiologic characteristics of Kawasaki syndrome cases and controls, with onset October-December, 1984

Epidemiologic characteristic		Cases Number	Cases Percent	Controls Number	Controls Percent
Antecedent illness	Yes	___	( )	___	( )
	No	___	( )	___	( )
		Odds ratio = ___, 95% CI = (,)			
		χ^2 = ___, p-value = ___			
Carpet shampoo exposure	Yes	___	( )	___	( )
	No	___	( )	___	( )
		Odds ratio = ___, 95% CI = (,)			
		χ^2 = ___, p-value = ___			

Creating Class Intervals

Some variables such as sex or "ate potato salad?" have a limited number of possible responses. These responses provide convenient categories for use in a table. When you study variables with a broader range of possible responses, such as time or systolic blood pressure, you must group the responses into a manageable number of categories (class intervals). In creating class intervals, keep the following guidelines in mind:

- Create class intervals that are mutually exclusive and that include all of the data. For example, if your first interval is 0-5, begin the next interval with 6, not 5. Also, consider what the *true* limits are. The true upper limit of 0.5 is 5.4999 . . . for most measures, but 5.999 . . . for age.
- Use a relatively large number of narrow class intervals for your initial analysis. You can always combine intervals later. In general, you will wind up with 4 to 8 intervals.
- Use natural or biologically meaningful intervals when possible. Try to use age groupings that are standard or are used most frequently in the particular field of study. If rates are to be calculated, the intervals for the numerator must be the same as the intervals used for the available population data.
- Create a category for unknowns. For example, in the standard age groupings shown in Table 8.7 the categories created for unknowns are "age not stated," "unknown," and "not stated."

TABLE 8.7 Some standard age groupings used at CDC

Notifiable Diseases	*Pneumonia and Influenza Mortality*	*Final Mortality Statistics*	*HIV/AIDS*
<1 year	<28 days	<1 year	<5 years
1-4	28 days-<1 year	1-4	5-12
5-9	1-14	5-14	13-19
10-14	15-24	15-24	20-24
15-19	25-44	25-34	25-29
20-24	45-64	35-44	30-34
25-29	65-74	45-54	35-39
30-39	75-84	55-64	40-44
40-49	⩾85	65-74	45-49
50-59	Unknown	75-84	50-54
⩾60		⩾85	55-59
Age not stated		Not stated	60-64
			⩾65
Total	Total	Total	Total

SOURCE: CDC, 1985; CDC, 1990a; NCHS, 1989.

Table 8.7 shows age groups commonly used by CDC for different purposes.

Keep a natural baseline group as a separate category, even if the rest of the distribution has no natural distinctions. For example, in creating categories for cigarette smoking in cigarettes per day, leave nonsmokers (0 cigarettes/day) as a separate category and group smokers according to any of the arbitrary methods described below.

If no natural or standard class intervals are apparent, several strategies are available for creating intervals. Three strategies are described below.

Strategy 1: Divide the Data into Groups of Similar Size

Using this strategy, you set out to create a manageable number of class intervals, with about the same number of observations in each interval. Initially, you might use 8 intervals, collapsing them later into 4 for presenting the data to others. In effect, the 4 intervals represent the 4 quartiles of the data distribution. This method is well-suited to creating categories for area maps.

To apply this strategy, divide your total number of observations by the number of intervals you wish to create. Next, develop a cumulative frequency column of a rank-ordered distribution of your data to find where each interval break would fall.

Strategy 2: Base Intervals on Mean and Standard Deviation

With this strategy, you can create 3, 4, or 6 class intervals. To use this strategy, you must first find the mean and standard deviation of your distribution. You then use the mean plus or minus different multiples of the standard deviation to establish the upper limits for your intervals:

Upper limit of interval 1 = mean − 2 standard deviations
Upper limit of interval 2 = mean − 1 standard deviation
Upper limit of interval 3 = mean
Upper limit of interval 4 = mean + 1 standard deviation
Upper limit of interval 5 = mean + 2 standard deviations
Upper limit of interval 6 = maximum value

For example, suppose you wanted to establish six intervals for data that had a mean of 50 and a standard deviation of 10. The minimum value was 19; the maximum value was 82. You would calculate the upper limits of the six intervals as follows:

Upper limit of interval 1 = 50 − 20 = 30
Upper limit of interval 2 = 50 − 10 = 40
Upper limit of interval 3 = 50
Upper limit of interval 4 = 50 + 10 = 60
Upper limit of interval 5 = 50 + 20 = 70
Upper limit of interval 6 = maximum value = 82

If you then select the obvious lower limit for each upper limit, you have your six intervals:

Interval 1 = 19 − 30
Interval 2 = 31 − 40
Interval 3 = 41 − 50
Interval 4 = 51 − 60
Interval 5 = 61 − 70
Interval 6 = 71 − 82

You can create three or four intervals by combining some of the adjacent six-interval limits:

Six Intervals	*Four Intervals*	*Three Intervals*
Interval 1 = 19 − 30 Interval 2 = 31 − 40	Interval 1 = 19 − 40	Interval 1 = 19 − 40
Interval 3 = 41 − 50	Interval 2 = 41 − 50	Interval 2 = 41 − 60
Interval 4 = 51 − 60	Interval 3 = 51 − 60	
Interval 5 = 61 − 70 Interval 6 = 71 − 82	Interval 4 = 61 − 82	Interval 3 = 61 − 82

Strategy 3: Divide the Range into Equal Class Intervals

This method is the simplest and most commonly used, and is most readily adapted to graphs. To apply this method, do the following:

TABLE 8.8 Mean annual age-adjusted cervical cancer mortality rates per 100,000 population, in rank order by state, United States, 1984-1986

Rank	State	Rate per 100,000	Rank	State	Rate per 100,000
1	SC	5.6	26	KS	3.6
2	WV	5.6	27	AR	3.6
3	AL	5.4	28	MD	3.5
4	LA	5.4	29	IA	3.4
5	AK	5.1	30	PA	3.4
6	TN	4.9	31	FL	3.4
7	ND	4.9	32	HI	3.4
8	KY	4.8	33	OR	3.3
9	MS	4.7	34	MI	3.3
10	NC	4.6	35	CA	3.2
11	GA	4.6	36	ID	3.1
12	ME	4.6	37	AZ	3.1
13	VT	4.3	38	MA	2.9
14	DE	4.3	39	NM	2.9
15	NH	4.3	40	WA	2.8
16	IN	4.1	41	NV	2.8
17	OK	4.1	42	CT	2.8
18	IL	4.0	43	RI	2.8
19	MT	4.0	44	WI	2.7
20	VA	3.9	45	CO	2.5
21	OH	3.8	46	NE	2.4
22	MO	3.8	47	SD	2.4
23	TX	3.7	48	MN	2.2
24	NY	3.7	49	WY	1.9
25	NJ	3.7	50	UT	1.8
			Total	U.S.	3.7

SOURCE: CDC, 1989a.

1. Find the range of the values in your data set. That is, find the difference between the maximum value (or some slightly larger convenient value) and zero (or the minimum value).
2. Decide how many class intervals (groups or categories) you want to have. For tables, we generally use 4 to 8 class intervals. For graphs and maps, we generally use 3 to 6 class intervals. The number will depend on what aspects of the data you want to disclose.
3. Find what size of class interval to use by dividing the range by the number of class intervals you have decided on.
4. Begin with the minimum value as the lower limit of your first interval and specify class intervals of whatever size you calculated until you reach the maximum value in your data.

Example In the example, we will demonstrate each strategy for creating categories using the cervical cancer mortality rates shown in Table 8.8. In each case, we will create four class intervals of rates.

Strategy 1: Divide the Data into Groups of Similar Size
(Note: If Table 8.8 had been arranged alphabetically, the first step would have been to sort the data into rank order by rate. Fortunately, this has already been done.)

1. Divide the list into four equal-sized groups of places:
   50 states ÷ 4 = 12.5 states per group. Because we can't cut a state in half, we will have to use two groups of 12 states and two groups of 13 states. Since Vermont (#13) could go into either the first or second group and Massachusetts (#38) could go into either the third or fourth group, we create the following groups:

   a. South Carolina through Maine (1 through 12)
   b. Vermont through New Jersey (13 through 25)
   c. Kansas through Arizona (26 through 37)
   d. Massachusetts through Utah (38 through 50)

   Notice that this arrangement puts Vermont with Delaware (both have rates of 4.3), and puts Massachusetts with New Mexico (both have rates of 1.8).
2. Identify the rate for the first and last state in each group:

States	*Rates per 100,000*
a. ME-SC	4.6-5.6
b. NJ-VT	3.7-4.3
c. AZ-KS	3.1-3.6
d. UT-MA	1.8-2.9

3. Adjust the limits of each interval so no gap exists between the end of one class interval and beginning of the next (compare the intervals below with those above):

States	*Rates per 100,000*	*Number of States*
a. ME-SC	**4.5**-5.6	12
b. NJ-VT	3.7-**4.4**	13
c. AZ-KS	**3.0**-3.6	12
d. UT-MA	1.8-**2.9**	13

Strategy 2: Base Intervals on Mean and Standard Deviation

1. Calculate the mean and standard deviation:

   Mean = 3.70
   Standard deviation = 0.96
2. Find the upper limits of 4 intervals (Note: We demonstrated creating 4 intervals by first creating 6 intervals and then combining the

upper and lower pairs of intervals. Here, however, we will simply use the appropriate upper limit of the pairs that would be combined.)

Upper limit of interval 1: mean − 1 standard deviation = 2.74
Upper limit of interval 2: mean = 3.70
Upper limit of interval 3: mean + 1 standard deviation = 4.66
Upper limit of interval 4: maximum value = 5.6

3. Select the lower limit for each upper limit to define four full intervals. Specify the states that fall into each interval (Note: To place the states with the highest rates first we have reversed the order of the intervals):

States	*Rates per 100,000*	*Number of States*
a. MS-SC	4.67-5.60	9
b. MO-NC	3.71-4.66	13
c. RI-TX	2.75-3.70	21
d. UT-WI	1.80-2.74	7

Strategy 3: Divide the Range into Equal Class Intervals

1. Divide the range from zero (or the minimum value) to the maximum value by 4:

$$(5.6 - 1.8) / 4 = 3.8 / 4 = 0.95$$

2. Use multiples of 0.95 to create four categories, starting with 1.8:
   1.80 through (1.8 + 0.95) = 1.8 through 2.75
   2.76 through (1.8 + 2 × 0.95) = 2.76 through 3.70
   3.71 through (1.8 + 3 × 0.95) = 3.71 through 4.65
   4.66 through (1.8 + 4 × 0.95) = 4.66 through 5.6
3. Final categories:

States	*Rates per 100,000*	*Number of States*
a. MS-SC	4.66-5.60	9
b. MO-NC	3.71-4.65	13
c. RI-TX	2.76-3.70	21
d. UT-WI	1.80-2.75	7

4. Alternatively, since 0.95 is close to 1.0, multiples of 1.0 might be used to create the four categories. Start at the center value (5.6 + 1.8)/2 = 3.7, subtract 1.0 to determine the upper limit of the first

interval (2.7). The upper limits of the third and fourth intervals will be 3.7 + 1.0 = 4.7, and 3.7 + 2 × 1.0 = 5.7.

Final categories:

States	*Rates per 100,000*	*Number of States*
a. KY-SC	4.71-5.70	8
b. MO-MS	3.71-4.70	14
c. RI-TX	2.71-3.70	21
d. UT-WI	1.71-2.70	7

GRAPHS

A graph is a way to show quantitative data visually, using a system of coordinates. It is a kind of statistical snapshot that helps us see patterns, trends, aberrations, similarities, and differences in the data. Also, a graph is an ideal way of presenting data to others. Your audience will remember the important aspects of your data better from a graph than from a table.

In epidemiology, we commonly use rectangular coordinate graphs, which have two lines, one horizontal and one vertical, that intersect at a right angle. We refer to these lines as the horizontal axis (or *x-axis*), and the vertical axis (or *y-axis*). We usually use the horizontal axis to show the values of the **independent** (or x) **variable,** which is the method of classification, such as time. We use the vertical axis to show the **dependent** (or y) **variable,** which, in epidemiology, is usually a frequency measure, such as number of cases or rate of disease. We label each axis to show what it represents (both the name of the variable and the units in which it is measured) and mark a scale of measurement along the line.

Table 8.9 shows the number of measles cases by year of report from 1950 to 1989. We have used a portion of these data to create the graph shown in Figure 8.2. The independent variable, years, is shown on the horizontal axis. The dependent variable, number of cases, is shown on the vertical axis. A grid is included in Figure 8.2 to illustrate how points are plotted. For example, to plot the point on the graph for the number of cases in 1953, draw a line up from 1953, then draw a line from 449 cases to the right. The point where these lines intersect is the point for 1953 on the graph. By using the data in Table 8.9, complete the graph in Figure 8.2 by plotting the points for 1955 to 1959.

Arithmetic-scale Line Graphs

An arithmetic-scale line graph shows patterns or trends over some variable, usually time. In epidemiology, we commonly use this type of graph to show a long series of data and to compare several series. It is the method of choice for plotting rates over time.

TABLE 8.9 Measles (rubeola) by year of report, United States, 1950-1989

Year	*Reported Cases (× 1,000)*	*Year*	*Reported Cases (× 1,000)*
1950	319	1970	47
1951	530	1971	75
1952	683	1972	32
1953	449	1973	27
1954	683	1974	22
1955	555	1975	24
1956	612	1976	41
1957	487	1977	57
1958	763	1978	27
1959	406	1979	14
1960	442	1980	13
1961	424	1981	3
1962	482	1982	2
1963	385	1983	1
1964	458	1984	3
1965	262	1985	3
1966	204	1986	6
1967	63	1987	4
1968	22	1988	3
1969	26	1989	18

SOURCE: CDC, 1989c.

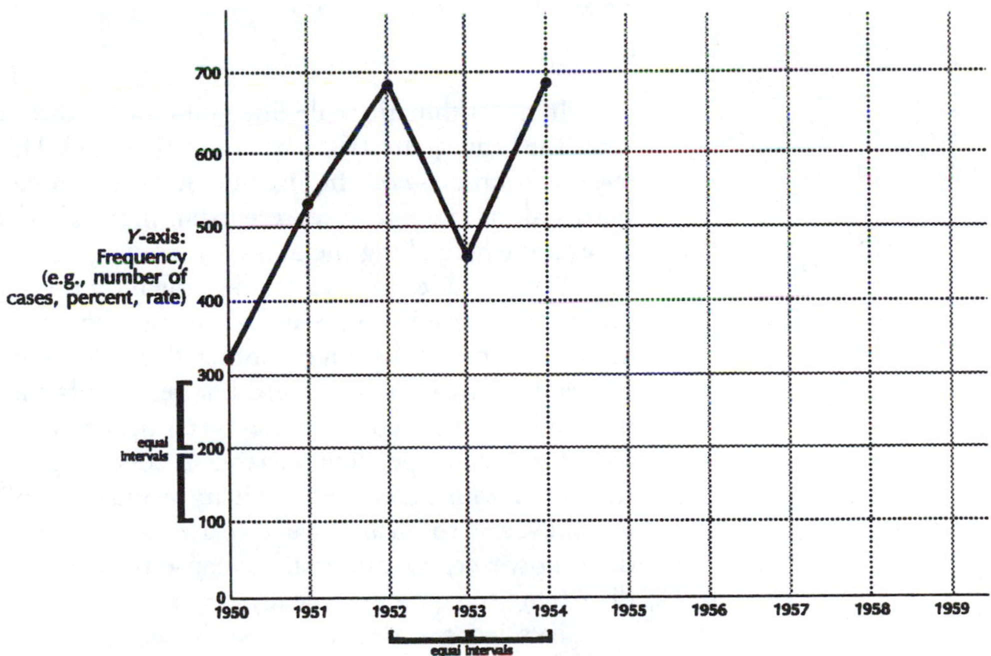

SOURCE: CDC, 1989c.

FIGURE 8.2 *Partial graph of measles (rubeola) by year of report, United States, 1950-1959*

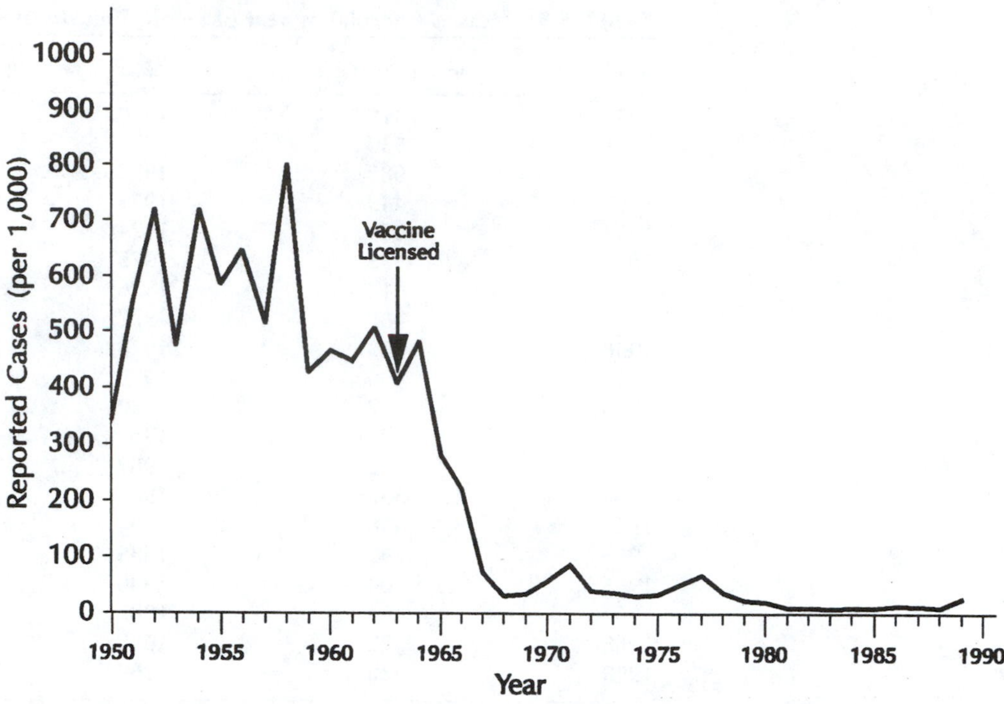

SOURCE: CDC, 1989c.

FIGURE 8.3 *Example of arithmetic-scale line graph: Measles (rubeola) by year of report, United States, 1950-1989*

In an arithmetic-scale line graph, a set distance along an axis represents the same quantity anywhere on that axis. This holds true for both the *x-axis* and the *y-axis*. In Figure 8.3, for example, the space between tick marks along the *y-axis* represents an increase of 100,000 (100 × 1,000) cases anywhere along the axis.

Several series of data can be shown on the same arithmetic-scale line graph. In Figure 8.4, one line represents the decline of rabies in domestic animals since 1955, while another line represents the concurrent rise of rabies in wild animals. A third line represents the total.

What scale we use on the *x-axis* depends on what intervals we have used for our independent variable in collecting the data. Usually, we plot time data with the same specificity we use to collect them, e.g., weekly, annually, and so forth. If we have used very small intervals in collecting the data, however, we can easily collapse those intervals into larger ones for displaying the data graphically.

To select a scale for the *y-axis*, do the following:

- Make the *y-axis* shorter than the *x-axis*, so that your graph is horizontal (i.e., the horizontal length is greater than the vertical length), and make the two axes in good proportion: an x:y ratio of about 5:3 is often recommended.

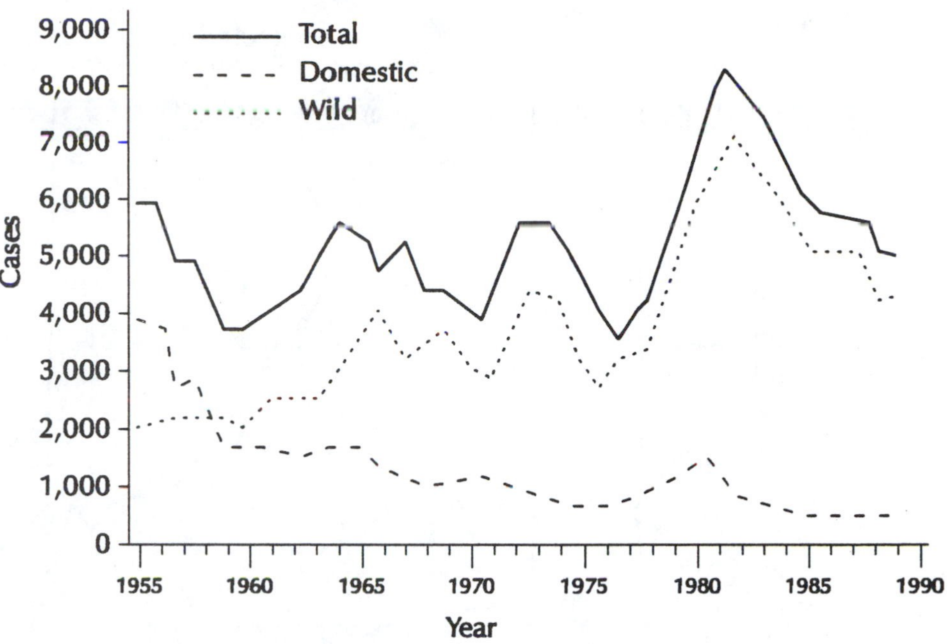

SOURCE: CDC, 1989c.

FIGURE 8.4 *Example of arithmetic-scale line graph: Rabies, wild and domestic animals by year of report, United States and Puerto Rico, 1955-1989*

- Always start the *y-axis* with 0.
- Determine the range of values you need to show on the *y-axis* by identifying the largest value you need to graph on the *y-axis* and rounding that figure off to a number slightly larger than that. For example, the largest y-value in Figure 8.3 is 763,094 in 1958. This value was rounded up to 1,000,000 for determining the range of values that were shown on the *y-axis*.
- Select an interval size that will give you enough intervals to show the data in enough detail for your purposes. In Figure 8.3, 10 intervals of 100,000 each were considered adequate to show the important details of the data.
- If the range of values to show on the *y-axis* includes a gap, that is, an area of the graph that will have no data points, a scale break may be appropriate. With a scale break the *y-axis* stops at the point where the gap begins and starts again where the gap ends. Scale breaks should be used only with scale line graphs.

Semilogarithmic-scale Line Graphs

In a semilogarithmic-scale line graph (a "semilog graph"), the divisions on the *y-axis* are logarithmical, rather than arithmetical as on arithmetic-scale line graphs. The *x-axis* has an arithmetic scale, as it does on arithmetic-scale line graphs.

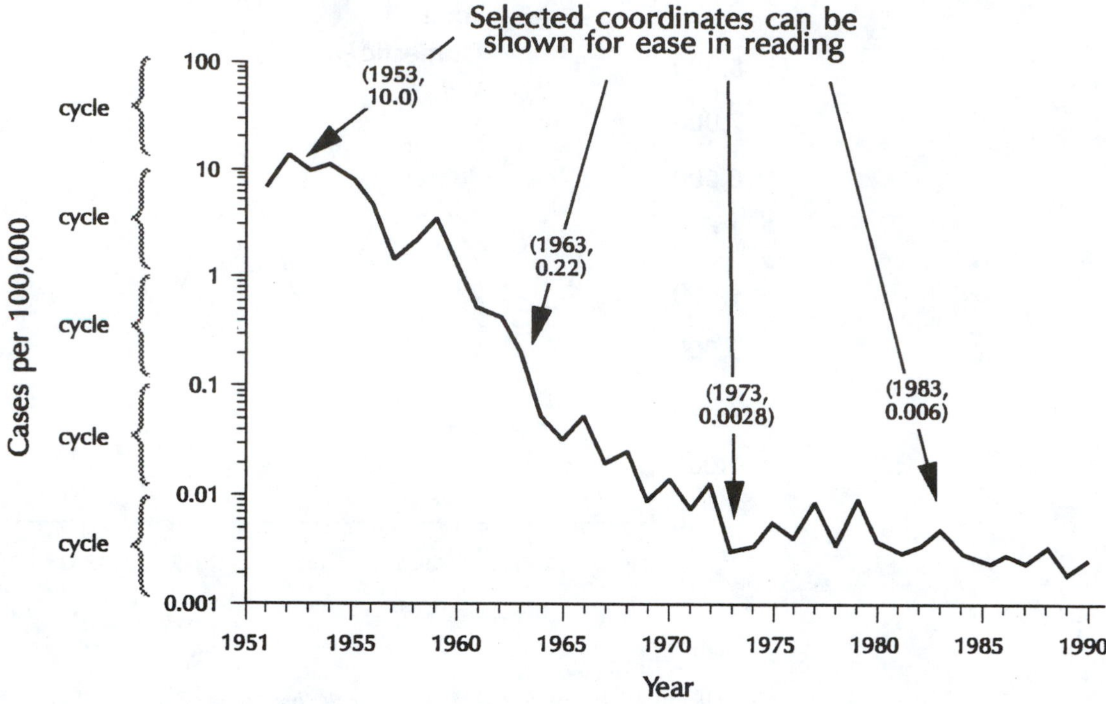

SOURCE: CDC, 1989c.

FIGURE 8.5 *Example of semilogarithmic-scale line graph: Reported cases of paralytic poliomyelitis per 100,000 population by year of occurrence, United States, 1951-1989*

Figure 8.5 shows an example of a semilog graph. Notice the following characteristics of the scale on the *y-axis*:

- There are five cycles of tick-marks along the axis; each cycle covers equal distance on the scale.
- Each cycle represents one order of magnitude greater than the one below it, that is, the values in each cycle are ten times greater than those in the preceding one. Notice, for example, that the values in the 4th cycle are 1 to 10 and in the 5th are 10 to 100 but the distances on the scale are the same.
- Within a cycle are ten tick-marks, with the space between tick marks becoming smaller and smaller as they move up the cycle. Thus the distance from 1 to 2 is not the same as the distance from 2 to 3.
- The axis covers a large range of *y*-values, which might have been difficult to show clearly on an arithmetic scale. Semilog graphs are useful when you must fit a wide range of values on a single graph, as here.

Because of the logarithmic scale, equal distances on the *y-axis* represent an *equal percentage* of change. This characteristic makes a semilog graph particularly useful for showing rates of change in data. To interpret data in a semilog graph, you must understand the following characteristics of the graph:

- A sloping straight line indicates a constant rate (not amount) of increase or decrease in the values.
- A horizontal line indicates no change.
- The slope of the line indicates the rate of increase or decrease.
- Two or more lines following parallel paths show identical rates of change.

Semilog graph paper is available commercially, and most include at least three cycles. To find how many cycles you need, do the following:

1. Find your smallest *y*-value and identify what order of magnitude it falls within. This establishes what your first cycle will represent.
   For example, if your smallest *y*-value is 47 your first cycle will begin with 10 and end with 100; if it is 352, your first cycle will begin with 100 and end with 1,000.
2. Find your largest *y*-value and identify what order of magnitude it falls within. This establishes what your last cycle will represent.
   For example, if your largest *y*-value is 134,826, your last cycle will begin with 100,000. Although a full cycle that begins with 100,000 ends with 1,000,000, you would not need to show the entire cycle. It would be sufficient to show only the first few tick-marks in your last cycle: 100,000, 200,000, and 300,000.
3. Identify how many cycles lie between your first and last cycles. You will need that number of cycles, plus two to include the first and last cycles.
   So, if your smallest *y*-value is 47, and your largest *y*-value is 134,826, you will need the following cycles:

   10–100
   100–1,000
   1,000–10,000
   10,000–100,000
   100,000–1,000,000

   Thus, with *y*-values ranging from 47 to 134,826, you will need four cycles and part of a fifth.

Figure 8.6 shows some of the ranges of values that could be shown on a four-cycle *y-axis* of a semilog graph.

The type of line graph you use depends primarily on whether you want to show the *actual changes* in a set of values or whether you want to emphasize *rates of change*. To show actual changes, use an arithmetic scale on the *y-axis* (an arithmetic-scale line graph). To show rates of change, use a logarithmic scale on the *y-axis* (a semilogarithmic-scale line graph).

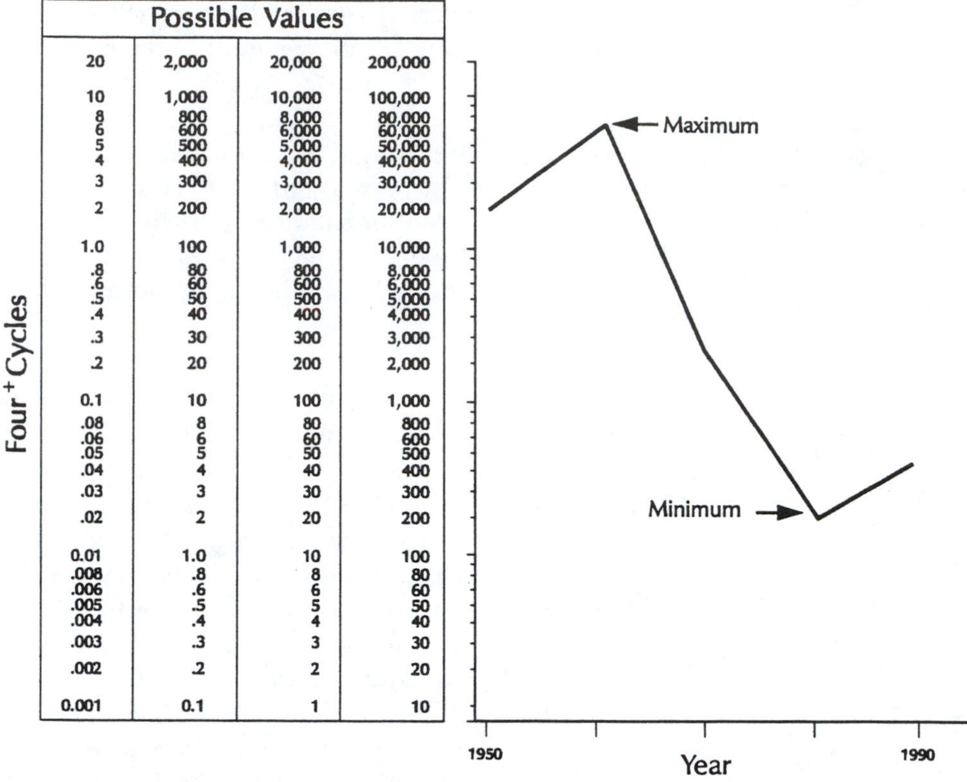

SOURCE: CDC, 1992.

FIGURE 8.6 *Possible values which could be assigned to the* y-axis *of a semilogarithmic-scale line graph*

However, you might also choose a semilog graph—even when you are interested in actual changes in the data—when the range of the values you must show on the *y-axis* is awkwardly large.

Histograms

A histogram is a graph of the frequency distribution of a continuous variable. It uses adjoining columns to represent the number of observations for each class interval in the distribution. The *area* of each column is proportional to the number of observations in that interval.

Figures 8.6, 8.7, and 8.8 show histograms of frequency distributions with equal class intervals. Since all class intervals are equal in these histograms, the height of each column is in proportion to the number of observations it depicts. Histograms with unequal class intervals are difficult to construct and interpret properly, and are not recommended. Neither should you use scale breaks in the *y-axis* of histograms, because they give a deceptive picture of relative frequencies.

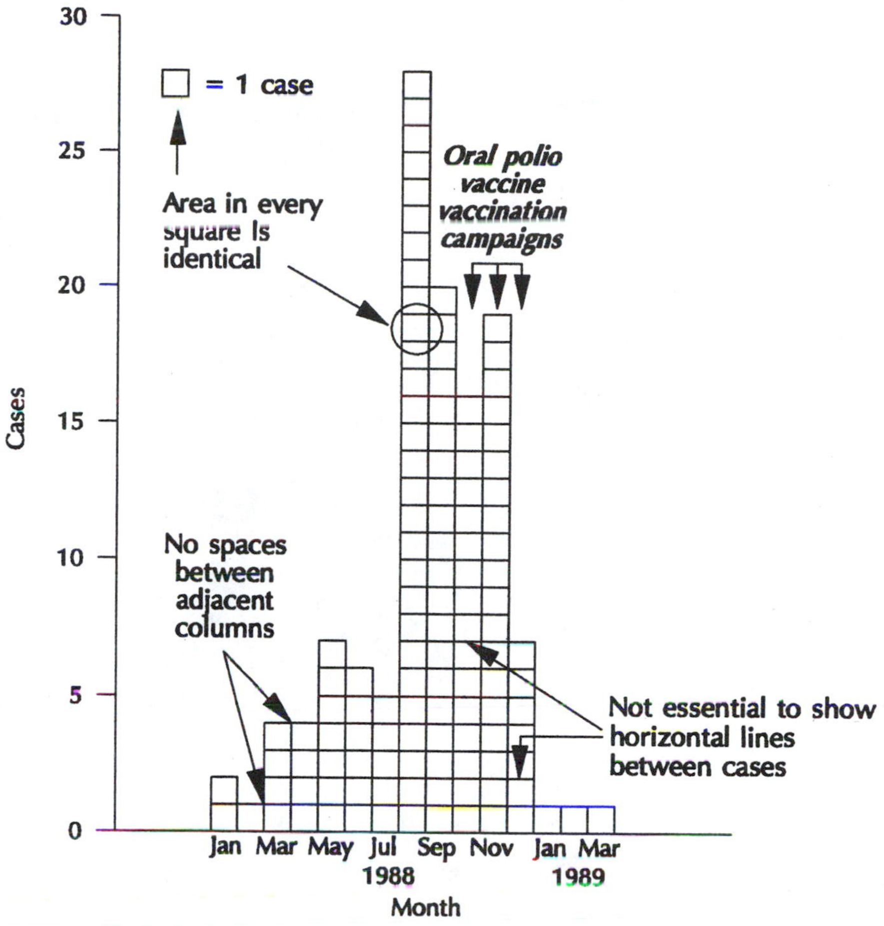

SOURCE: Sutter et al., 1991.

FIGURE 8.7 *Example of histogram: Reported cases of paralytic poliomyelitis by month of occurrence, Oman, January 1988-March 1989*

The most common *x-axis* variable is time, as shown in figures 8.7, 8.9, and 8.10. However, other continuous variables such as cholesterol level or blood pressure level may be used on the *x-axis*. Figure 8.8 shows the frequency of observations by cholesterol level in class intervals.

You may show a second variable with a histogram by shading each column into the component categories of the second variable. Suppose, for example, that we wanted to show the number of hepatitis A cases by date of onset and residency status. In Figure 8.9 the appropriate number of nonresidents are shaded at the bottom of each column. When you show data in this format, however, it is difficult to compare the upper component from column to column because it does not have a flat baseline. Therefore, you should put the component that is of most interest at the bottom of the columns. Alternatively, instead of shading columns, you can create a separate histogram for each component of the second variable, stacking them for display, as in Figure 8.10.

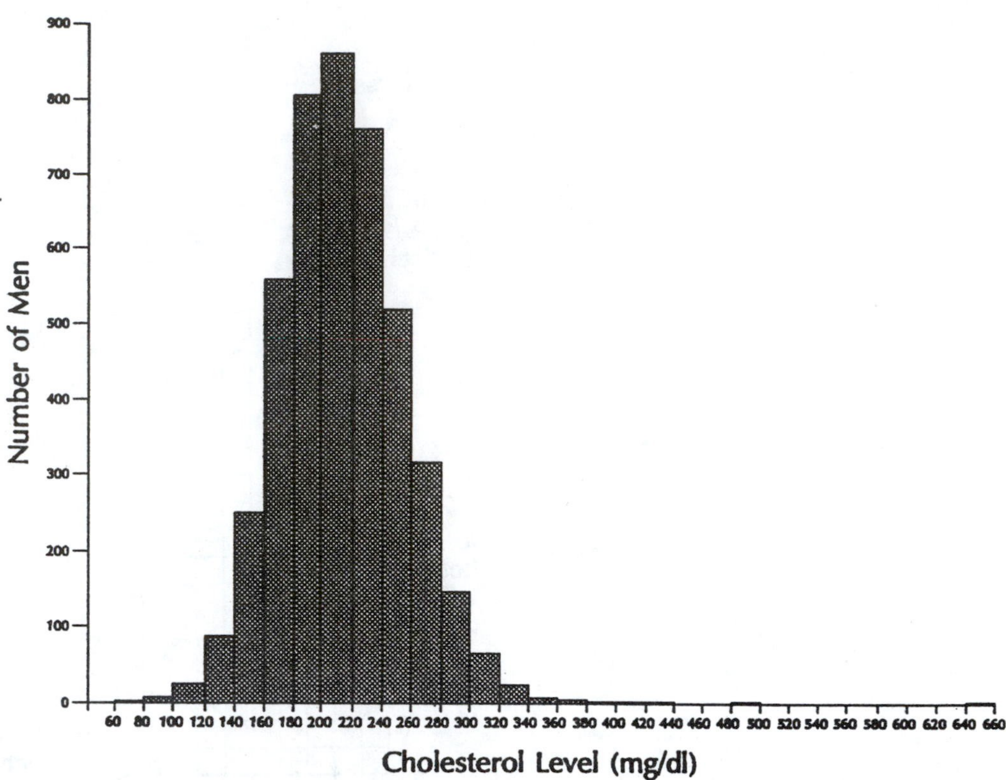

SOURCE: CDC, 1989d.

FIGURE 8.8 *Example of histogram: Reported cholesterol levels among 4,462 men, Men's Health Study, United States, 1985-1986*

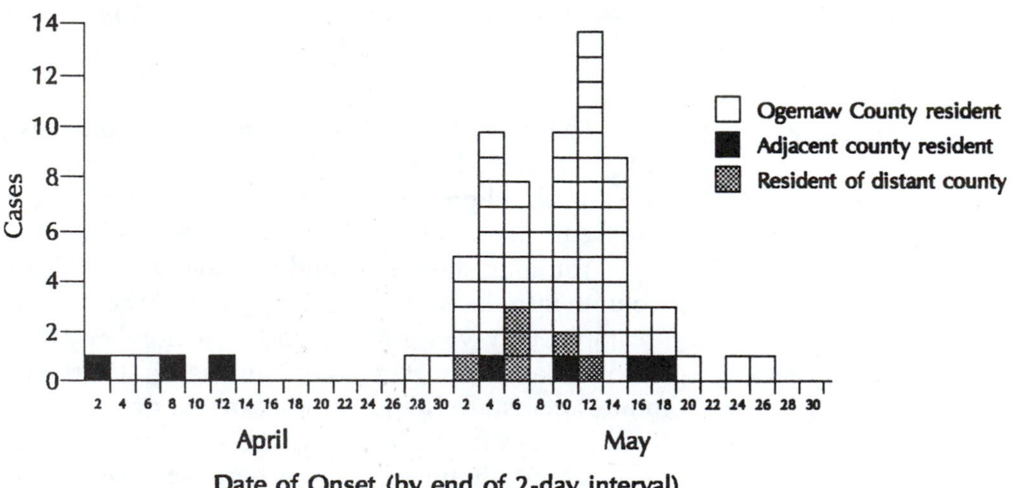

SOURCE: Schoenbaum, Baker, and Jezek, 1976.

FIGURE 8.9 *Example of histogram: Number of reported cases of hepatitis A by date of onset and residency status, Ogemaw County, April-May 1968*

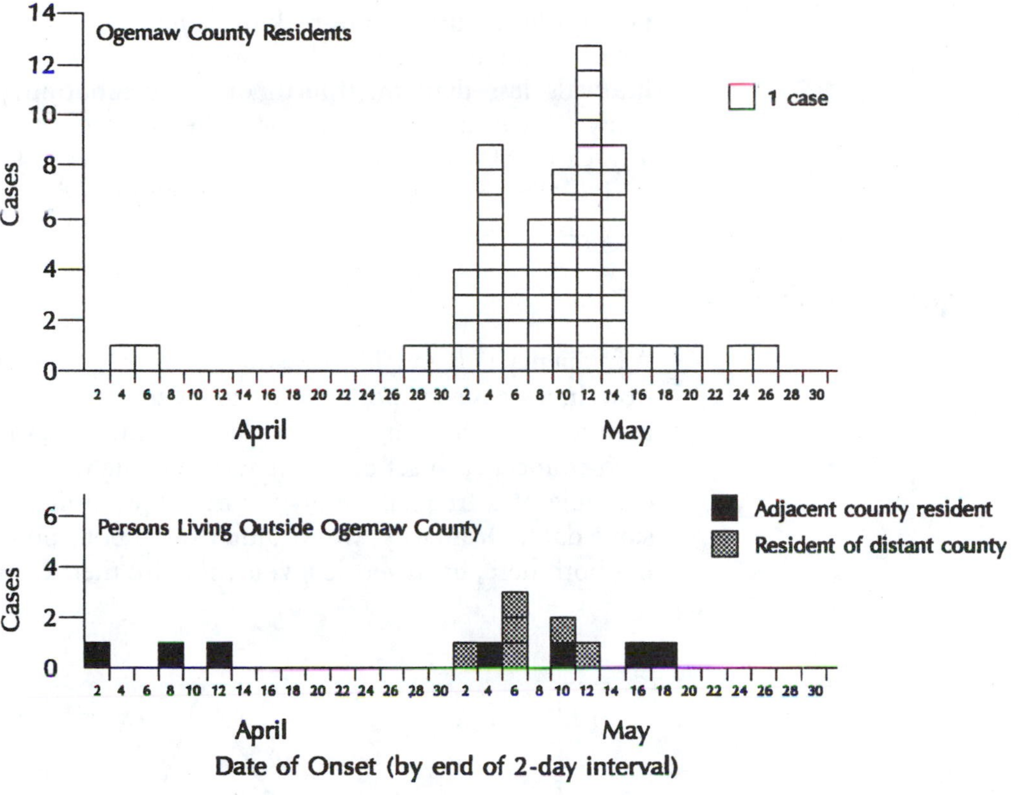

SOURCE: Schoenbaum, Baker, and Jezek, 1976.

FIGURE 8.10 *Example of histogram: Number of reported cases of hepatitis A by date of onset and residency status, Ogemaw County, April-May 1968*

Compare Figures 8.9 and 8.10. They contain the same data, but in different formats. Which format do you prefer for comparing the time pattern of cases among residents and nonresidents?

It is sometimes helpful to include a box or rectangle to show how many values of *y* (usually cases) that a given height of a column represents. We make this legend as wide as a single column, and as high as some convenient number of values on the *y-axis*—1, 5, 10, . . . etc. We note beside the square or rectangle what it represents, e.g., 1 case or 5 cases.

Epidemiologists frequently create and discuss *epidemic curves*. An epidemic curve isn't a curve at all, but a histogram that shows cases of disease during a disease outbreak or epidemic by their date of onset. As shown in Figure 8.8, we often draw the columns as stacks of squares, with each square representing one case. Figure 8.8 shows us that one person had the onset of symptoms between April 27 and 28, one more person had the onset on April 29 or 30, and between May 1 and 2 five additional individuals had the onset of symptoms. We show the duration of the epidemic along the *x-axis* in equal time periods. On an epidemic curve, each number should be centered between the tick marks of the appropriate interval. We use whatever interval of time is appropriate for the disease in question:

perhaps hours for an outbreak of *C. perfringens* gastroenteritis, or 3 to 5 days for an outbreak of hepatitis A. As a general rule, we make the intervals less than one-fourth of the incubation period of the disease shown. We begin the *x-axis* before the first case of the outbreak, and show any cases of the same disease which occurred during the preepidemic period. These cases may represent background or unrelated cases. They may also represent the source of the outbreak!

Frequency Polygons

A frequency polygon, like a histogram, is the graph of a frequency distribution. In a frequency polygon, we mark the number of observations within an interval with a single point placed at the midpoint of the interval, and then connect each set of points with a straight line. Figure 8.11 shows an example of a frequency polygon over the outline of a histogram for the same data. Ordinarily, we wouldn't show both on the same graph. Showing both here, however, lets you compare their construction.

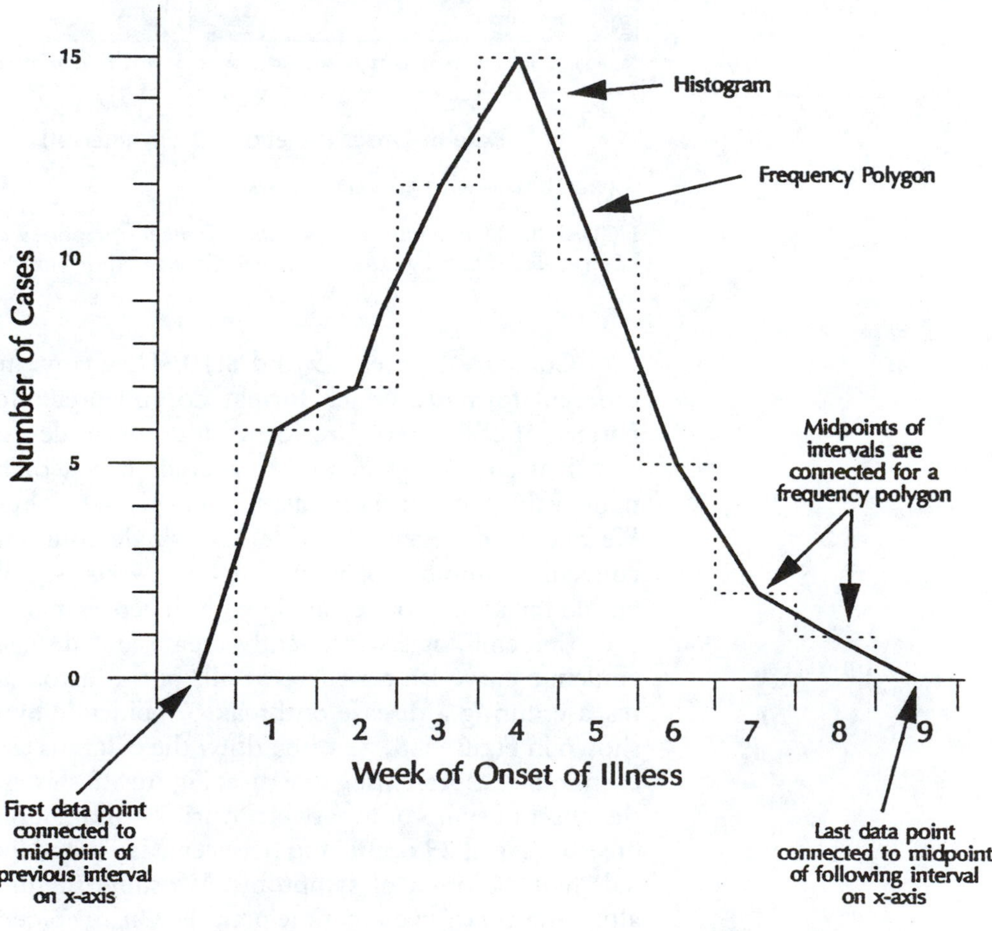

SOURCE: CDC, 1992.

FIGURE 8.11 *Number of reported cases of influenza-like illness by week of onset*

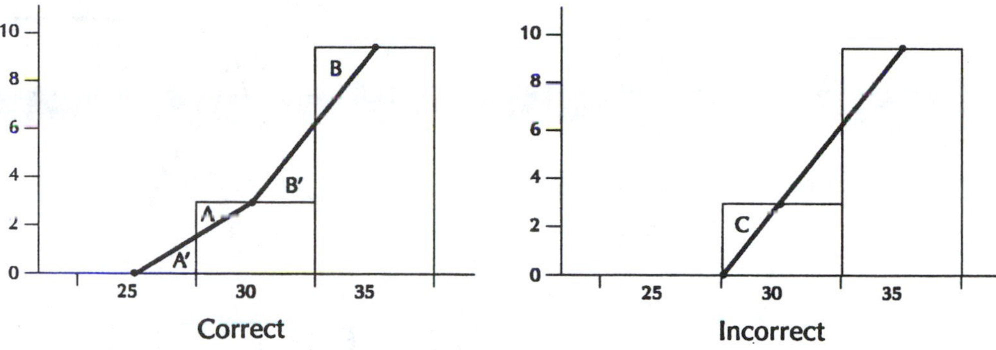

SOURCE: CDC, 1992.

FIGURE 8.12 *Correct method of closing a frequency polygon at left; incorrect method for closing a frequency polygon at right*

Notice how the histogram and the line of the frequency polygon—as it moves from midpoint to midpoint—create a series of equal-sized pairs of triangles—one that lies outside the histogram and one that lies inside it. This is a necessary aspect of frequency polygons: a frequency polygon of a set of data must enclose the same area as a histogram of that data: for every area of histogram that the polygon leaves out, it must import an area of equal size.

To maintain an equal total area you must pay special attention to how you "close" a frequency polygon. Figure 8.12 shows the correct method at the left and the incorrect method at the right—again superimposed on a corresponding segment of a histogram. In the correct method, notice that the line of the frequency polygon begins in the interval below the first interval that contains any observations, completely outside the histogram. It begins at the midpoint of that interval (with a y value of 0) and connects with the midpoint of the first interval that contains observations. This extension of the line beyond the values observed in the data serves to create an area A′ under the polygon that equals area A that is cut out of the corresponding histogram. Notice in Figure 8.11 that the right side of a frequency polygon is closed in a similar way.

In contrast, the incorrect but unfortunately common method of closing a frequency polygon is shown at the right in Figure 8.12. Here, the line has been brought to the baseline at the beginning of the first interval that contains observations, cutting off an area, C, from inside the histogram without enclosing an equal area from outside the histogram. As a consequence, the area under the polygon would not be in proportion to the total number of observations in the data set.

Frequency polygons make it easy to depict and compare two or more distributions on the same set of axes. Figure 8.13 shows a graph in which three frequency polygons are compared with each other and to the normal distribution.

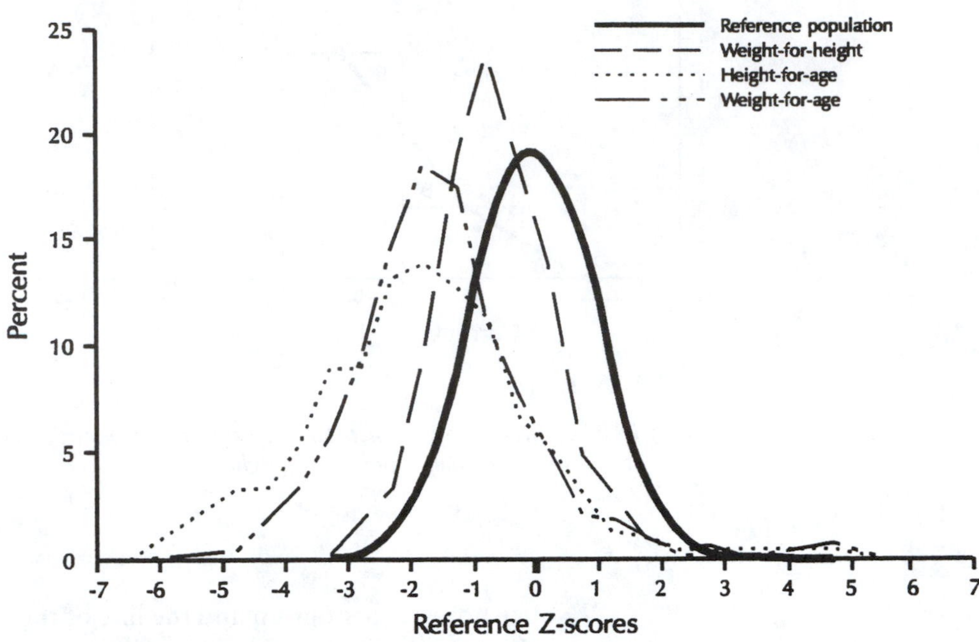

SOURCE: CDC, 1991b.

FIGURE 8.13 *Anthropometry of Haitian children ages 24.0 to 59.9 months compared with CDC's National Center for Health Statistics/World Health Organization reference population, northern departments of Haiti, 1990*

A frequency polygon differs from an arithmetic-scale line graph in several ways. We use a frequency polygon (or histogram) to display the entire frequency distribution (counts) of a continuous variable. We use an arithmetic-scale line graph to plot a series of observed data points (counts or rates), usually over time. A frequency polygon must be closed at both ends because the area under the curve is representative of the data; an arithmetic-scale line graph simply plots the data points.

Cumulative Frequency and Survival Curves

As its name implies, a cumulative frequency curve plots the cumulative frequency rather than the actual frequency for each class interval of a variable. Figure 8.14 shows a graph with four cumulative frequency curves. This type of graph is useful for identifying medians, quartiles, and other percentiles. The *x-axis* records the class intervals and the *y-axis* shows the cumulative frequency either on an absolute scale (e.g., number of cases) or as proportions of 100%. We plot each cumulative frequency at the upper limit of the interval it applies to, rather than at the midpoint. This practice allows the graph to represent visually the number or percentage of observations above and below the particular value.

A survival curve is used with follow-up studies to display the proportion of one or more groups still alive at different time periods. Similar to

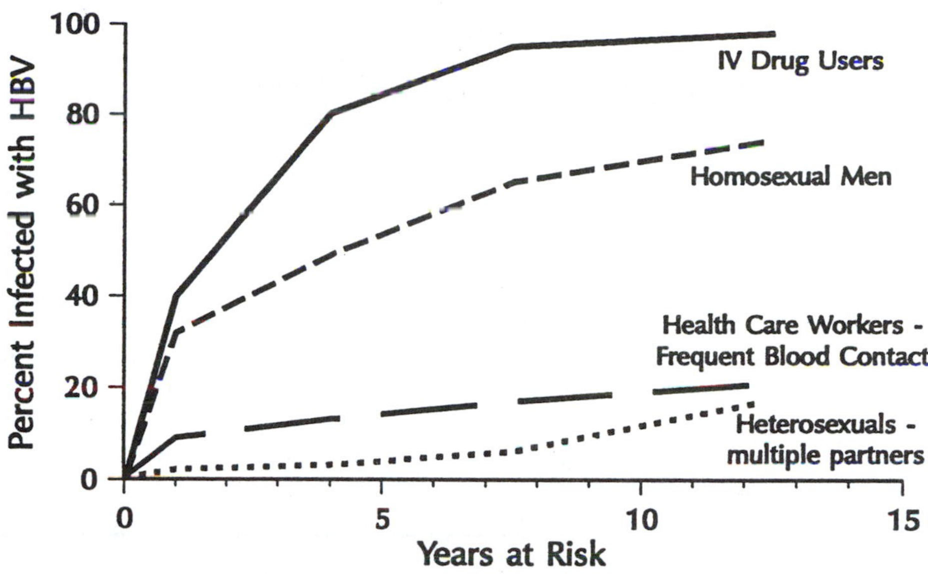

SOURCE: Alter et al., 1986; Hadler et al., 1985; Lettau et al., 1987; Schreeder, 1982.

FIGURE 8.14 *Cumulative incidence of hepatitis B virus infection by duration of high-risk behavior*

the axes of the cumulative frequency curve, the *x-axis* records the time periods and the *y-axis* shows percentages, from 0% to 100%, still alive. The most striking difference is in the plotted curves themselves. Whereas a cumulative frequency starts at zero in the lower left corner of the graph and approaches 100% in the upper right corner, a survival curve begins at 100% in the upper left corner and proceeds toward the lower right corner as members of the group die. The survival curve in Figure 8.15 compares the percentage of survival by those with peripheral arterial disease (PAD) with those without PAD. Which group has the higher survival percentage (or survival experience)? By Year 10 the survival experience for those without PAD was substantially better than those with PAD.

Scatter Diagrams

A scatter diagram (or "scattergram") is a graph used for plotting the relationship between two continuous variables, with the *x-axis* representing one variable and the *y-axis* representing the other. To create a scatter diagram we must have a pair of values for every person, group, or other entity in our data set, one value for each variable. We then plot each pair of values by placing a point on the graph where the two values intersect. Figure 8.16 shows a scatter diagram that plots serum tetrachlorodibenzo-*p*-dioxin (TCDD) levels by years of exposure for a group of workers.

In interpreting a scatter diagram, we look at the overall pattern made by the plotted points. A fairly compact pattern indicates a high degree of correlation. Widely scattered points indicate little correlation. If we want

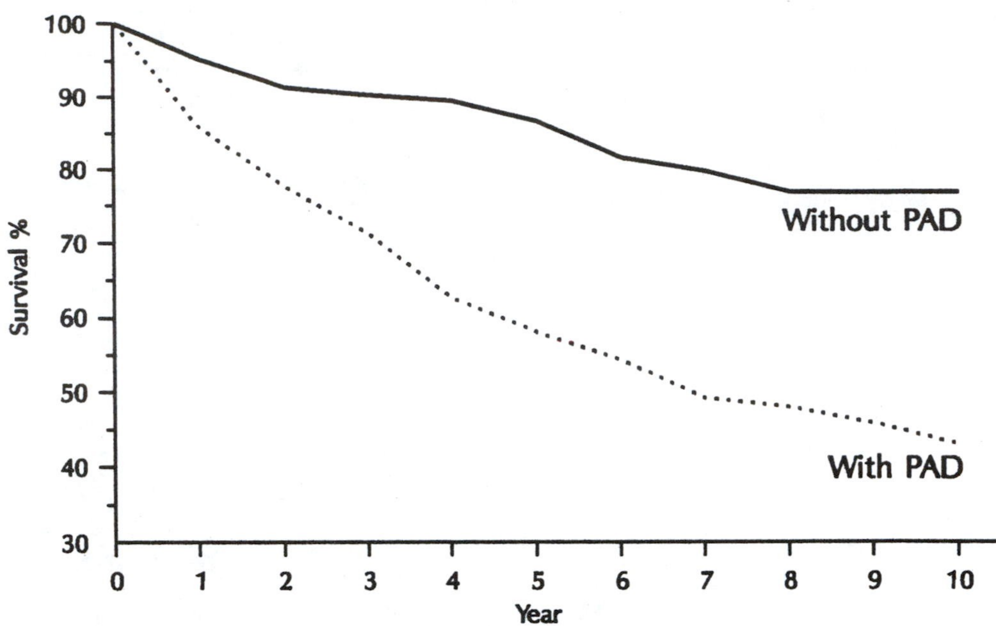

SOURCE: McKenna, Wolfson, and Kuller, 1991.

FIGURE 8.15 *Survival curves for a cohort of patients with peripheral arterial disease (PAD) (n = 482) and without PAD (n = 262), Pittsburgh, Pennsylvania, 1977-1985*

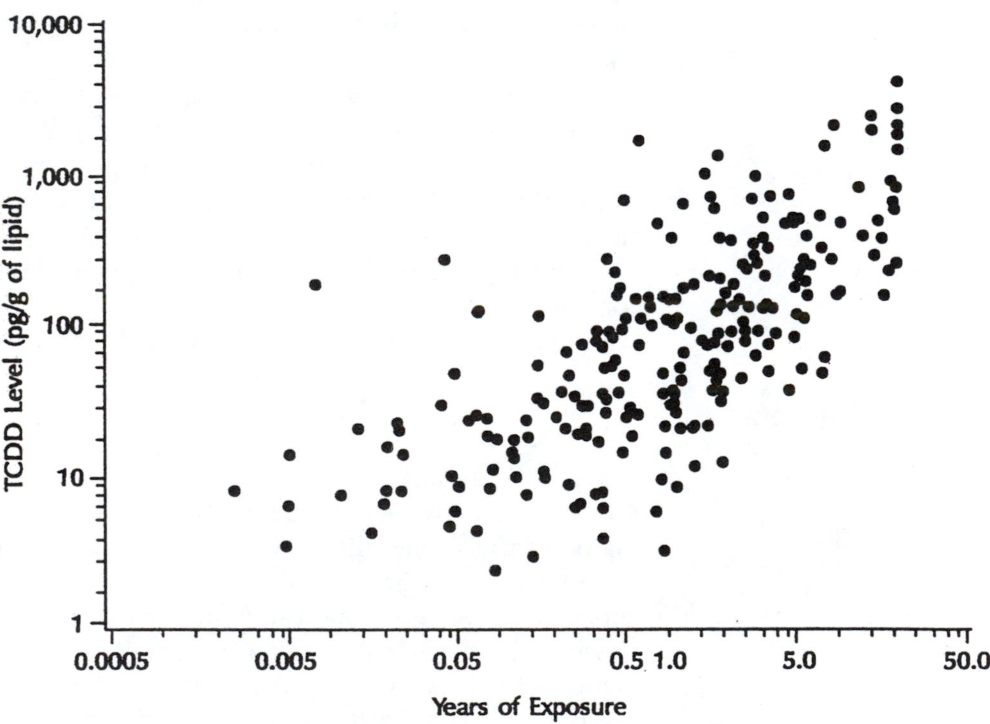

SOURCE: Fingerhut et al., 1991. Reprinted by permission of The New England Journal of Medicine.

FIGURE 8.16 *Example of scattergram: Serum levels of tetrachlorodibenzo-*p*-dioxin (TCDD), as adjusted for lipids, in 253 workers, according to years of exposure, 12 chemical plants, United States, 1987*

a more exact, quantitative measure of the relationship between the variables in a scatter diagram, we can use formal statistical methods, such as linear regression. We will not cover those methods in this chapter.

CHARTS

Charts are methods of illustrating statistical information using only *one* coordinate. They are most appropriate for comparing data with discrete categories other than place, but have many other uses as well.

Bar Charts

The simplest bar chart is used to display the data from a one-variable table. Each value or category of the variable is represented by a bar. The length of the bar is proportional to the number of persons or events in that category. Figure 8.17 shows the number of infant deaths by cause in the United States. This presentation of the data makes it very easy to compare the relative size of the different causes and to see that birth defects are the most common cause of infant mortality.

Variables shown in bar charts are either discrete and noncontinuous (e.g., race; sex) or are treated as though they were discrete and noncontinuous (e.g., age groups rather than age intervals along an axis).

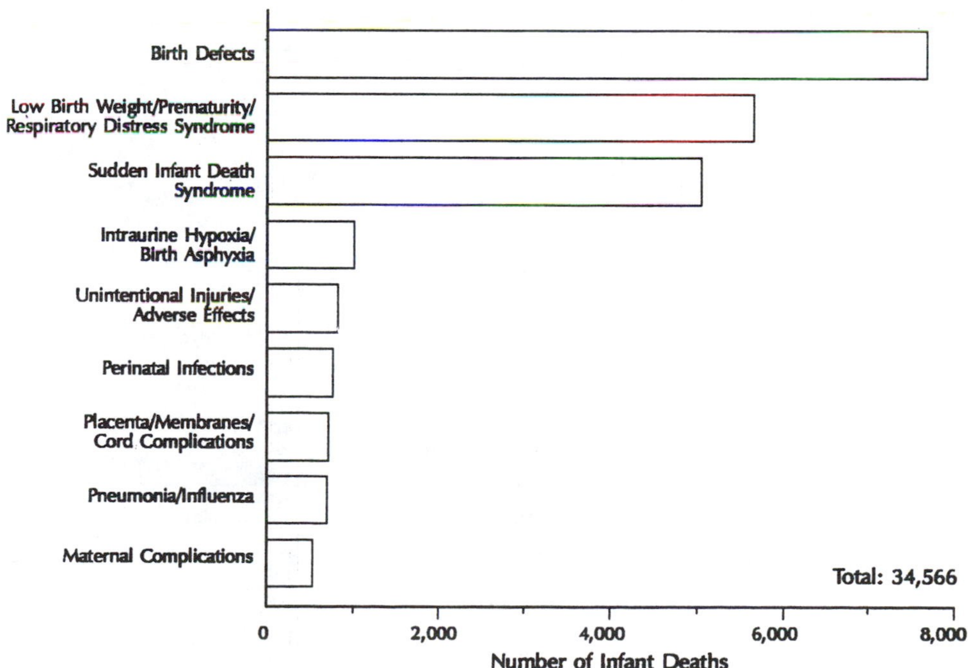

SOURCE: CDC, 1990b.

FIGURE 8.17 *Example of horizontal bar chart: Number of infant deaths by leading causes, United States, 1983*

Bars can be presented either horizontally or vertically. The length or height of each bar is proportional to the frequency of the event in that category. For this reason, *a scale break should not be used with a bar chart* since this could lead to misinterpretation in comparing the magnitude of different categories.

A vertical bar chart differs from a histogram in that the bars of a bar chart are separated while the bars of a histogram are joined. This distinction follows from the type of variable used on the *x-axis*. A histogram is used to show the frequency distribution of a continuous variable such as age or serum cholesterol or dates of onset during an epidemic. A bar chart is used to show the frequency distribution of a variable with discrete, noncontinuous categories such as sex or race or state.

Grouped Bar Charts

A grouped bar chart is used to illustrate data from two-variable or three-variable tables, when an outcome variable has only two categories. Bars within a group are usually adjoining. The bars must be illustrated distinctively and described in a legend. It is best to limit the number of bars within a group to no more than three. As you can see in Figure 8.18, it is difficult to interpret the data when the chart contains so many bars.

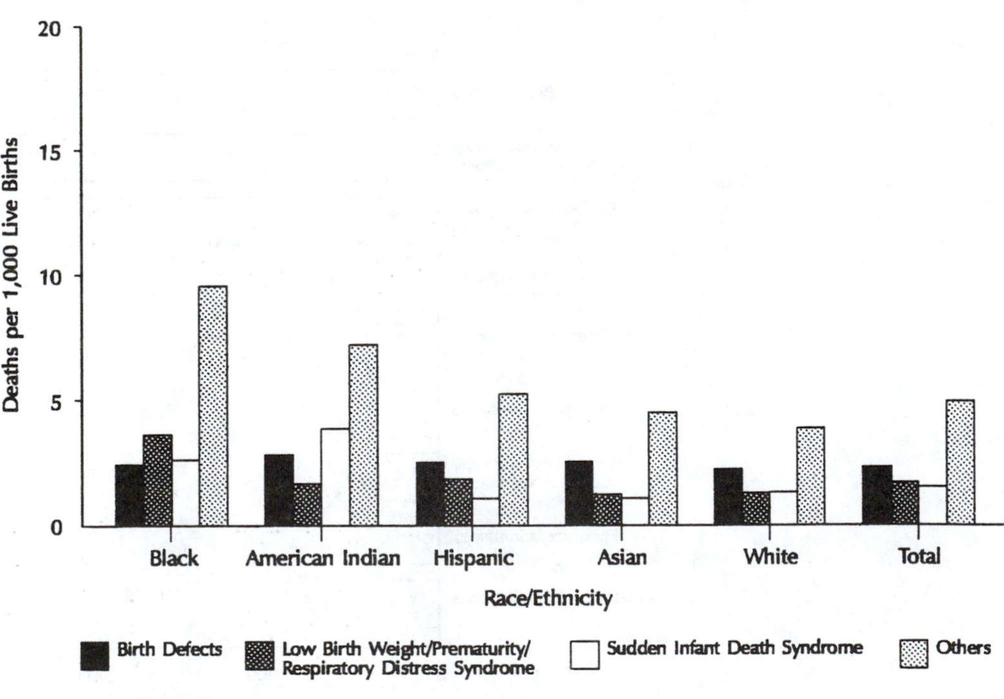

SOURCE: CDC, 1990b.

FIGURE 8.18 *Underlying cause of infant mortality among racial/ethnic groups, United States, 1983*

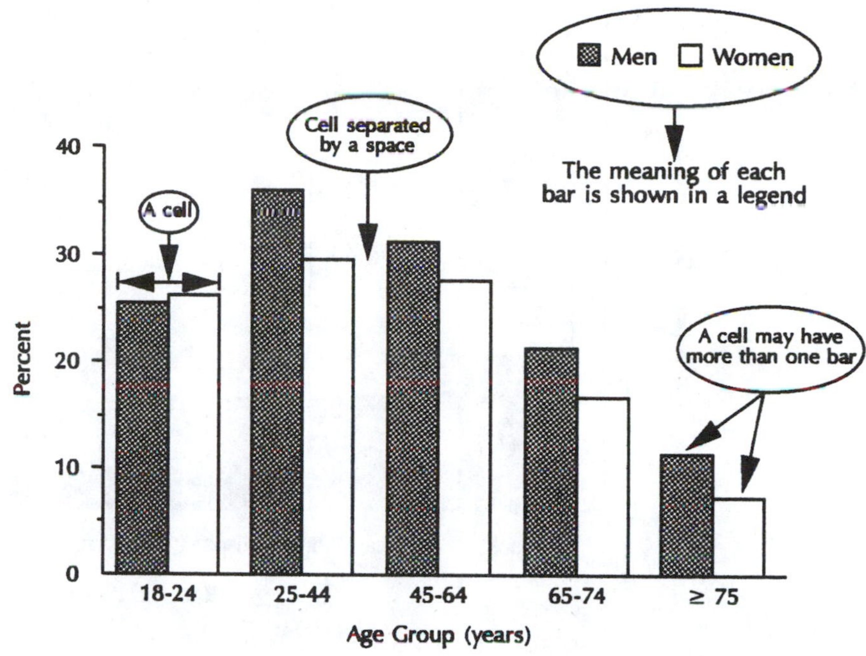

SOURCE: CDC, 1988.

FIGURE 8.19 *Example of vertical bar chart with annotation: Percentage of adults who were current cigarette smokers (persons ≥ 18 years of age who reported having smoked at least 100 cigarettes and who were currently smoking) by sex and age, United States, 1988*

The bar chart in Figure 8.19 represents three variables: age, sex, and current smoking status. Current smoking status is the outcome variable and has two categories: yes or no. The bars represent the 10 age-sex categories. The height of each bar is proportional to the percentage of current smokers in each age-sex category.

Stacked Bar Charts

You can also show categories of a second variable as components of the bars that represent the first variable, as in Figure 8.20. Notice that a stacked bar chart can be difficult to interpret because, except for the bottom component, the components do not rest on a flat baseline.

Deviation Bar Charts

We can also use bar charts to show deviations in a variable, both positive and negative, from a baseline. Figure 8.21 shows such a deviation bar chart of selected reportable diseases in the United States. A similar chart appears weekly in CDC's *Morbidity and Mortality Weekly Report*. In this chart, the number of cases reported during the past 4 weeks are compared to the number reported during comparable periods of the past few years.

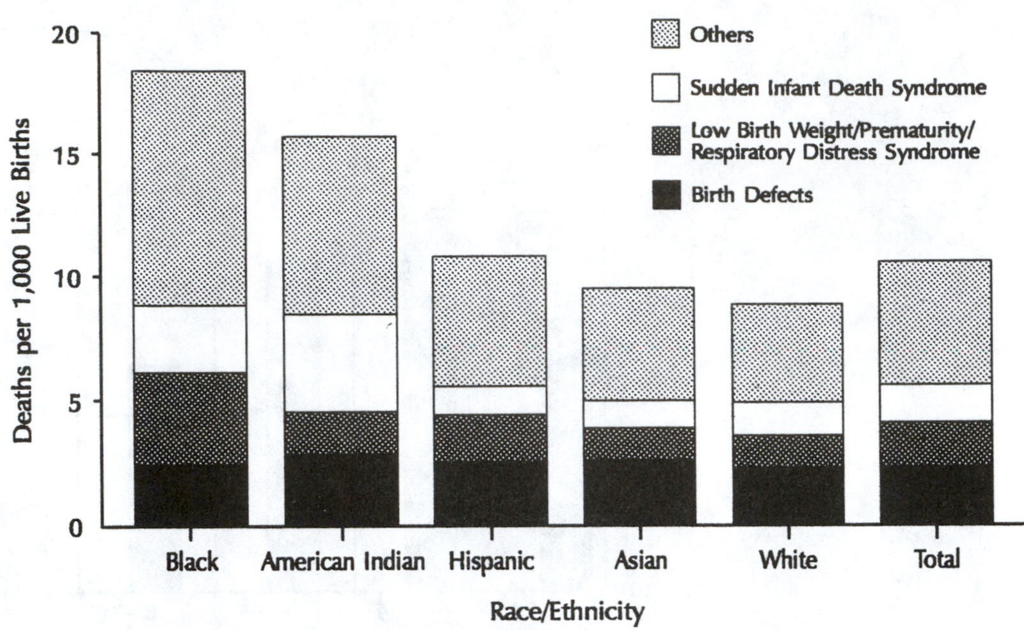

SOURCE: CDC, 1990b.

FIGURE 8.20 *Underlying causes of infant mortality among racial/ethnic groups, United States, 1983*

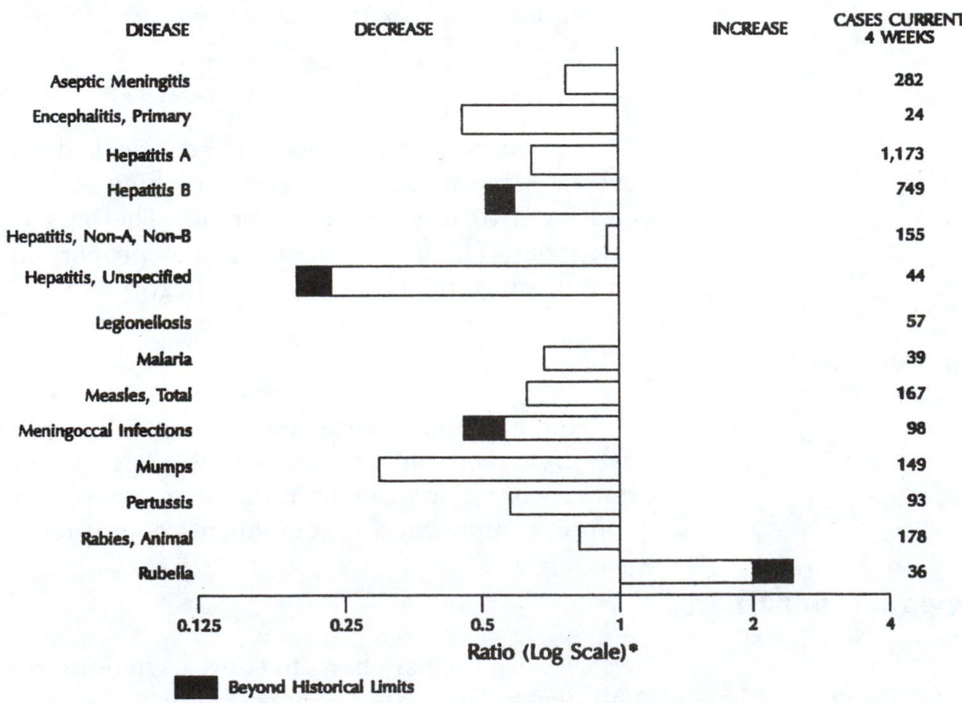

SOURCE: CDC, 1991a.

FIGURE 8.21 *Notifiable disease reports, comparisons of 4-week totals ending January 26, 1991 with historical data, United States, 1991*

The deviation to the right for rubella indicates an increase over historical levels. The deviations to the left indicate declines in reported cases compared to past levels. In this particular chart, the *x-axis* is on a logarithmic scale, so that a 50% reduction (one-half of the cases) and a doubling (50% increase) of cases would be represented by bars of the same length, though in opposite directions. Values beyond historical limits (comparable to 95% confidence limits) are highlighted for special attention.

100% Component Bar Charts

In a variant of a stacked bar chart, we make all of the bars the same height (or length) and show the components as percents of the total rather than as actual values. This type of chart is useful for comparing the contribution of different components to each of the categories of the main variable. Figure 8.22 shows a 100% component bar chart. Notice that this type of bar chart is not useful for comparing the relative sizes of the various categories of the main variable (in this case, race/ethnicity); only the totals given above the bars indicate that the categories differed in size.

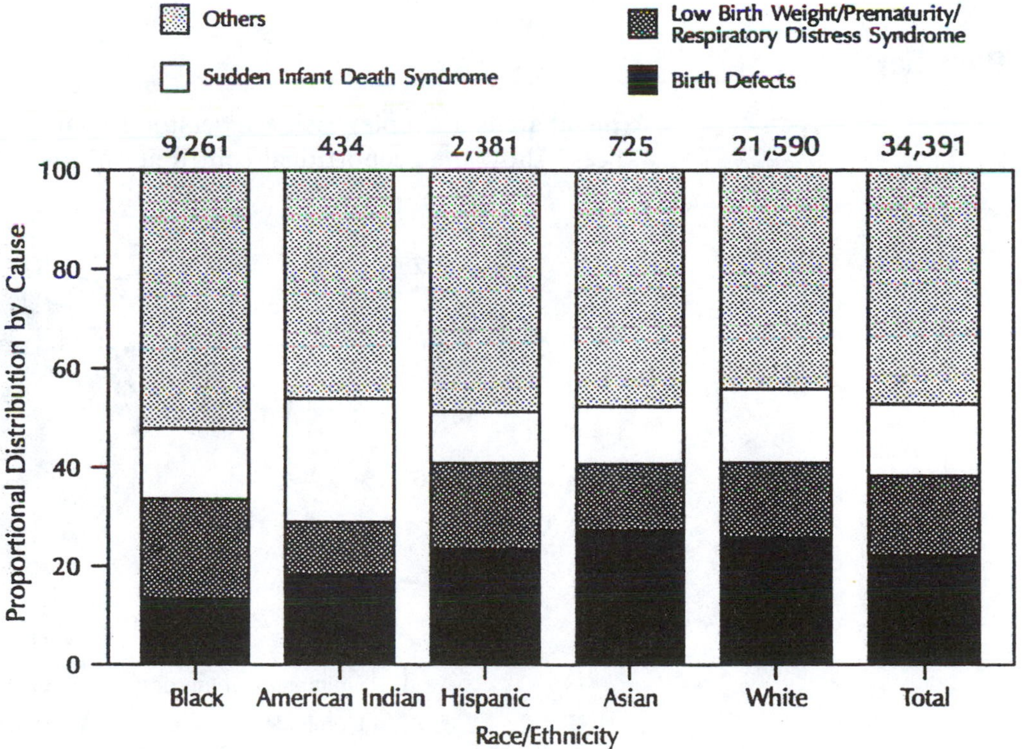

SOURCE: CDC, 1990b.

FIGURE 8.22 *Underlying cause of infant mortality among racial/ethnic groups, United States, 1983*

How to Construct a Bar Chart

To construct a bar chart, observe the following guidelines:

- Arrange the categories that define the bars, or groups of bars, in a natural order, such as alphabetical or by increasing age, or in an order that will produce increasing or decreasing bar lengths
- Position the bars either vertically or horizontally as you prefer, except for deviation bar charts, in which the bars are usually positioned horizontally
- Make all of the bars the same width (which can be whatever looks in good proportion to you)
- Make the length of bars in proportion to the frequency of the event. Do not use a scale break, because it could lead to misinterpretation in comparing the size of different categories
- Show no more than three bars within a group of bars
- Leave a space between adjacent groups of bars, but not between bars within a group (see Figure 8.19)
- Code different variables by differences in bar color, shading, cross-hatching, etc. and include a legend that interprets your code

Pie Charts

A pie chart is a simple, easily understood chart in which the size of the "slices" show the proportional contribution of each component part. Pie

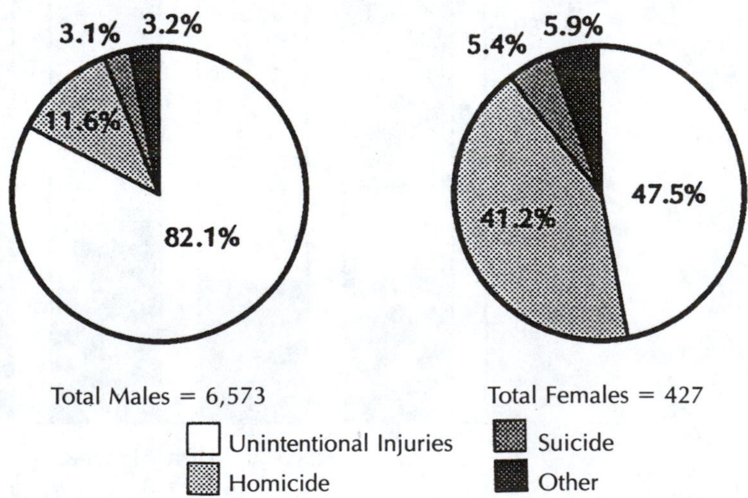

SOURCE: CDC, National Institute of Occupational Safety and Health, National Traumatic Occupational Fatalities Database.

FIGURE 8.23 *Manner of traumatic deaths for male and female workers in the United States, 1980-1985*

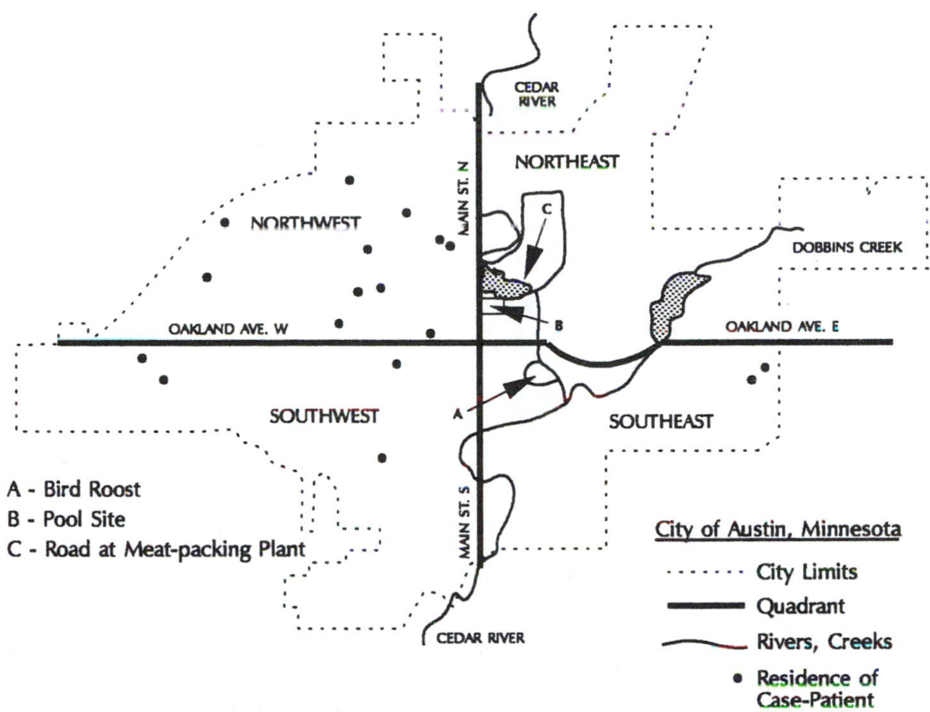

SOURCE: CDC, unpublished data, 1985.

FIGURE 8.24 *Example of spot map: Histoplasmosis by residence, Austin, Minnesota, October-November 1984*

charts are useful for showing the component parts of a single group or variable.

Graph paper is available commercially that has the circumference of a circle marked into 100 equal parts. This type of graph paper is called polar coordinate graph paper and an example is provided in Appendix C. Conventionally, you begin at 12 o'clock and arrange your component slices from largest to smallest, proceeding clockwise, although you may put the categories "other" and "unknown" last. You may use differences in shading to distinguish between slices. You should show somewhere on the graph what 100% represents, and because our eyes do not accurately gauge the area of the slices, you should indicate what percentage each slice represents either inside or near each slice.

Multiple pie charts as in Figure 8.23 are not optimal for comparing the same components in more than one group or variable, because it is difficult to compare components between two or more pie charts. When we want to compare the components of more than one group or variable, we use a 100% component bar chart.

Maps (Geographic Coordinate Charts)

Maps or geographic coordinate charts are used to show the location of events or attributes. **Spot maps** and **area maps** are commonly used examples

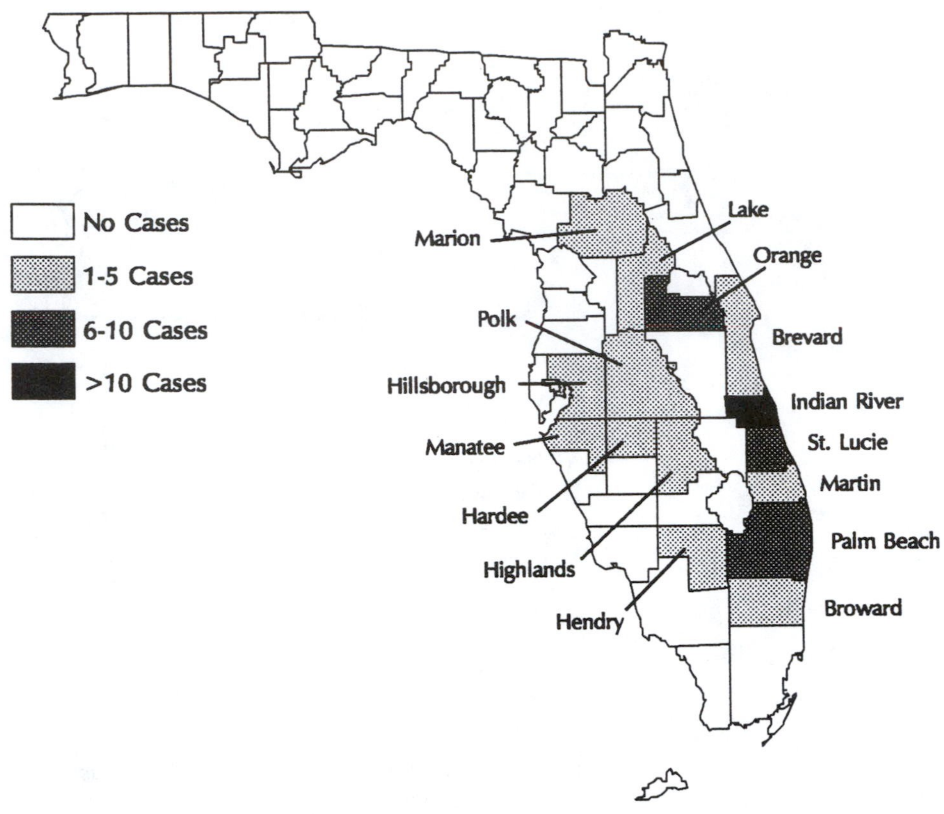

SOURCE: CDC, 1990c.

FIGURE 8.25 *Confirmed and presumptive cases of St. Louis encephalitis by county of residence, Florida, July-October 1990*

of this type of chart. Spot maps use dots or other symbols to show where an event took place or a disease condition exists. Figure 8.24 is an example of a spot map.

To make a **spot map**, place a dot or other symbol on the map at the site where the event occurred or the condition exists. If events are clustered at one location, making it difficult to distinguish between dots, you can use coded symbols (e.g., ● = 1 case, ■ = 2 cases, ▲ = 3 cases, etc.) that indicate the occurrence of more than one event.

A spot map is useful for showing the geographic distribution of an event, but—because it does not take into consideration the size of the population at risk—it does not show the **risk** of the event occurring in that particular place, for example, the risk of a resident acquiring a particular disease. Even when a spot map shows a large number of dots in the same area, the risk of acquiring the disease plotted may not be great there if that area is densely populated.

An area map uses shaded or coded areas to show either the incidence of an event in subareas, or the distribution of some condition over a geographic area. Figure 8.25 is an example of an area map.

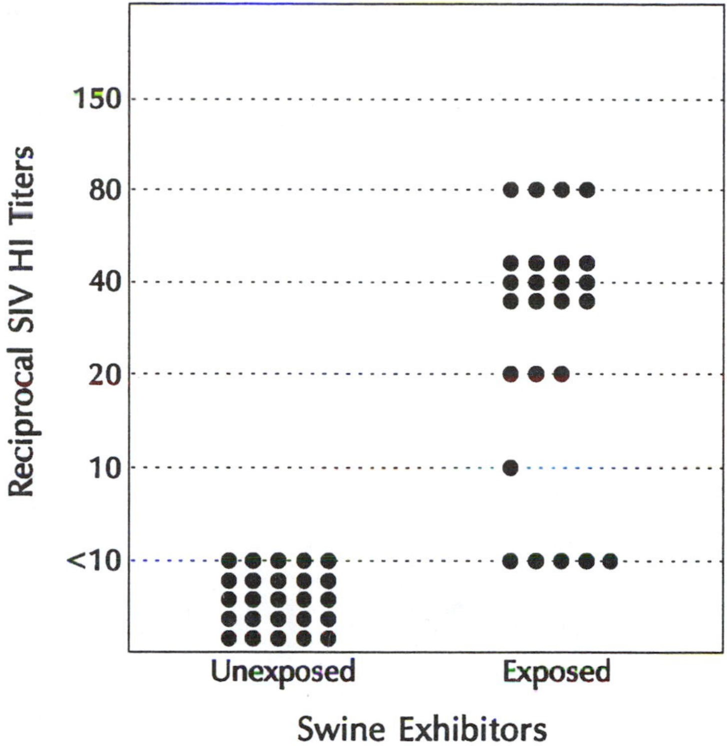

SOURCE: Wells et al., 1991. Reprinted by permission; © 1991, American Medical Association.

FIGURE 8.26 *Example of dot plot: Results of swine influence virus (SIV) hemagglutination-inhibition (HI) antibody testing among exposed and unexposed swine exhibitors, Wisconsin, 1988*

We can show either numbers of rates with an **area map**. Figure 8.25 shows the numbers of cases of St. Louis encephalitis in different Florida counties in 1990. As with a spot map, this does not show the risk to persons living in these counties of acquiring St. Louis encephalitis. By showing *rates* in an area map, however, we *can* illustrate the differences in the risk of an event occurring in different areas. When we use rates, we must calculate a specific rate for each area—that is, we must divide the number of cases in each area by the population at risk in the same area.

Dot Plots and Box Plots

A **dot plot** is similar to a scatter diagram because it plots one variable against another. In a dot plot, however, the variable on the *x-axis* is not continuous—it represents discrete categories of a noncontinuous variable. As shown in Figure 8.26, we plot an observation by entering a dot over the appropriate *x* category at the level of the appropriate *y* value; and we show as many dots at that position as there are observations with those same values. Notice in Figure 8.26 that the different vertical positions of the 12 dots at the intersection of "Exposed" and "40" do not indicate their

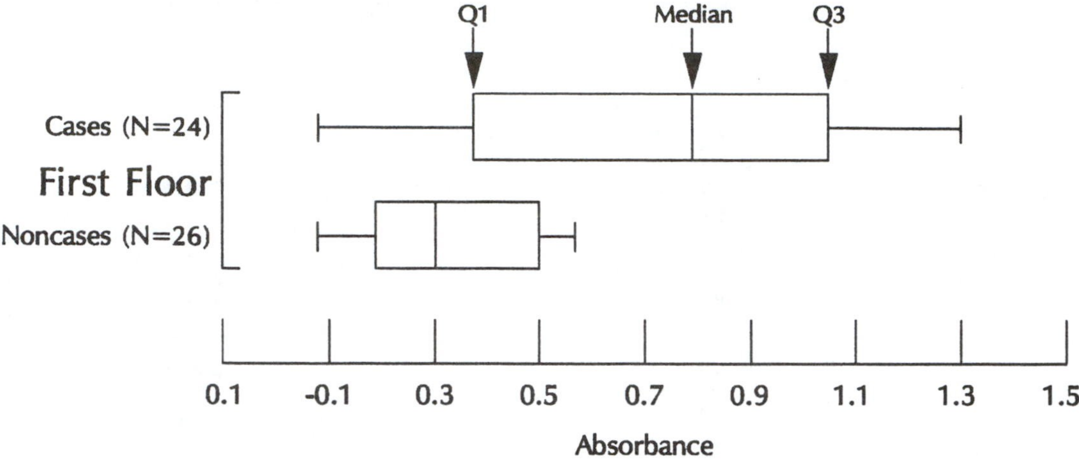

SOURCE: CDC, unpublished data, 1990.

FIGURE 8.27 *Example of box plot: Results of indirect ELISA for IgG antibodies to parainfluenza type I virus in convalescent phase serum specimens from cases to noncases, Baltimore County, Maryland, January 1990*

titer levels: they all have titer levels of 40. The dots are placed on different lines to facilitate showing them as a unit. Similarly, the 25 dots at "Unexposed" all represent a titer level of <10.

We use a dot plot to make a visual comparison of the actual data points of two noncontinuous variables. If we instead want to compare the *distributions* of noncontinuous variables, we use a **box plot**. In a box plot, we show the distributions of data as "box and whiskers" diagrams, shown in Figure 8.27. The "box" represents the middle 50% or interquartile range of the data, and the "whiskers" extend to the minimum and maximum values. We mark the position of the median with a vertical line inside the box. Thus, with a box plot we can show (and compare) the central location (median), dispersion (interquartile range and range), and any tendency toward skewness, which is indicated if the median line is not centered in the box.

A COMMENT ABOUT USING COMPUTER TECHNOLOGY

A large number of software packages for the personal computer are available that can help us make tables, graphs, and charts. Most of these packages are quite useful, particularly in letting us redraw a graph with only a few keystrokes. With these packages, finding the best epidemic curve is no longer an onerous and tedious task: We can now quickly and easily draw a number of curves with different class intervals on the *x-axis*.

On the other hand, we are sometimes tempted to let the software dictate the graph. For example, many packages can draw bar charts and

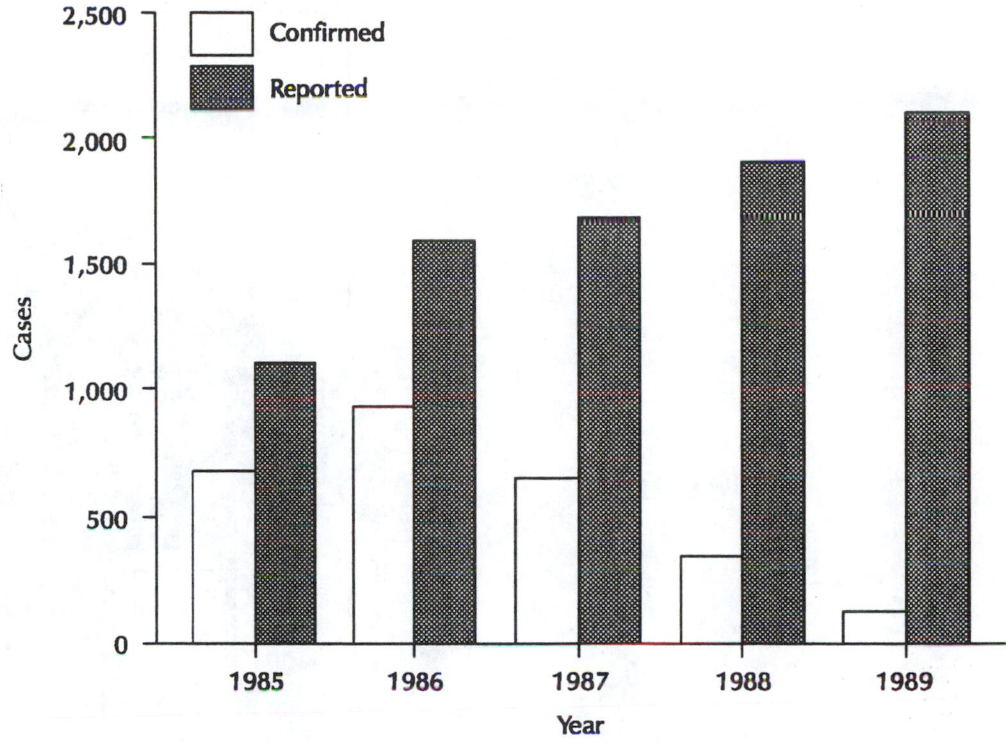

SOURCE: CDC, 1989b.

FIGURE 8.28a *Example of two-dimensional bar chart: Reported and confirmed polio cases by year, the Americas, 1985-1989*

pie charts that appear three-dimensional. Does that mean we should develop three-dimensional charts? We need to keep our purpose in mind: to communicate information to others. Will three-dimensional charts communicate the information better than a two-dimensional chart?

Decide for yourself: Does the three-dimensional chart in Figure 8.28b provide any more information than the two-dimensional bar chart in Figure 8.28a? Which is easier to interpret?

If we wanted to focus on the trends over time for confirmed and for reported cases, perhaps the three-dimensional chart is preferable. However, an arithmetic-scale line graph with two lines might be best of all. A problem common to three-dimensional bar charts is that a bar in the front row may block a bar in the back row. Suppose that we are interested in the ratio of confirmed to reported cases each year. We see immediately from the two-dimensional bar chart that the number of confirmed cases in 1985 is approximately two-thirds of the number of reported cases in 1985. How long do you have to look at the three-dimensional chart to reach that same conclusion? Now compare that ratio of confirmed to reported cases for all five years. If you need to communicate this information with a slide in 20 seconds during a 10-minute oral presentation, which figure would you show?

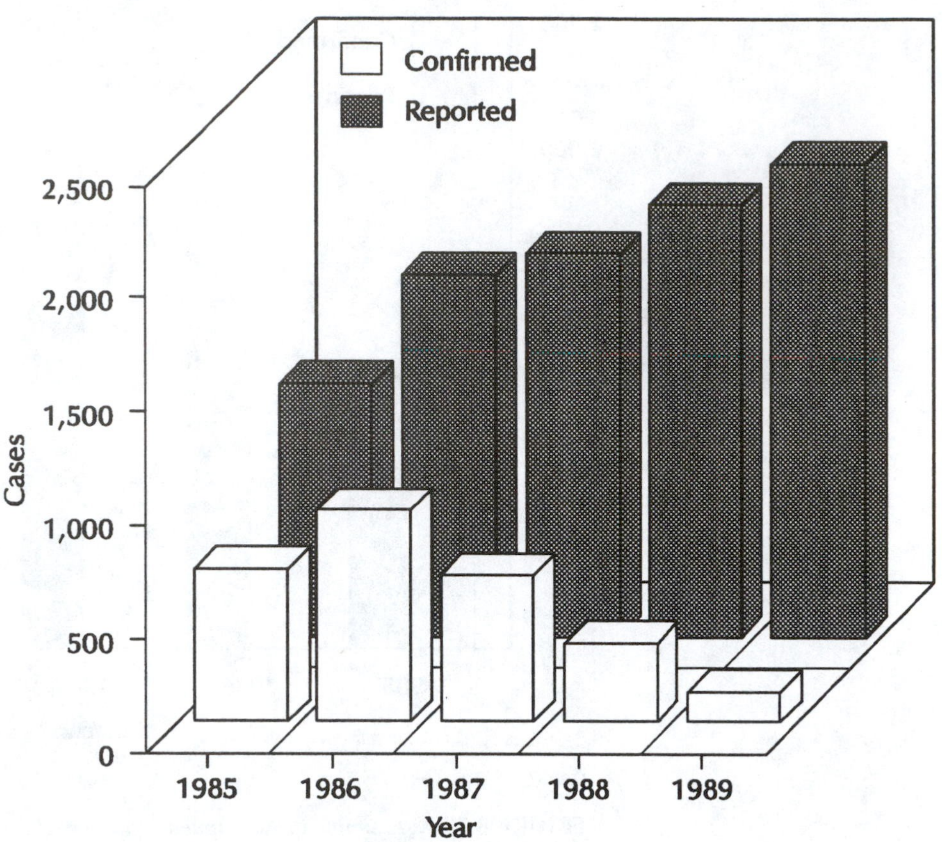

SOURCE: CDC, 1989b.

FIGURE 8.28b *Example of three-dimensional bar chart: Reported and confirmed polio cases by year, the Americas, 1985-1989*

Does the three-dimensional pie chart in Figure 8.29b provide any more information than the two-dimensional chart in Figure 8.29a? Can you judge the relative sizes of the components as well in the three-dimensional version? Look at the three-dimensional pie and block out the percentages for Hispanics and Asian/Pacific Islanders. Can you really tell which wedge is bigger and by how much? We think you can't. Can you tell from the two-dimensional pie? Remember that size is the whole purpose of a pie chart.

The addition of gimmicky features to a figure which adds no information and which may even promote misinterpretation has been termed **chartjunk** (Tufte, 1983).

Many people misuse technology in selecting color, particularly for slides that accompany oral presentations. If you use colors at all, follow these recommendations:

- Select colors so that all components of the graph—title, axes, data plots, legends—stand out clearly from the background, and so that each plotted series of data can be distinguished from the others.

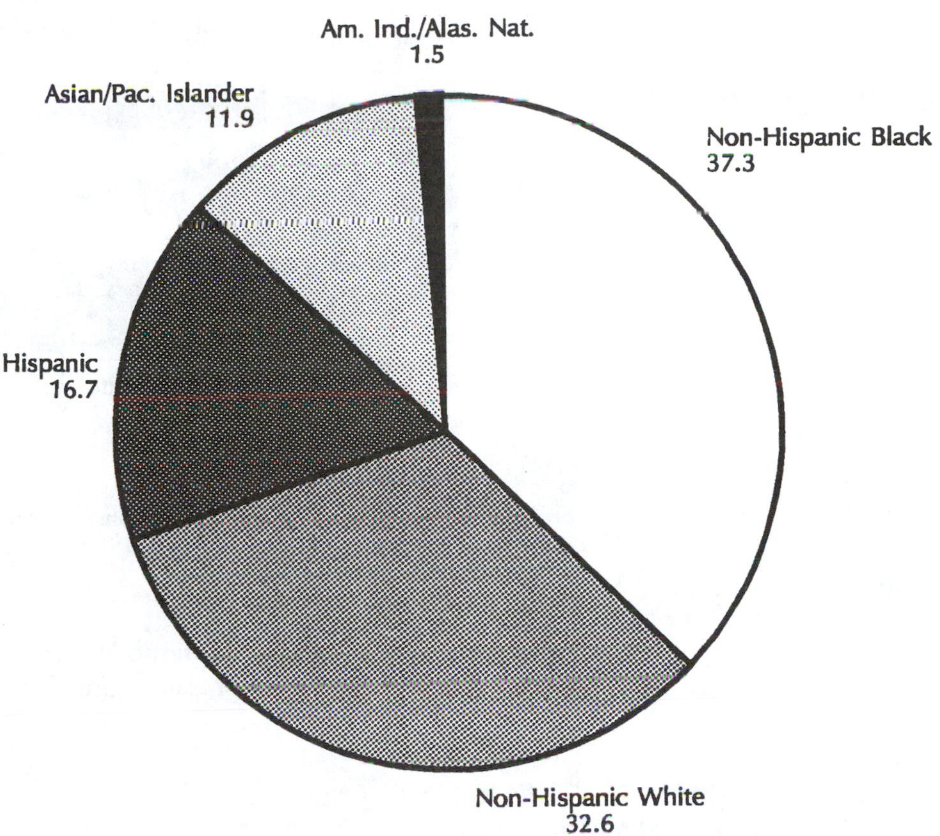

SOURCE: CDC, 1989c.

FIGURE 8.29a *Example of two-dimensional pie chart: Percentage of tuberculosis cases by race and ethnicity, United States, 1989 (N = 23,495)*

- Avoid contrasting red and green, because up to 10% of males in the audience may have some degree of color blindness.
- When possible, select colors so that they communicate information. For example, consider an area map in which states are divided into four groups according to their rates for a particular disease. Rather than choosing colors solely for appearance, you might use a light color or shade for the states with the lowest rates and progressively darker colors or shades for the groups with progressively higher rates. In this way, the colors contribute to, rather than distort or distract from, the information you want to convey.

Finally, with some software packages you cannot produce some of the types of graphs covered in this manual. In particular, some software packages cannot create a histogram; instead they produce a bar chart. Your graphs should be dictated by your data and the relationships you want to communicate visually, not by the technology at hand. If the

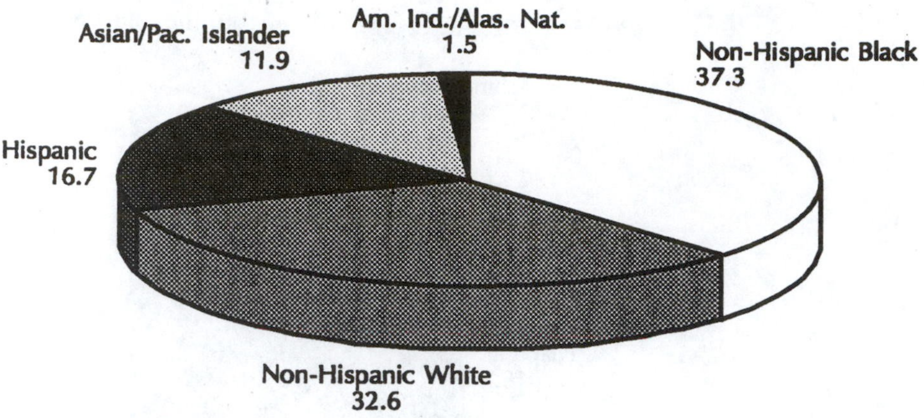

SOURCE: CDC, 1989c.

FIGURE 8.29b *Example of three-dimensional pie chart: Percentage of tuberculosis cases by race and ethnicity, United States, 1989 (N = 23,495)*

software you have cannot accommodate your data, don't compromise the integrity of the data or its presentation. Use different software!

SELECTING AND CONSTRUCTING TABLES, GRAPHS, AND CHARTS

To convey the messages of epidemiologic findings, you must first select the best illustration method. But even the best method must be constructed properly or the message will be lost. The tables in this section provide guidance in the selection of illustration methods and construction of tables, graphs, and charts.

TABLE 8.10 Guide to selecting a graph or chart to illustrate epidemiologic data

Type of Graph or Chart	*When to Use*
Arithmetic-scale line graph	Trends in numbers or rates over time
Semilogarithmic-scale line graph	1. Emphasize rate of change over time 2. Display values ranging over more than 2 orders of magnitude
Histogram	1. Frequency distribution of continuous variable 2. Number of cases during epidemic (epidemic curve) or over time
Frequency polygon	Frequency distribution of continuous variable, especially to show components
Cumulative frequency	Cumulative frequency for continuous variables

Continued

TABLE 8.10 *Continued*

Type of Graph or Chart	*When to Use*
Scatter diagram	Plot association between two variables
Simple bar chart	Compare size or frequency of different categories of a single variable
Grouped bar chart	Compare size or frequency of different categories of 2-4 series of data
Stacked bar chart	Compare totals and illustrate component parts of the total among different groups
Deviation bar chart	Illustrate differences, both positive and negative, from baseline
100% component bar chart	Compare how components contribute to the whole in different groups
Pie chart	Show components of a whole
Spot map	Show location of cases or events
Area map	Display events or rates geographically
Box plot	Visualize statistical characteristics (median, range, skewness) of a variable

SOURCE: CDC, 1992.

TABLE 8.11 Selecting a method of illustrating epidemiologic data

<table>
<tr><th colspan="2">If Data Are:</th><th colspan="2">And These Conditions Apply:</th><th>Then Choose:</th></tr>
<tr><td colspan="2" rowspan="4">Time series</td><td rowspan="2">Numbers of cases (epidemic or secular trend)</td><td>1 or 2 sets</td><td>Histogram</td></tr>
<tr><td>2 or more sets</td><td>Frequency polygon</td></tr>
<tr><td rowspan="2">Rates</td><td>Range of values ≤ 2 orders of magnitude</td><td>Arithmetic scale line graph</td></tr>
<tr><td>Range of values ≥ 2 orders of magnitude</td><td>Semilogarithmic scale line graph</td></tr>
<tr><td colspan="2">Continuous data other than time series</td><td colspan="2">Frequency distribution</td><td>Histogram or frequency polygon</td></tr>
<tr><td colspan="2">Data with discrete categories (other than place)</td><td colspan="2"></td><td>Bar chart or pie chart</td></tr>
<tr><td rowspan="4">Place</td><td rowspan="3">Number of cases</td><td colspan="2">Not readily identified on map</td><td>Bar chart</td></tr>
<tr><td rowspan="2">Readily identified on map</td><td>Specific site important</td><td>Spot map</td></tr>
<tr><td>Specific site unimportant</td><td>Area map</td></tr>
<tr><td colspan="3">Rates</td><td>Area map</td></tr>
</table>

SOURCE: CDC, 1992.

TABLE 8.12 Checklist for construction of tables, graphs, charts, and visuals

Checklist for Tables

1. Title
   - Does the table have a title?
   - Does the title describe the content, including subject, person, place, and time?
   - Is the title preceded by the designation "Table #"? ("Table" is used for typed text; "Figure" for graphs, charts, and maps. Separate numerical sequences are used for tables and figures in the same document [e.g., Table 1, Table 2, Figure 1, Figure 2]).
2. Rows and columns
   - Is each row and each column labeled clearly and concisely?
   - Are the specific units of measurement shown? (e.g., years, mm Hg, mg/dl, rate per 100,000, etc.)
   - Are the categories appropriate for the data?
   - Are the row and column totals provided?
3. Footnotes
   - Are all codes, abbreviations, or symbols explained?
   - Are all exclusions noted?
   - If the data are not original, is the source provided?

Checklist for Graphs and Charts

1. Title
   - Does the graph or chart have a title?
   - Does the title describe the content, including subject, person, place, and time?
   - Is the title preceded by the designation "Figure #"? ("Table" is used for typed text; "Figure" for graphs, charts, and maps. Separate numerical sequences are used for tables and figures in the same document [e.g., Table 1, Table 2, Figure 1, Figure 2]).
2. Axes
   - Is each axis labeled clearly and concisely?
   - Are the specific units of measurement included as part of the label? (e.g., years, mm Hg, mg/dl, rate per 100,000, etc.)
   - Are the scale divisions on the axes clearly indicated?
   - Are the scales for each axis appropriate for the data?
   - Does the y-axis start at zero?
   - If a scale break is used with a scale line graph, is it clearly identified?
   - Has a scale break been used with a histogram, frequency polygon, or bar chart? (Answer should be **NO**!)
   - Are the axes drawn heavier than the other coordinate lines?
3. Coordinate lines
   - Does the figure include only as many coordinate lines as are necessary to guide the eye? (Often, these are unnecessary.)
4. Data plots
   - Are the plots drawn clearly?
   - If more than one series of data or components are shown, are they clearly distinguishable on the graph?
   - Is each series or component labeled on the graph, or in a legend or key?
   - If color or shading is used on an area map, does an increase in color or shading correspond to an increase in the variable being shown?

Continued

TABLE 8.12 *Continued*

5. Footnotes
   - Are all codes, abbreviations, or symbols explained?
   - Are all exclusions noted?
   - If the data are not original, is the source provided?
6. Visual Display
   - Does the figure include any information that is not necessary?
   - Is the figure positioned on the page for optimal readability?
   - Do font sizes and colors improve readability?

Checklist for Effective Visuals (Creech, 1988)

1. Legibility (make sure your audience can easily read your visuals)
   - Can your overhead transparencies be read easily from 6 feet when not projected?
   - Can your 35 mm slides be read easily from 1 foot when not projected?
   - When projected, can your visuals be read from the farthest parts of the room?
2. Simplicity (keep the message simple)
   - Have you used plain words?
   - Is the information presented in the language of the audience?
   - Have you used only "key" words?
   - Have you omitted conjunctions, prepositions, etc.?
   - Is each visual limited to only one major idea/concept/theme?
   - Does each visual have no more than 3 colors?
   - Are there no more than 35 letters and numbers on each visual?
   - Are there no more than 6 lines of narration and 6 words per line?
3. Colorfulness
   - The colors you select for your visuals will have an impact on the effect of your visuals. You should use warm/hot colors to emphasize, to highlight, to focus, or to reinforce key concepts. You should use cool/cold colors for background or to separate items. Use the table below to select the appropriate color for the effect you desire.

	Hot	*Warm*	*Cool*	*Cold*
Colors:	Reds Bright orange Bright yellow Bright gold	Light orange Light yellow Light gold Browns	Light blue Light green Light purple Light gray	Dark blue Dark green Dark purple Dark gray
Effect:	Exciting	Mild	Subdued	Somber

   - Are you using the best color combinations? The most important item should be in the most important color and have the greatest contrast with its background. The most legible color combinations are:

     Black on Yellow
     Black on White
     Dark Green on White

Continued

TABLE 8.12 *Continued*

Dark Blue on White
White on Dark Blue

4. Accuracy
Visuals become distractions when mistakes are spotted. Have someone who has not seen the visual before check for typos, inaccuracies, and errors in general.
5. Durability
Transparencies and 35mm slides are the most durable of the visual aids. However, both require some protection from scratches. A clear sheet of acetate or Mylar will protect a transparency. Keep 35mm slides in a cool, dark place. If left in the light, colors will fade.

CHAPTER SUMMARY

Tables, graphs, and charts are effective tools for summarizing and communicating data. Tables are commonly used to display numbers, rates, proportions, and cumulative percents. Because tables are intended to communicate information, most tables should have no more than two variables and no more than eight categories (class intervals) of any variable. Tables are sometimes used out of context by others, so they should be properly titled, labeled, and referenced.

Tables can be used with either nominal or continuous ordinal data. Nominal variables such as sex and state of residence have obvious categories. Continuous variables do not; class intervals must be created. For some diseases, standard class intervals for age have been adopted. Otherwise a variety of methods are available for establishing reasonable class intervals. These include class intervals with an equal number of people or observations in each; class intervals with a constant width; and class intervals based on the mean and standard deviation.

Graphs and charts are even more effective tools for communicating data rapidly. Although some people use the terms *graph* and *chart* interchangeably, in this chapter *graph* refers to a figure with two coordinates, a horizontal *x-axis* and a vertical *y-axis*. In other words, both variables are continuous. For example, the *y-axis* commonly features number of cases or rate of disease; the *x-axis* usually represents time. In contrast, a *chart* refers to a figure with one continuous and one nominal variable. For example, the chart may feature number of cases (a continuous variable) by sex (a nominal variable).

Arithmetic-scale line graphs have traditionally been used to show trends in disease *rates* over time. Semilogarithmic-scale line graphs are preferred when the disease rates vary over two or more orders of magnitude. Histograms and frequency polygons are used to display frequency distributions. A special type of histogram known as an epidemic curve shows the *number* of cases by time of onset of illness or time of diagnosis during an epidemic period. The cases may be represented by squares which are stacked to form the columns of the histogram; the squares may be shaded to distinguish important characteristics of cases, such as fatal outcome.

Simple bar charts and pie charts are used to display the frequency distribution of a single variable. Grouped and stacked bar charts can display two or even three variables.

Spot maps pinpoint the location of each case or event. An area map uses shading or coloring to show different levels of disease numbers or rates in different areas.

When using these tools, it is important to remember their purpose: to summarize and to communicate. Glitzy and colorful are not necessarily better; sometimes less is more!

REFERENCES

Alter MJ, Ahtone J, Weisfuse I, Starko K, Vacalis TD, Maynard JE: Hepatitis B virus transmission between heterosexuals. *Journal of the American Medical Association* 1986; 256:1307-1310.

Centers for Disease Control: Chronic Disease Supplement, 1987. Deaths from cervical cancer—U.S., 1984-1986. *MMWR* 1989;38:38. (1989a)*

Centers for Disease Control: HIV/AIDS Surveillance Report. November 1990. (1990a)

Centers for Disease Control: Manual of reporting procedures for national morbidity reporting and public health surveillance activities. July 1985.

Centers for Disease Control: Progress toward eradicating poliomyelitis from the Americas. *MMWR* 1989;39:33. (1989b)

Centers for Disease Control: Infant mortality among racial/ethnic minority groups, 1983-1984. *MMWR* 1990;39:SS-3. (1990b)

Centers for Disease Control: St. Louis encephalitis—Florida and Texas, 1990. *MMWR* 1990;39:42. (1990c)

Centers for Disease Control: *MMWR* 1991;40:4. (1991a)

Centers for Disease Control: Nutritional assessment of children in drought-affected areas—Haiti, 1990. *MMWR* 1991;40:13. (1991b)

Centers for Disease Control: Cigarette smoking among adults—United States, 1988. *MMWR* 1988;40:44.

Centers for Disease Control: National Institute of Occupational Safety and Health. National Traumatic Occupational Fatalities Database.

Centers for Disease Control: Summary of notifiable diseases, United States, 1989. *MMWR* 1989;38(54). (1989c)

---

*Numbers in parentheses after a reference citation refer to sources cited for Tables and Figures in Chapter 8.

Centers for Disease Control: Health status of Vietnam veterans. Volume 3: Medical Examination. 1989. (1989d)

Creech JW: Effective oral presentations. Epi in Action Course, Centers for Disease Control, 1988.

Dicker RC, Webster LA, Layde PM, Wingo PA, Ory HW: Oral contraceptive use and the risk of ovarian cancer: The Centers for Disease Control Cancer and Steroid Hormone Study. *Journal of the American Medical Association* 1983;249:1596-1599.

Fingerhut MA, et al.: Cancer mortality in workers exposed to 2,3,7,8-tetrachlorodibenzo-*p*-dioxin. *New England Journal of Medicine* 1991;324:212-218.

Hadler SC, et al.: Occupational risk of hepatitis B infection in hospital workers. *Infectious Control* 1985;6:24-31.

Kleinman JC, Donahue RP, Harris MI, Finucane FF, Madans JH, Brock DB: Mortality among diabetics in a national sample. *American Journal of Epidemiology* 1988;128:389-401.

Lettau LA, et al.: Outbreak of severe hepatitis due to delta and hepatitis F viruses in parenteral drug abusers and their contacts. *New England Journal of Medicine* 1987;317:1256-1262.

McKenna M, Wolfson S, Kuller L: The ratio of ankle and arm arterial pressure as an independent predictor of mortality. *Athero* 1991;87:119-128.

National Center for Health Statistics: Advance report of final mortality statistics, 1987. Monthly vital statistics report; vol 38, no 5 supp. Hyattsville, MD: Public Health Service. 1989.

Schoenbaum SC, Baker O, Jezek Z: Common source epidemic of hepatitis due to glazed and iced pastries. *American Journal of Epidemiology* 1976; 104:74-80.

Schreeder MT, et al.: Hepatitis B in homosexual men: prevalence of infection and factors related to transmission. *Journal of Infectious Diseases* 1982; 146:1.

Sutter RW, Patriarca PA, Brogran S, et al.: Outbreak of paralytic poliomyelitis in Oman. Evidence for widespread transmission among fully vaccinated children. *Lancet* 1991;338:715-20.

Tufte ER: *The visual display of quantitative information*. Cheshire, CT: Graphics Press, 1983.

Wells DL, Hopfensperger DJ, Arden NH, et al.: Swine influenza virus infections. *Journal of the American Medical Association* 1991;265:478-481.

Williamson DF, Parker RA, Kendrick JS: The box plot: A simple visual method to interpret data. *Annals of Internal Medicine* 1989;110:916-921.

PROBLEMS

1. The data in Table 8.13 describe characteristics of the 36 residents of a nursing home during an outbreak of diarrheal disease.

   A. Construct a table of the illness (diarrhea) by menu type. Use diarrhea status as column labels and menu types as row labels.

   B. Construct a two-by-two table of the illness (diarrhea) by exposure to menu A.

TABLE 8.13 Characteristics of residents of Nursing Home A during outbreak of diarrheal disease, January 1989

Resident No.	*Age*	*Sex*	*Room*	*Menu*	*Diarrhea?*	*Date of Onset*
1	71	F	103	A	Yes	1/15
2	72	F	105	A	Yes	1/23
3	74	F	105	A	No	
4	86	F	107	B	No	
5	83	F	107	B	No	
6	68	F	109	A	Yes	1/18
7	69	F	109	C	No	
8	64	F	111	A	Yes	1/16
9	66	M	111	A	Yes	1/18
10	68	M	104	A	Yes	1/20
11	70	M	106	A	No	
12	86	M	110	A	No	
13	73	M	112	B	No	
14	82	M	219	C	No	
15	72	M	221	C	No	
16	70	M	221	B	No	
17	77	M	227	D	No	
18	80	M	227	D	No	
19	71	F	231	A	Yes	1/14
20	68	F	231	D	Yes	1/15
21	64	F	233	A	No	
22	73	F	235	A	Yes	1/13
23	75	F	235	B	No	
24	78	F	222	C	No	
25	72	F	222	A	No	
26	66	M	224	B	No	
27	69	M	226	A	Yes	1/16
28	75	M	228	E	No	
29	71	M	230	A	Yes	1/13
30	83	M	232	F	No	
31	84	M	232	D	No	
32	79	M	234	A	Yes	1/12
33	72	M	234	D	Yes	1/14
34	77	M	236	A	Yes	1/13
35	78	M	236	B	No	
36	80	M	238	D	No	

SOURCE: CDC, 1992.

2. With the data on cervical cancer mortality rates presented in Table 8.8, use each strategy to create **three** class intervals for the rates.

TABLE 8.8 REVISITED Mean annual age-adjusted cervical cancer mortality rates per 100,000 population, in rank order by state, United States, 1984-1986

Rank	*State*	*Rate per 100,000*	*Rank*	*State*	*Rate per 100,000*
1	SC	5.6	26	KS	3.6
2	WV	5.6	27	AR	3.6
3	AL	5.4	28	MD	3.5
4	LA	5.4	29	IA	3.4
5	AK	5.1	30	PA	3.4
6	TN	4.9	31	FL	3.4
7	ND	4.9	32	HI	3.4
8	KY	4.8	33	OR	3.3
9	MS	4.7	34	MI	3.3
10	NC	4.6	35	CA	3.2
11	GA	4.6	36	ID	3.1
12	ME	4.6	37	AZ	3.1
13	VT	4.3	38	MA	2.9
14	DE	4.3	39	NM	2.9
15	NH	4.3	40	WA	2.8
16	IN	4.1	41	NV	2.8
17	OK	4.1	42	CT	2.8
18	IL	4.0	43	RI	2.8
19	MT	4.0	44	WI	2.7
20	VA	3.9	45	CO	2.5
21	OH	3.8	46	NE	2.4
22	MO	3.8	47	SD	2.4
23	TX	3.7	48	MN	2.2
24	NY	3.7	49	WY	1.9
25	NJ	3.7	50	UT	1.8
			Total	U.S.	3.7

SOURCE: CDC, 1989a.

3. In both graphs, be sure to use intervals on the *y-axis* that are appropriate for the range of data you are graphing. Graph paper is provided in Appendix C.

   A. Construct an arithmetic-scale line graph of the measles data in Table 8.14, showing measles rates from 1955-1990 with a single line.

B. Construct an arithmetic-scale line graph of the measles data for 1980-1990.

TABLE 8.14 Measles (rubeola) rate per 100,000 population, United States, 1955-1990

Year	Rate	Year	Rate	Year	Rate
1955	336.3	1967	31.7	1979	6.2
1956	364.1	1968	11.1	1980	6.0
1957	283.4	1969	12.8	1981	1.4
1958	438.2	1970	23.2	1982	0.7
1959	229.3	1971	36.5	1983	0.6
1960	246.3	1972	15.5	1984	1.1
1961	231.6	1973	12.7	1985	1.2
1962	259.0	1974	10.5	1986	2.6
1963	204.2	1975	11.4	1987	1.5
1964	239.4	1976	19.2	1988	1.4
1965	135.1	1977	26.5	1989	7.3
1966	104.2	1978	12.3	1990	10.7

SOURCE: CDC, 1989c.

4. Graph the measles data in Table 8.14 with a semilogarithmic-scale line graph. Semilog graph paper with five cycles is provided in Appendix C.

5. Using the data from the nursing home outbreak in Problem 1, draw an epidemic curve. Describe the features of this graph as if you were speaking over the telephone to someone who cannot see the graph. Graph paper is provided in Appendix C.

6. Use the data in Table 8.15 to draw a stacked bar chart, a grouped bar chart, and a 100% component bar chart to illustrate the differences in the age distribution of syphilis cases among white males, white females, black males, and black females. What information is best conveyed by each chart? Graph paper is provided in Appendix C.

TABLE 8.15 Number of primary and secondary syphilis cases by age, sex, and race, United States, 1989

	White		*Black*		
Age Group (years)	*Males*	*Females*	*Males*	*Females*	*Total*
<20	90	267	1,443	2,422	4,222
20-29	957	908	8,180	8,093	18,138
30-39	931	478	6,893	3,676	11,978
⩾40	826	160	3,860	941	5,787
Total	2,804	1,813	20,376	15,132	40,125

SOURCE: CDC, 1989c.

7. Using the cervical cancer mortality data in Table 8.8 on page 294, construct two area maps based on the first two strategies for categorizing data into four class intervals as described on pages 250-256. Maps of the United States are provided in Appendix C.

ANSWERS

1. A.

Occurrence of diarrhea by menu, residents of Nursing Home A, 1989

Menu	Diarrhea Status Yes	No	Total
A	12	5	17
B	0	7	7
C	0	4	4
D	2	4	6
E	0	1	1
F	0	1	1
Total	14	22	36

1. B.

Occurrence of diarrhea by exposure to menu A, residents of Nursing Home A, 1989

		Diarrhea Yes	No	Total
Menu A	Yes	12	5	17
	No	2	17	19
Total		14	22	36

2. Strategy 1: Divide the data into groups of similar size

Divide the list into three equal-sized groups of states:

50 states ÷ 3 = 16.67 states per group. Thus, two groups will contain 17 states and one group will contain 16 states.

Oklahoma (#17) could go in either group 1 or group 2, but since it has the same rate as Indiana (#16), it makes sense to put Oklahoma in group 1. Similarly, since Michigan (#34) could go in either group 2 or group 3 but has the same rate as Oregon (#33), Michigan should go in group 2.

Final categories:

States	Range of Rates per 100,000	Number of States
1. OK-SC	4.1-5.6	17
2. MI-IL	3.3-4.0	17
3. UT-CA	1.8-3.2	16

Strategy 2: Base categories on the mean and standard deviation

Create 3 categories based on mean (3.70) and standard deviation (0.96):

upper limit of category 1 = mean − 1 standard deviation = 3.70 − 0.96 = 2.74
upper limit of category 2 = mean + 1 standard deviation = 3.70 + 0.96 = 4.66
upper limit of category 3 = maximum value = 5.6

Final categories:

States	Rates per 100,000	Number of States
1. MS-SC	4.67-5.60	9
2. RI-NC	2.75-4.66	34
3. UT-WI	1.80-2.74	7

Strategy 3: Divide the range into equal class intervals

Divide the range by 3: (5.60 − 1.80) ÷ 3 = 1.267

Use multiples of 1.27 to create three categories, starting with 1.8:

1. 1.80 through (1.80 + 1.27) = 1.80 through 3.07
2. 3.08 through (1.80 + 2 × 1.27) = 3.08 through 4.34
3. 4.35 through (1.80 + 3 × 1.27) = 4.35 through 5.61

Final categories:

States	Range of Rates per 100,000	Number of States
1. ME-SC	4.35-5.61	12
2. AZ-VT	3.08-4.34	25
3. UT-MA	1.80-3.07	13

Or rounding categories:

States	Range of Rates per 100,000	Number of States
1. ME-SC	4.4-5.6	12
2. AZ-VT	3.1-4.3	25
3. UT-MA	1.8-3.0	13

3. A. and B.

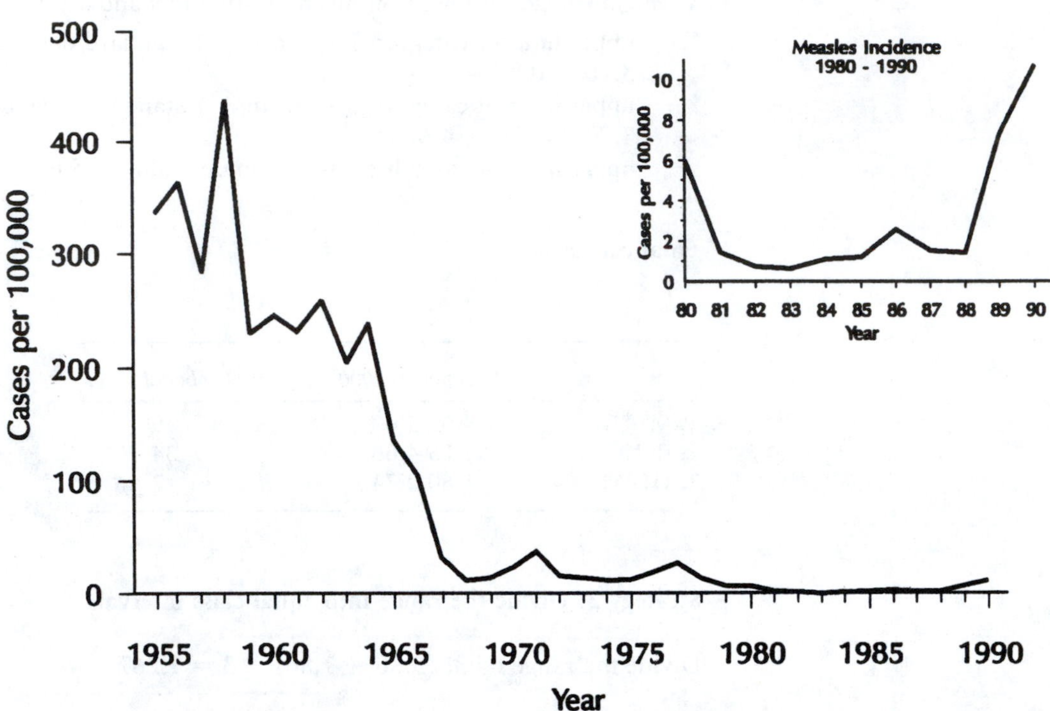

SOURCE: CDC, 1989c.

FIGURE 8.30 *Annual measles incidence rates per 100,000, United States, 1955-1990; with inset of 1980-1990*

4.

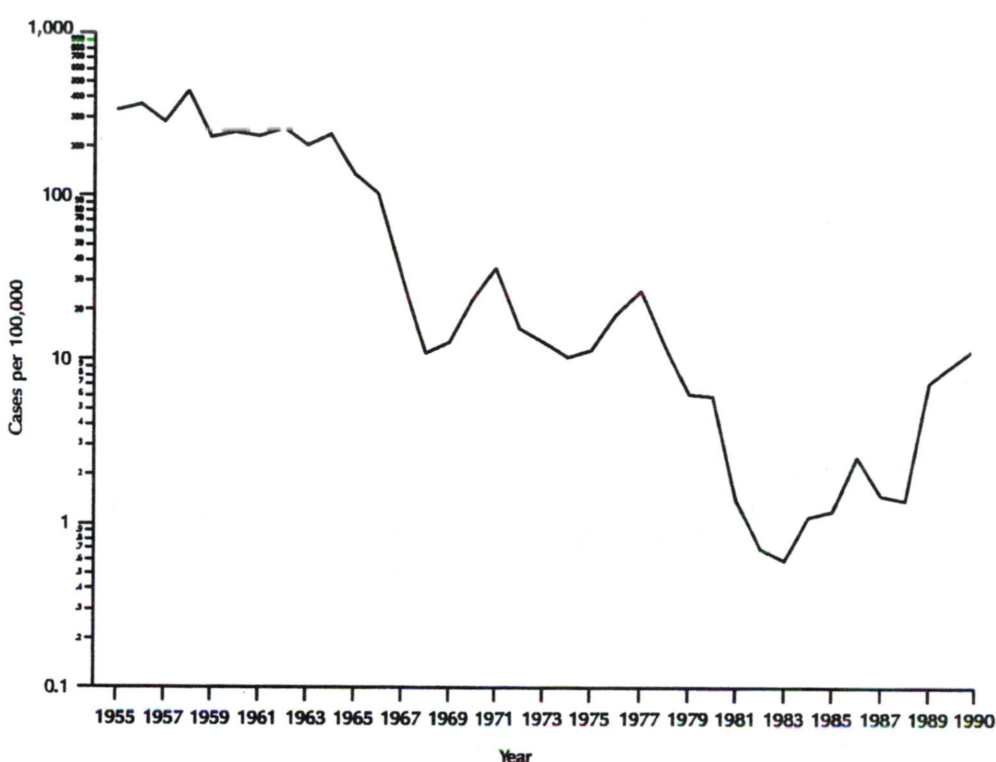

SOURCE: CDC, 1989c.

FIGURE 8.31 *Annual measles incidence rates per 100,000, United States, 1955-1990*

5.

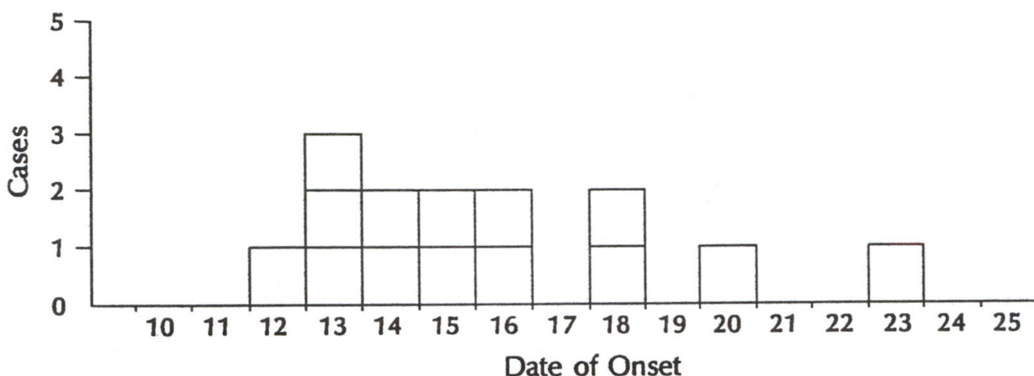

This outbreak appeared to last just under two weeks, from January 12 to January 23. After the initial case on January 12th, the peak occurred the following day, with three cases on January 13. The curve was relatively flat after that, with two cases each on four of the next five days. Single cases occurred in January 20 and January 23.

SOURCE: CDC, 1992.

FIGURE 8.32 *Outbreak of diarrheal disease in Nursing Home A, January 1989*

6.

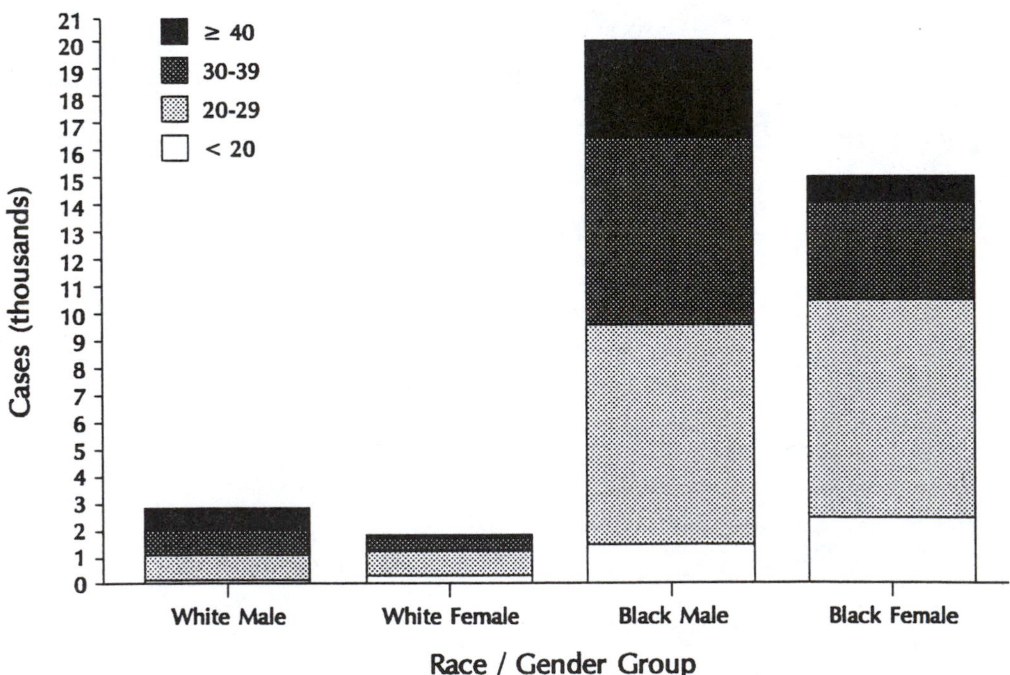

SOURCE: CDC, 1989c.

FIGURE 8.33a *Stacked bar chart: Number of primary and secondary syphilis cases by age, sex, and race, 1989*

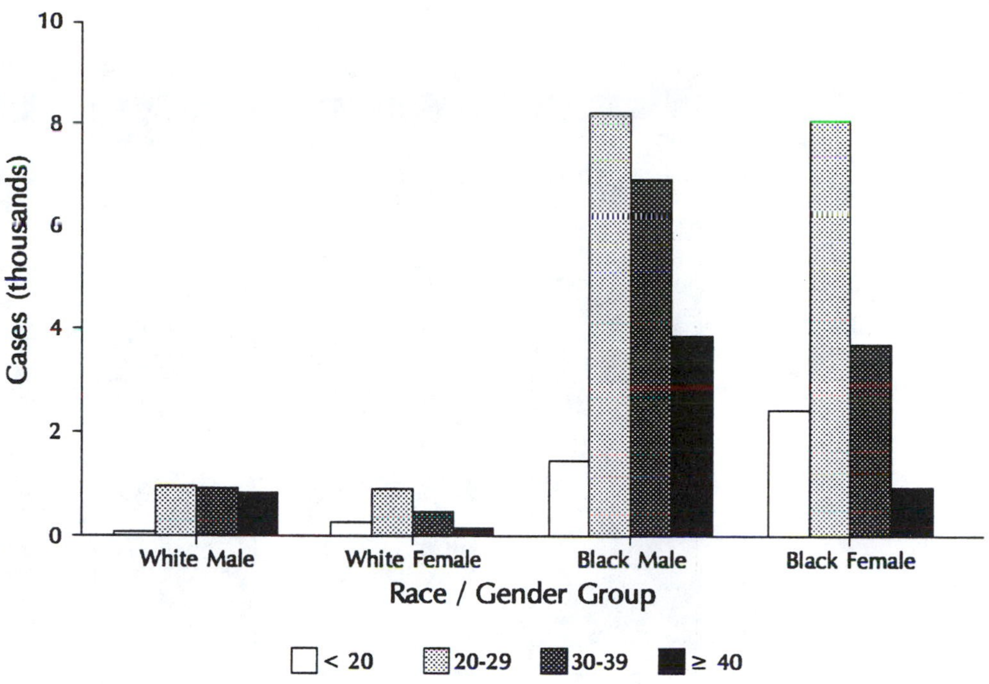

SOURCE: CDC, 1989c.

FIGURE 8.33b *Grouped bar chart: Number of primary and secondary syphilis cases by age, sex, and race, 1989*

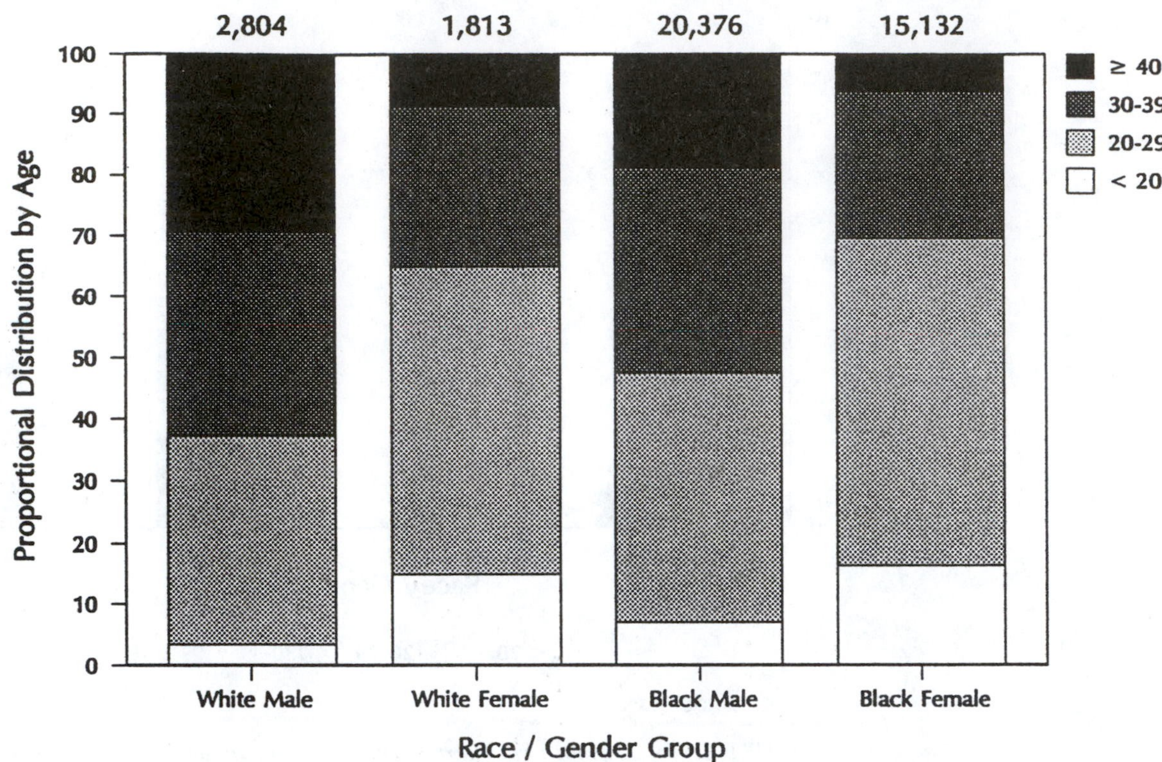

SOURCE: CDC, 1989c.

FIGURE 8.33c *100% component bar chart: Number of primary and secondary syphilis cases by age, sex, and race, 1989*

7.

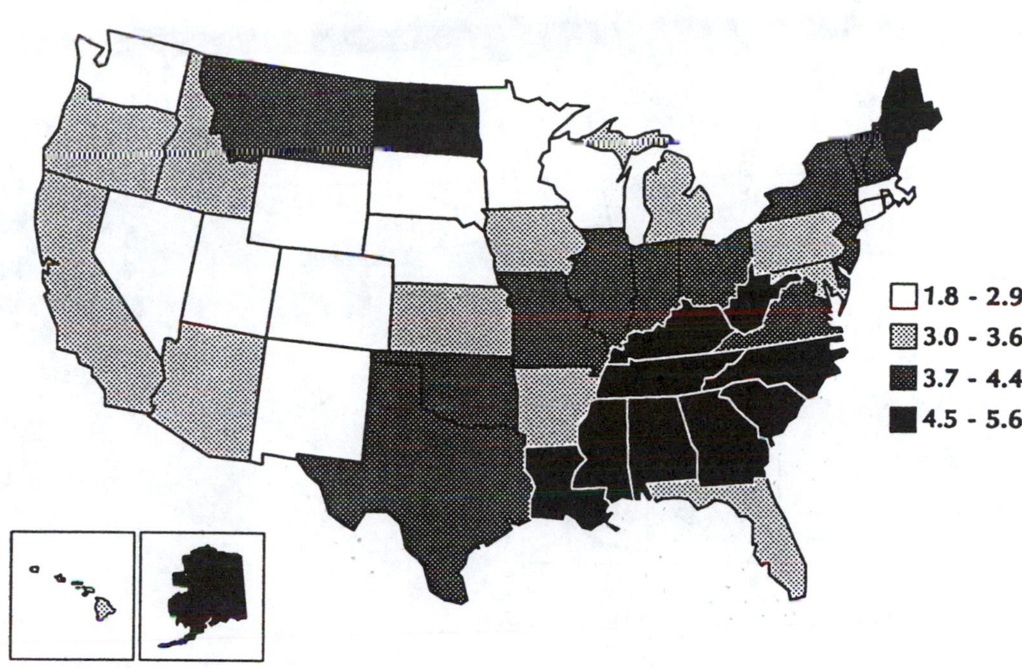

SOURCE: CDC, 1989a.

FIGURE 8.34a *Strategy 1: Mean annual age-adjusted cervical cancer mortality rates per 100,000 population by state, United States, 1984-1986*

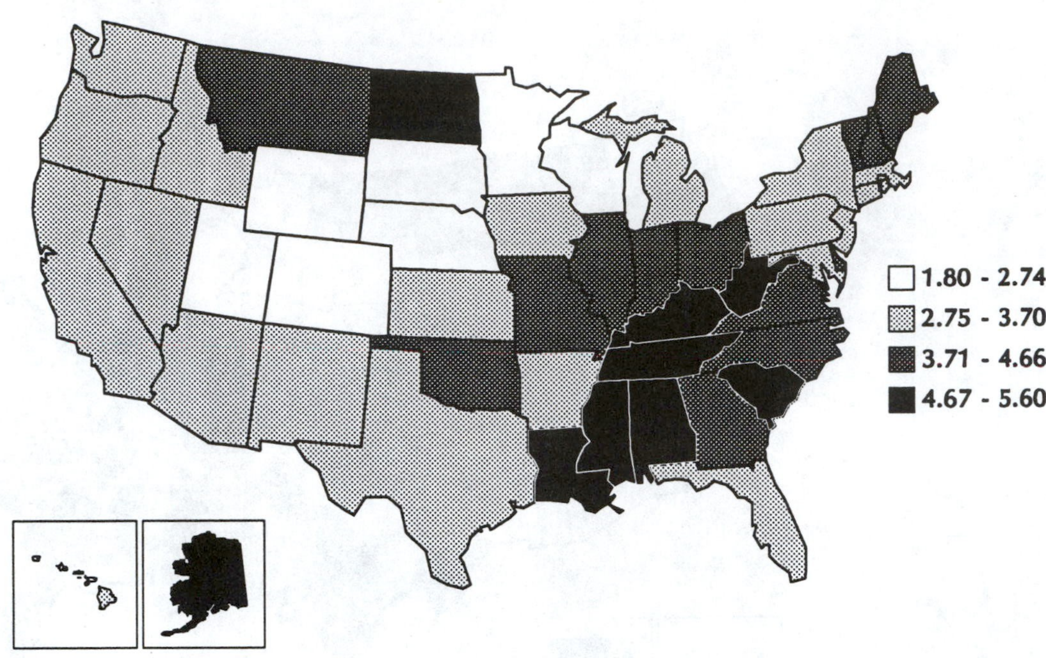

SOURCE: CDC, 1989a.

FIGURE 8.34b *Strategy 2: Mean annual age-adjusted cervical cancer mortality rates per 100,000 population by state, United States, 1984-1986*

9 Investigating an Outbreak

OBJECTIVES

On completion of this chapter, you will be able to:

- List the reasons that health agencies investigate reported outbreaks
- List the steps in the investigation of an outbreak
- Define the terms **cluster**, **outbreak**, **epidemic**
- Given the initial information of a possible disease outbreak, describe how to determine whether an epidemic exists
- State what a line listing is and what it is used for
- Given information about a community outbreak of disease, execute the initial steps of an investigation and develop biologically plausible hypotheses
- Draw a traditional epidemic curve
- Given data in a two-by-two table, calculate the appropriate measure of association and chi-square test

One of the most exciting and challenging tasks facing an epidemiologist working in a public health department is investigating an outbreak. Frequently, the cause and source of the outbreak are unknown. Sometimes large numbers of people are affected. Often, the people in the community are concerned because they feel more people, including themselves, may be stricken unless the cause is found soon. There may be hostilities and defensiveness if an individual, product, or company has been accused of being the cause. Into this pressure-packed situation comes the epidemiologist, sometimes from the local health department, more often from "the outside." In this setting the epidemiologist must remain calm, professional, and scientifically objective. Fortunately, epidemiology provides the scientific basis, the systematic approach, and the population and prevention orientations that are needed.

NOTE: This chapter is adapted from Centers for Disease Control and Prevention: *Principles of epidemiology: An introduction to applied epidemiology and biostatistics*. Atlanta, GA: CDC, 1992.

INTRODUCTION TO INVESTIGATING AN OUTBREAK

Uncovering Outbreaks

One of the uses of surveillance is the detection of outbreaks. Outbreaks may be detected when routine, timely analysis of surveillance data reveals an increase in reported cases or an unusual clustering of cases. In a health department, we may detect increases in or unusual patterns of disease from the weekly tabulations of case reports by time and place or from the examination of the exposure information on the case reports themselves. For example, health department staff detected an outbreak of hepatitis B that was transmitted by a dentist because they regularly reviewed and compared the dental exposures reported for hepatitis B cases (Rimland, Parkin, Miller, and Schrack, 1977). Similarly, in a hospital, weekly analysis of microbiologic isolates from patients by organism and ward may reveal an increased number of apparent nosocomial (hospital-acquired) infections in one part of the hospital.

Nonetheless, most outbreaks come to the attention of health authorities because an alert clinician is concerned enough to call the health department. The nationwide epidemic of eosinophilia-myalgia syndrome (EMS) was first detected when a physician in New Mexico called a consultant in Minnesota and realized that, together, they had seen three patients with a highly unusual clinical presentation. All three patients said they used L-tryptophan. The local physician promptly called the New Mexico State Health and Environment Department, which set into motion a chain of public health actions leading to the recall of L-tryptophan throughout the country (Hertzman et al., 1990; Swygert et al., 1990).

Members of affected groups are another important reporting source for apparent clusters of both infectious and noninfectious disease. For example, someone may call a health department and report that he and several co-workers came down with severe gastroenteritis after attending a banquet several nights earlier. Similarly, a local citizen may call about several cases of cancer diagnosed among his neighbors and express concern that these are more than coincidental. Most health departments have routine procedures for handling calls from the public regarding potential communicable disease outbreaks, and a few states have developed guidelines for how to respond to noninfectious disease cluster reports (Bender et al., 1990; Devier et al., 1990; Fiore et al., 1990).

Why Investigate Possible Outbreaks?

Health departments investigate suspected outbreaks for a variety of reasons. These include the need to institute control and prevention measures; the opportunity for research and training; program considerations; and public relations, political concerns, and legal obligations.

Control/Prevention

The primary public health reason to investigate an outbreak is to control and prevent further disease. Before we can develop control strategies for an

TABLE 9.1 Relative priority of investigative and control efforts during an outbreak, based on level of knowledge of the source, mode of transmission, and causative agent

		Source/Mode of Transmission: Known	Source/Mode of Transmission: Unknown
Causative Agent	Known	Investigation + Control + + +	Investigation + + + Control +
	Unknown	Investigation + + + Control + + +	Investigation + + + Control +

+ + + = highest priority
+ = lower priority

SOURCE: Goodman, Buehler, and Koplan, 1990.

outbreak, however, we must identify where the outbreak is in its natural course: Are cases occurring in increasing numbers or is the outbreak just about over? Our goal will be different depending on the answers to these questions.

If cases are continuing to occur in an outbreak, our goal may be to prevent additional cases. Therefore, the objective of our investigation would be to assess the extent of the outbreak and the size and characteristics of the population at risk in order to design and implement appropriate control measures.

On the other hand, if an outbreak appears to be almost over, our goal may be to prevent outbreaks in the future. In that case, the objective of our investigation is more likely to be to identify factors which contributed to the outbreak in order to design and implement measures that would prevent similar outbreaks in the future.

The balance between control measures versus further investigation depends on how much is known about the cause, the source, and the mode of transmission of the agent (Goodman et al., 1990). Table 9.1 illustrates the relative emphasis as influenced by how much we know about these factors.

If we know little about the source and mode of transmission, as indicated in the right-hand column of the table, we must investigate further before we can design appropriate control measures. In contrast, if we know the source and mode of transmission, as indicated in the left-hand column, control measures can be implemented immediately. However, if we don't know what the agent is, as indicated in the bottom row of the table, we must investigate further to identify the agent.

The public health response to the outbreak of EMS described earlier illustrates this point. Since investigators quickly determined that EMS was associated with the ingestion of L-tryptophan, that product was immediately withdrawn from the market, and persons were warned to avoid taking any they had on hand. However, officials continued the investigation for quite some time until they were certain they had identified the specific contaminant and reason that contamination occurred.

The decisions regarding whether and how extensively to investigate an outbreak are influenced by characteristics of the problem itself: the severity of the illness, the source or mode of transmission, and the availability of prevention and control measures. It is particularly urgent to investigate an outbreak when the disease is severe (serious illness with high risk of hospitalization, complications, or death) and has the potential to affect others unless prompt control measures are taken. For example, in the United States, every case of plague and botulism is investigated immediately to identify and eradicate the source. Cases of syphilis, tuberculosis, and measles are investigated promptly to identify contacts and interrupt further transmission.

Research Opportunities

Another important objective of outbreak investigations is, simply, to gain additional knowledge. Each outbreak may be viewed as an experiment of nature waiting to be analyzed and exploited. Each presents a unique opportunity to study the natural history of the disease in question. For a newly recognized disease, field investigation provides an opportunity to define the natural history—including agent, mode of transmission, and incubation period—and the clinical spectrum of disease. Investigators also attempt to characterize the populations at greatest risk and to identify specific risk factors. Acquiring such information was an important motivation for investigators studying such newly recognized diseases as Legionnaires' disease in Philadelphia in 1976, toxic shock syndrome in 1980, acquired immunodeficiency syndrome in the early 1980s and EMS in 1989.

Even for diseases that are well characterized, an outbreak may provide opportunities to gain additional knowledge by assessing the impact of control measures and the usefulness of new epidemiology and laboratory techniques. For example, an outbreak of measles in a highly immunized community provides a setting for investigators to study vaccine efficacy, the effect of age at vaccination, and the duration of vaccine-induced protection (Hutchins et al., 1990). An outbreak of giardiasis was used to study the appropriateness of a new clinical case definition (Hopkins and Juranek, 1991), while an outbreak of pertussis was used to study the performance of a new culture medium (CDC, 1985).

Training

Investigating an outbreak requires a combination of diplomacy, logical thinking, problem-solving ability, quantitative skills, epidemiologic know-how, and judgment. These skills improve with practice and experience. Thus many investigative teams pair a seasoned epidemiologist with an epidemiologist-in-training. The latter gains valuable on-the-job training and experience while providing assistance in the investigation and control of the outbreak.

Public, Political, or Legal Concerns

Public, political, or legal concerns sometimes override scientific concerns in the decision to conduct and investigation. Increasingly, the public has taken an interest in disease clusters and potential environmental exposures, and has called upon health departments to investigate. Such investigations almost never identify a causal link between exposure and disease (Caldwell, 1990; Schulte et al., 1987). Nevertheless, many health departments have learned that it is essential to be "responsibly responsive" to public concerns, even if the concern has little scientific basis (Bender et al., 1990; Fiore et al., 1990; Neutra, 1990). Thus several states, recognizing their need to be responsive and an opportunity to educate the public, have adopted protocols for investigating disease clusters reported by its citizens. Some investigations are conducted because the law requires an agency to do so. For example, CDC's National Institute of Occupational Safety and Health (NIOSH) is required to evaluate the risks to health and safety in a workplace if requested to do so by three or more workers.

Program Considerations

Many health departments routinely offer a variety of programs to control and prevent illnesses such as tuberculosis, vaccine-preventable diseases, and sexually transmitted diseases. An outbreak of a disease targeted by a public health program may reveal a weakness in that program and an opportunity to change or strengthen the program's efforts. Investigating the causes of an outbreak may identify populations which have been overlooked, failures in the intervention strategy, changes in the agent, or events beyond the scope of the program. By using an outbreak to evaluate the program's effectiveness, program directors can improve the program's future directions and strategies.

STEPS OF AN OUTBREAK INVESTIGATION

In the investigation of an ongoing outbreak, working quickly is essential. Getting the right answer is essential, too. Under such circumstances, epidemiologists find it useful to have a systematic approach to follow, such as the sequence listed in Table 9.2. This approach ensures that the investigation proceeds forward without missing important steps along the way.

The steps described in Table 9.2 are in conceptual order. In practice, however, several steps may be done at the same time, or the circumstances of the outbreak may dictate that a different order be followed. For example, control measures should be implemented as soon as the source and mode of transmission are known, which may be early or late in any particular outbreak investigation.

TABLE 9.2 Steps of an outbreak investigation

1. Prepare for field work
2. Establish the existence of an outbreak
3. Verify the diagnosis
4. Define and identify cases
   a. establish a case definition
   b. identify and count cases
5. Perform descriptive epidemiology
6. Develop hypotheses
7. Evaluate hypotheses
8. As necessary, reconsider/refine hypotheses and execute additional studies
   a. additional epidemiologic studies
   b. other types of studies—laboratory, environmental
9. Implement control and prevention measures
10. Communicate findings

SOURCE: CDC, 1992.

Step 1: Preparing for Field Work

Anyone about to embark on an outbreak investigation should be well prepared before leaving for the field. Preparations can be grouped into three categories: (a) investigation, (b) administration, and (c) consultation. Good preparation in all three categories will facilitate a smooth field experience.

a. *Investigation*
   First, as a field investigator, you must have the appropriate scientific knowledge, supplies, and equipment to carry out the investigation. You should discuss the situation with someone knowledgeable about the disease and about field investigations, and review the applicable literature. You should assemble useful references such as journal articles and sample questionnaires.
   Before leaving for a field investigation, consult laboratory staff to ensure that you take the proper laboratory material and know the proper collection, storage, and transportation techniques. Arrange for a portable computer, dictaphone, camera, and other supplies.
b. *Administration*
   Second, as an investigator, you must pay attention to administrative procedures. In a health agency, you must make travel and other arrangements and get them approved. You may also need to take care of personal matters before you leave, especially if the investigation is likely to be lengthy.
c. *Consultation*
   Third, as an investigator, you must know your expected role in the field. Before departure, all parties should agree on your role, particularly if you are coming from "outside" the local area. For example, are you expected to lead the investigation, provide

consultation to the local staff who will conduct the investigation, or simply lend a hand to the local staff? In addition, you should know who your local contacts will be. Before leaving, you should know when and where you are to meet with local officials and contacts when you arrive in the field.

Step 2: Establishing the Existence of an Outbreak

An **outbreak** or an **epidemic** is the occurrence of more cases of disease than expected in a given area or among a specific group of people over a particular period of time. In contrast, a **cluster** is an aggregation of cases in a given area over a particular period without regard to whether the number of cases is more than expected. In an outbreak or epidemic, we usually presume that the cases are related to one another or that they have a common cause.

Many epidemiologists use the terms "outbreak" and "epidemic" interchangeably, but the public is more likely to think that "epidemic" implies a crisis situation. Some epidemiologists restrict the use of the term "epidemic" to situations involving larger numbers of people over a wide geographic area.

Most outbreaks come to the attention of health departments in one of two ways. One way is by regular analysis of surveillance data. Unusual rises or patterns of disease occurrence can be detected promptly if surveillance data collection and analysis are timely. The second, and probably more common, way is through calls from a health care provider or citizen who knows of "several cases." For example, a member of the public may report three infants born with birth defects within a 1-month period in the same community. This aggregation of cases *seems* to be unusual, but frequently the public does not know the denominator—e.g., the total number of births—or the expected incidence of birth defects.

One of your first tasks as a field investigator is to verify that a purported outbreak is indeed an outbreak. Some will turn out to be true outbreaks with a common cause, some will be sporadic and unrelated cases of the same disease, and others will turn out to be unrelated cases of similar but unrelated diseases. Often, you must first determine the expected number of cases before deciding whether the observed number exceeds the expected number, i.e., whether a cluster is indeed an outbreak.

Thus, as in other areas of epidemiology, you compare the **observed with the expected**. How then, do you determine what's expected? Usually we compare the current number of cases with the number from the previous few weeks or months, or from a comparable period during the previous few years.

- For a notifiable disease, you can use health department surveillance records.
- For other diseases and conditions, you can usually find existing data locally—hospital discharge records, mortality statistics, cancer or birth defect registries.

- If local data are not available, you can apply rates from neighboring states or national data, or, alternatively, you may conduct a telephone survey of physicians to determine whether they have seen more cases of the disease than usual.
- Finally, you may conduct a survey of the community to establish the background or historical level of disease.

Even if the current number of reported cases exceeds the expected number, the excess may not necessarily indicate an outbreak. Reporting may rise because of changes in local reporting procedures, changes in the case definition, increased interest because of local or national awareness, or improvements in diagnostic procedures. A new physician, infection control nurse, or health care facility may see referred cases and more consistently report cases, when in fact there has been no change in the actual occurrence of the disease. Finally, particularly in areas with sudden changes in population size such as resort areas, college towns, and migrant farming areas, changes in the numerator (number of reported cases) may simply reflect changes in the denominator (size of the population).

Whether you should investigate an apparent problem further is not strictly tied to your verifying that an epidemic exists (observed numbers greater than expected). As noted earlier, the severity of the illness, the potential for spread, political considerations, public relations, available resources, and other factors all influence the decision to launch a field investigation.

Step 3: Verifying the Diagnosis

Closely linked to verifying the existence of an outbreak is establishing what disease is occurring. In fact, as an investigator, you frequently will be able to address these two steps at the same time. Your goals in verifying the diagnosis are (a) to ensure that the problem has been properly diagnosed and (b) to rule out laboratory error as the basis for the increase in diagnosed cases.

In verifying the diagnosis you should review the clinical findings and laboratory results. If you have any question about the laboratory findings, i.e., if the laboratory tests are inconsistent with the clinical and epidemiologic findings, you should have a qualified laboratorian review the laboratory techniques being used. If you plan specialized laboratory work such as confirmation in a reference laboratory, DNA or other chemical or biological fingerprinting, or polymerase chain reaction, you must secure the appropriate specimens, isolates, and other laboratory material as soon as possible, and from a sufficient number of patients.

You should always summarize the clinical findings with frequency distributions. Such frequency distributions are useful in characterizing the spectrum of illness, verifying the diagnosis, and developing case definitions. Many investigators consider these clinical frequency distributions so important that they routinely present these findings in the first table of their report or manuscript.

Finally, you should visit several patients with the disease. If you do not have the clinical background to verify the diagnosis, a qualified clinician should do so. Nevertheless, regardless of background, you should see and talk to some patients to gain a better understanding of the clinical features, and to develop a mental image of the disease and the patients affected by it. In addition, you may be able to gather critical information from these patients: What were their exposures before becoming ill? What do *they* think caused their illness? Do they know anyone else with the disease? Do they have anything in common with others who have the disease? Conversations with patients are very helpful in generating hypotheses about disease etiology and spread.

Step 4a: Establishing a Case Definition

Your next task as an investigator is to establish a case definition. A case definition is a standard set of criteria for deciding whether an individual should be classified as having the health condition of interest. A case definition includes clinical criteria and—particularly in the setting of an outbreak investigation—restrictions by time, place, and person. You should base the clinical criteria on simple and objective measures such as elevated antibody titers, fever ≥101°F, three or more loose bowel movements per day, or myalgias severe enough to limit the patient's usual activities. You may restrict the case definition by time (for example, to persons with onset of illness within the past 2 months), by place (for example, to residents of the nine-county area or to employees of a particular plant) and by person (for example, to persons with no previous history of musculo-skeletal disease, or to pre-menopausal women). Whatever your criteria, you must apply them consistently and without bias to all persons under investigation.

Be careful that the case definition does not include an exposure or risk factor you want to test. This is a common mistake. For example, do not define a case as "illness X among persons who were in homeless shelter Y" if one of the goals of the investigation is to determine whether the shelter is associated with illness.

Ideally, your case definition will include most if not all of the actual cases, but very few or none of what are called "false-positive" cases (persons who actually do not have the disease in question but nonetheless meet the case definition). Recognizing the uncertainty of some diagnoses, investigators often classify cases as confirmed, probable, or possible.

To be classified as confirmed, a case usually must have laboratory verification. A case classified as probable usually has typical clinical features of the disease without laboratory confirmation. A case classified as possible usually has fewer of the typical clinical features. For example, in an outbreak of bloody diarrhea and hemolytic-uremic syndrome caused by infection with *E. coli* O157:H7, investigators defined cases in the following three classes:

- **Definite** case: *E. coli* O157:H7 isolated from a stool culture or development of hemolytic-uremic syndrome in a school-age child resident of the county with gastrointestinal symptoms beginning between November 3 and November 8, 1990
- **Probable** case: Bloody diarrhea, with the same person, place, and time restrictions
- **Possible** case: Abdominal cramps and diarrhea (at least three stools in a 24-hour period) in a school-age child with onset during the same period (CDC, unpublished data, 1991)

As an investigator, you will find such classifications useful in several situations. First, they will allow you to keep track of a case even if the diagnosis is not confirmed. For example, you might temporarily classify a case as probable or possible while laboratory results are pending. Alternatively, the patient's physician or you may have decided not to order the laboratory test required to confirm the diagnosis because the test is expensive, difficult to obtain, or unnecessary. For example, during a community outbreak of measles, which has a characteristic clinical picture, investigators might follow the usual practice of confirming only a few cases and then relying on clinical features to identify the rest of the cases. Similarly, while investigating an outbreak of diarrhea on a cruise ship, investigators usually try to identify an agent from stool samples from a few afflicted persons. If those few cases are confirmed to be infected with the same agent, the other persons with compatible clinical illness are all presumed to be part of the same outbreak.

Early in an investigation, investigators often use a sensitive or "loose" case definition which includes confirmed, probable, and even possible cases. Later on, when hypotheses have come into sharper focus, the investigator may "tighten" the case definition by dropping the possible category. You will find this is a useful strategy in investigations that require you to travel to different hospitals, homes, or other sites to gather information, because it is better to collect extra data while you're there than to have to go back. This illustrates an important axiom of field epidemiology: "Get it while you can."

A "loose" case definition is used early in the investigation to identify the extent of the problem and the populations affected. Important hypotheses may arise from this process. However, in analytic epidemiology, inclusion of false-positive cases can produce misleading results. Therefore, to test these hypotheses using analytic epidemiology, specific or "tight" case definitions must be used.

Step 4b: Identifying and Counting Cases

As noted earlier, many outbreaks are brought to the attention of health authorities by concerned health care providers or citizens. However, the cases which prompted the concern are often only a small and nonrepresentative fraction of the total number of cases. Public health workers must therefore "cast the net wide" to determine the geographic extent of the problem and the populations affected by it.

When you need to identify cases, use as many sources as you can. You may have to be creative, aggressive, and diligent in identifying these sources. Your methods for identifying cases must be appropriate for the setting and disease in question.

First, direct your case finding at health care facilities where the diagnosis is likely to be made: physicians' offices, clinics, hospitals, and laboratories. If you send out a letter describing the situation and asking for reports, that is called "stimulated or enhanced passive surveillance." Alternatively, if you telephone or visit the facilities to collect information on cases, that is called "active surveillance."

In some outbreaks, public health officials may decide to alert the public directly, usually through the local media. For example, in outbreaks caused by a contaminated food product such as salmonellosis caused by contaminated milk (Ryan et al., 1987) or L-tryptophan-induced EMS (Hertzman et al., 1990) announcements in the media alerted the public to avoid the implicated product and to see a physician if they had symptoms compatible with the disease in question.

If an outbreak affects a restricted population, such as on a cruise ship, in a school, or at a worksite, and if a high proportion of cases are unlikely to be diagnosed (if, for example, many cases are mild or asymptomatic), you may want to conduct a survey of the entire population. You could administer a questionnaire to determine the true occurrence of clinical symptoms, or you could collect laboratory specimens to determine the number of asymptomatic cases.

Finally, you can ask case-patients if they know anyone else with the same condition. Frequently, one person with an illness knows or hears of others with the same illness.

Regardless of the particular disease you are investigating, you should collect the following types of information about every case:

- identifying information
- demographic information
- clinical information
- risk factor information
- reporter information

Identifying information—name, address, and telephone number—allows you and other investigators to contact patients for additional questions, and to notify them of laboratory results and the outcome of the investigation. Names will help you in checking for duplicate records, while the addresses allow you to map the geographic extent of the problem.

Demographic information—age, sex, race, and occupation—provides the "person" characteristics of descriptive epidemiology you need to characterize the populations at risk.

Line Listing of reported suspect cases, page 1

Case #	Initials	Date of Report	Date of Onset	Diagnostic							Lab		Age	Sex
				MD Dx	Signs and Symptoms									
					N	V	A	F	DU	J	HA IgM	Other		
1	JG	10/12	10/6	Hep A	+	+	+	+	+	+	+	SGOT↑	37	M
2	BC	10/12	10/5	Hep A	+	–	+	+	+	+	+	ALT ↑	62	F
3	HP	10/13	10/4	Hep A	±	–	+	+	+	S*	+	SGOT↑	30	F
4	MC	10/15	10/4	Hep A	–	–	+	+	?	–	+	HBs Ag-	17	F
5	NG	10/15	10/9	NA	–	–	+	–	+	+	NA	NA	32	F
6	RD	10/15	10/8	Hep A	+	+	+	+	+	+	+		38	M
7	KR	10/16	10/13	Hep A	±	–	+	+	+	+	+	SGOT= 240	43	M
8	DM	10/16	10/12	Hep A	–	–	+	+	+	–	+		57	M
9	PA	10/18	10/7	Hep A	±	–	+	±	+	+	+		52	F
10	SS	10/11	10/11	r/o Hep A Hep [illegible]	+	+	+	[illegible]	+	–	pending	hbsAg [illegible]	[illegible]	[illegible]

S* = scleral
N = nausea
V = vomiting
A = anorexia
F = fever
DU = dark urine
J = jaundice
HA IgM = hepatitis A IgM antibody test

SOURCE: CDC, 1992.

FIGURE 9.1 *Example of line listing for an outbreak of hepatitis A*

Clinical information allows you to verify that the case definition has been met. Date of onset allows you to chart the time course of the outbreak. Supplementary clinical information, including whether hospitalization or death occurred, will help you describe the spectrum of illness.

You must tailor risk factor information to the specific disease in question. For example, in an investigation of hepatitis A, you would ascertain exposure to food and water sources.

Finally, by identifying the person who provided the case report, you will be able to seek additional clinical information or report back the results of your investigation.

Traditionally, we collect the information described above on a standard case report form, questionnaire, or data abstraction form. We then abstract selected critical items on a form called a line listing. An example of a line listing is shown in Figure 9.1.

In a line listing, each column represents an important variable, such as name or identification number, age, sex, case classification, etc., while each row represents a different case. New cases are added to a line listing as they are identified. Thus, a line listing contains key information on every case, and can be scanned and updated as necessary. Even in the era of microcomputers, many epidemiologists still maintain a handwritten line listing of key data items, and turn to their computers for more complex manipulations, cross-tabulations, and the like.

Step 5: Performing Descriptive Epidemiology

Once you have collected some data, you can begin to characterize an outbreak by time, place, and person. In fact, you may wind up performing this step several times during the course of an outbreak. Characterizing an outbreak by these variables is called **descriptive epidemiology**, because you describe what has occurred in the population under study. This step is critical for several reasons. First, by looking at the data carefully, you become familiar with them. You can learn what information is reliable and informative (such as if many cases report the same unusual exposure) and learn what may not be as reliable (for example, many missing or "don't know" responses to a particular question). Second, you provide a comprehensive description of an outbreak by portraying its trend over time, its geographic extent (place), and the populations (persons) affected by the disease. You can assess your description of the outbreak in light of what is known about the disease (usual source, mode of transmission, risk factors and populations affected, etc.) to develop causal hypotheses. You can, in turn, test these hypotheses using the techniques of analytic epidemiology, described under Step 7.

Note that you should begin descriptive epidemiology early, and should update it as you collect additional data. To keep an investigation moving quickly and in the right direction, you must discover both errors and clues in the data as early as possible.

Time

Traditionally, we depict the time course of an epidemic by drawing a histogram of the number of cases by their date of onset. This graph, called an **epidemic curve**, or **epi curve** for short, gives us a simple visual display of the outbreak's magnitude and time trend. Figure 9.2 shows a typical epidemic curve. This visual display can be understood by both epidemiologists and nonepidemiologists alike.

An epidemic curve will provide you with a great deal of information about an epidemic. First, you will usually be able to tell where you are in the time course of an epidemic, and what the future course might be. Second, if you have identified the disease and know its usual incubation period, you usually can deduce a probable time period of exposure and can develop a questionnaire focusing on that time period. Finally, you may be able to draw inferences about the epidemic pattern—whether it is common source or propagated, or both. For a review of epidemic patterns see Chapter 1.

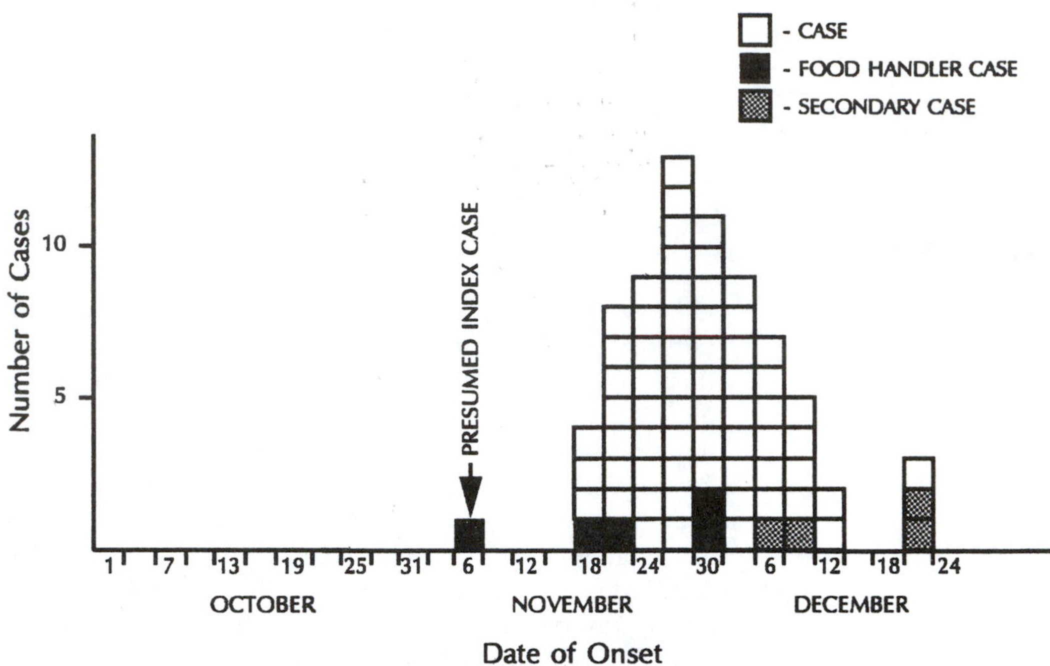

SOURCE: CDC, unpublished data, 1978.

FIGURE 9.2 *Typical epidemic curve: Hepatitis A cases by date of onset, Fayetteville, Arkansas, November-December 1978*

How to Draw an Epidemic Curve To draw an epidemic curve, you first must know the time of onset of illness for each case. For most diseases, date of onset is sufficient; for a disease with a very short incubation period, hours of onset may be more suitable.

Next, select the unit of time on the x-axis. We usually base these units on the incubation period of the disease (if known) and the length of time over which cases are distributed. As a rule of thumb, select a unit that is one-eighth to one-third, i.e., roughly one-quarter as long as the incubation period. Thus, for an outbreak of *Clostridium perfringens* food poisoning (usual incubation period 10 to 12 hours), with cases confined to a few days, you could use an x-axis unit of 2 or 3 hours. Unfortunately, we often need to draw an epidemic curve when we don't know the disease and/or its incubation time. In that circumstance, it is useful to draw several epidemic curves with different units on the x-axis to find one that seems to portray the data best. For example, Figure 9.3 shows an epidemic curve of the same data as in Figure 9.2; in Figure 9.2 the x-axis unit is 3 days and in Figure 9.3 the x-axis unit is 6 days. Which unit seems to provide the most useful information about the course of the epidemic?

The units used for the x-axis in Figures 9.2 and 9.3 are both useful. They both demonstrate a point-source epidemic. The unit selected for Figure 9.2 is preferred because (1) it distributes the cases more clearly, and (2) it separates out the presumed index case more clearly.

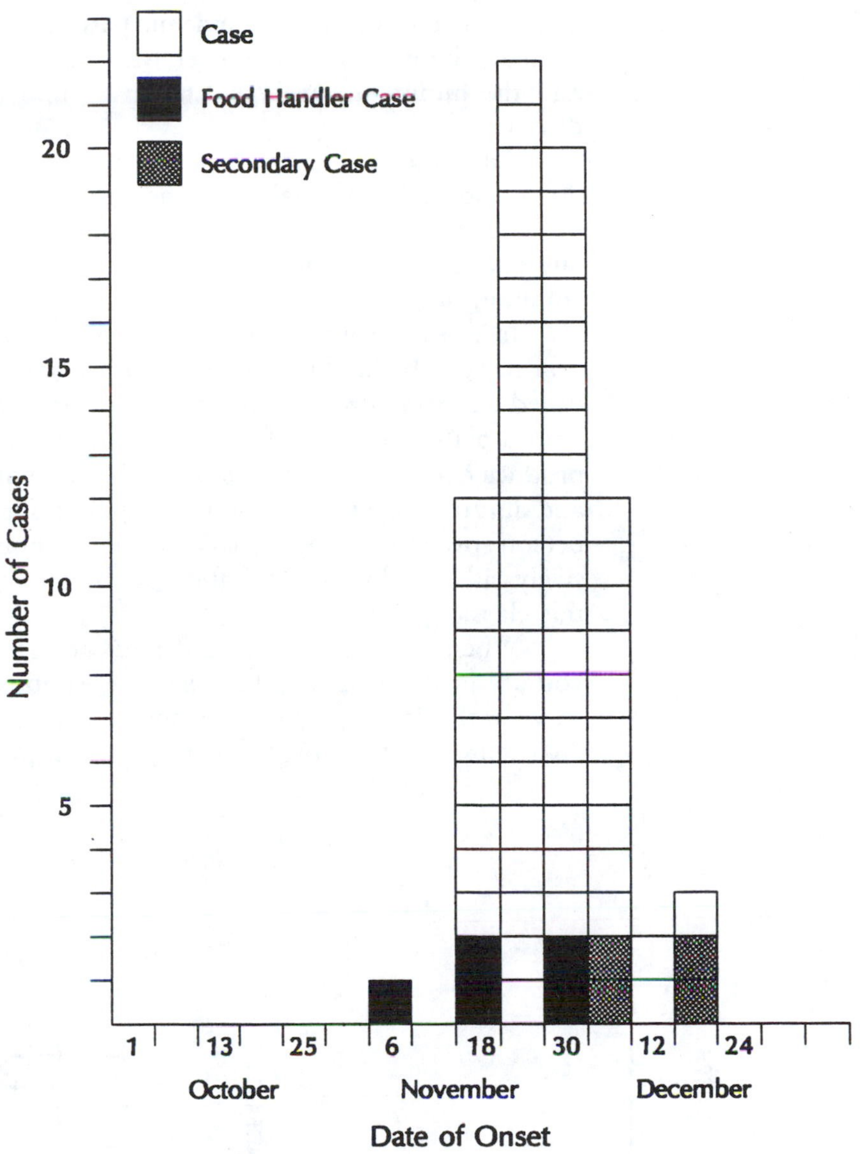

SOURCE: CDC, unpublished data, 1978

FIGURE 9.3 *Epidemic curve with different units on x-axis: Hepatitis A cases by date of onset, Fayetteville, Arkansas, November-December 1978*

Finally, show the pre-epidemic period on your graph to illustrate the background or "expected" number of cases. (Remember, an epidemic is defined as more cases than expected.) For a disease with a human host, such as hepatitis A, one of the early cases may be a foodhandler who is the source of the epidemic! Notice that both figures 9.2 and 9.3 show a relatively long pre-epidemic period.

Interpreting an Epidemic Curve The first step in interpreting an epidemic curve is to consider its overall shape. The shape of the epidemic curve is determined by the epidemic pattern (common source versus propagated), the period of time over which susceptible persons are exposed, and the minimum, average, and maximum incubation periods for the disease.

An epidemic curve which has a steep upslope and a more gradual downslope (a log-normal curve) indicates a **point source** epidemic in which persons are exposed to the same source over a relative brief period. In fact, any sudden rise in the number of cases suggests sudden exposure to a common source.

In a point source epidemic, all the cases occur within one incubation period. If the duration of exposure was prolonged, the epidemic is called a **continuous common source** epidemic, and the epidemic curve will have a plateau instead of a peak. Intermittent common source epidemics produce irregularly jagged epidemic curves which reflect the intermittency and duration of exposure, and the number of persons exposed. Person-to-person spread—a **propagated** epidemic—should have a series of progressively taller peaks one incubation period apart, but in reality few produce this classic pattern.

When you examine an epidemic curve, you should determine where you are in the epidemic. For example, suppose you plotted an epidemic curve of the data in Figure 9.4 when you had only data through November 26—that is, only through point A. At that point, it should seem clear to

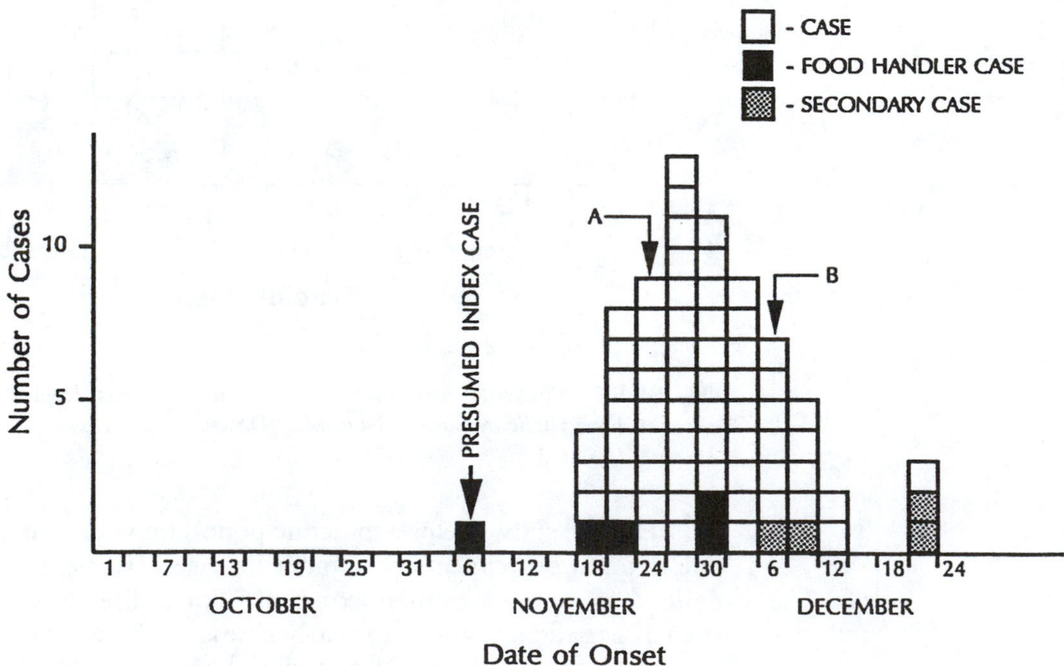

SOURCE: CDC, 1992.

FIGURE 9.4 *Typical epidemic curve with point A on upslope and point B on downslope*

you that the outbreak is still on the upswing, and you could safely predict that new cases would continue to occur. On the other hand, if you plotted an epidemic curve using the data through point B, you should realize that the outbreak has peaked and may soon be over, although, depending on the disease, a few late or secondary cases might still occur.

The cases that stand apart may be just as informative as the overall pattern. An early case may represent a background or unrelated case, a source of the epidemic, or a person who was exposed earlier than most of the cases (the cook who tasted her dish hours before bringing it to the big picnic!). Similarly, late cases may represent unrelated cases, long-incubation-period cases, secondary cases, or persons exposed later than most of the cases. On the other hand, these outliers sometimes represent miscoded or erroneous data. All outliers are worth examining carefully because if they are part of the outbreak, their unusual exposures may point directly to the source.

In a point-source epidemic of a known disease with a known incubation period, you can use the epidemic curve to identify a likely period of exposure. This is critical to asking the right questions to identify the source of the epidemic.

To identify the likely period of exposure from an epidemic curve,

1. Look up the average and minimum incubation periods of the disease. This information can be found in *Control of Communicable Diseases in Man* (Benenson, 1990).
2. Identify the peak of the outbreak or the median case and count back on the x-axis one average incubation period. Note the date.
3. Start at the earliest case of the epidemic and count back the minimum incubation period, and note this date as well.

Ideally, the two dates are similar, and represent the probable period of exposure. This technique is not precise, however, and you usually should widen the period of exposure by 10–20% on either side of these dates. You should then ask about exposures during the wider period in an attempt to identify the source.

For example, consider the outbreak of hepatitis A illustrated by the epidemic curve in Figure 9.5. The incubation period for hepatitis A ranges from 15 to 50 days, with an average incubation period of 28 to 30 days (roughly one month). First, is this epidemic curve consistent with a point source? That is, do all 48 cases fall within one incubation period?

The epidemic *is* consistent with a point source because the last case is within 35 days (50 − 15) of the first case. Therefore, we can use the epidemic curve to identify the likely period of exposure by making the following determinations:

1. What is the peak of the outbreak or the median date of onset?

   The peak of the outbreak occurred during the 4-day interval beginning on October 28. The median date of onset of the 48 cases

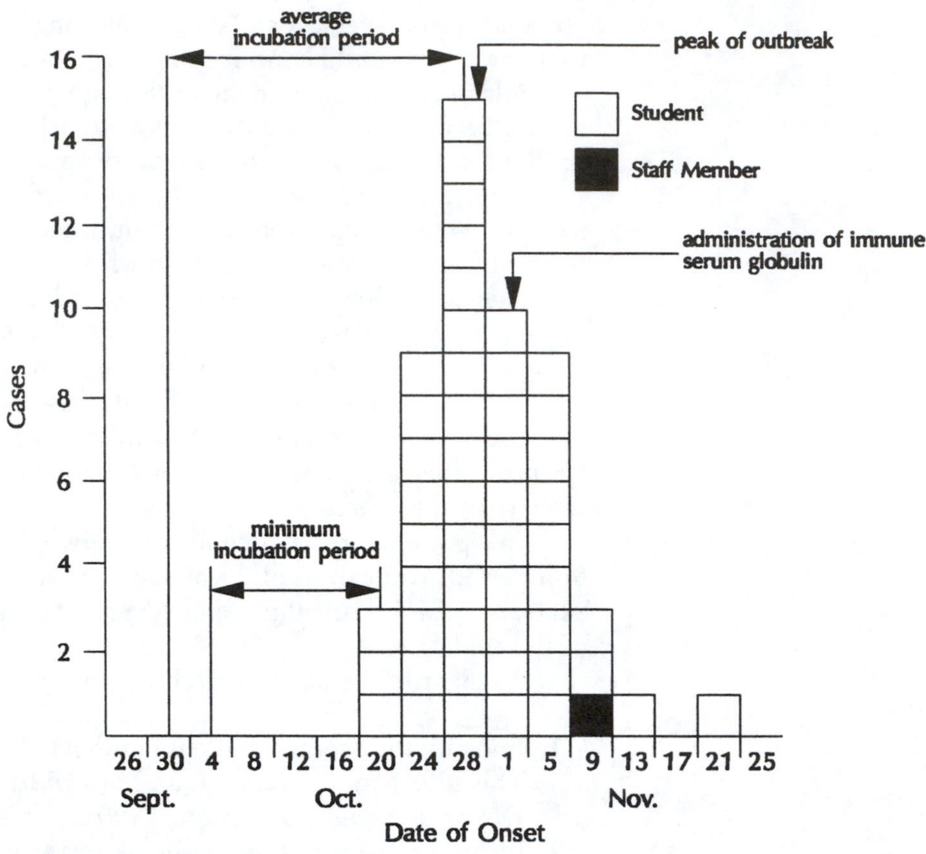

SOURCE: CDC, 1992.

FIGURE 9.5 *Hepatitis A cases in Colbert County, Alabama, October-November 1972*

lies between the 24th and 25th case. Both of these occurred during the same 4-day period.

2. What would be the beginning of one average incubation period prior to the peak (median date) of the outbreak?

   Since the interval containing both the peak and the median of the outbreak includes the last four days of October, one month earlier would fall during the last few days of September.

3. What would be the beginning of one minimum incubation period before the first case?

   The earliest case occurred on October 20. Subtracting 15 days from October 20 points us to October 5.

Thus we would look for exposures around the end of September and the beginning of October. This turned out to be the exact period during which there had been a temporary lapse in chlorination of the school's water supply (Caldwell, 1990)!

Place

Assessment of an outbreak by place not only provides information on the geographic extent of a problem, but may also demonstrate clusters or patterns that provide important etiologic clues. A spot map is a simple and useful technique for illustrating where cases live, work, or may have been exposed.

On a spot map of a community, clusters or patterns may reflect water supplies, wind currents, or proximity to a restaurant or grocery. In Figure 9.6, for example, the homes of patients with Legionnaires' disease are shown in relation to the cooling tower at plant A (Addiss et al., 1989).

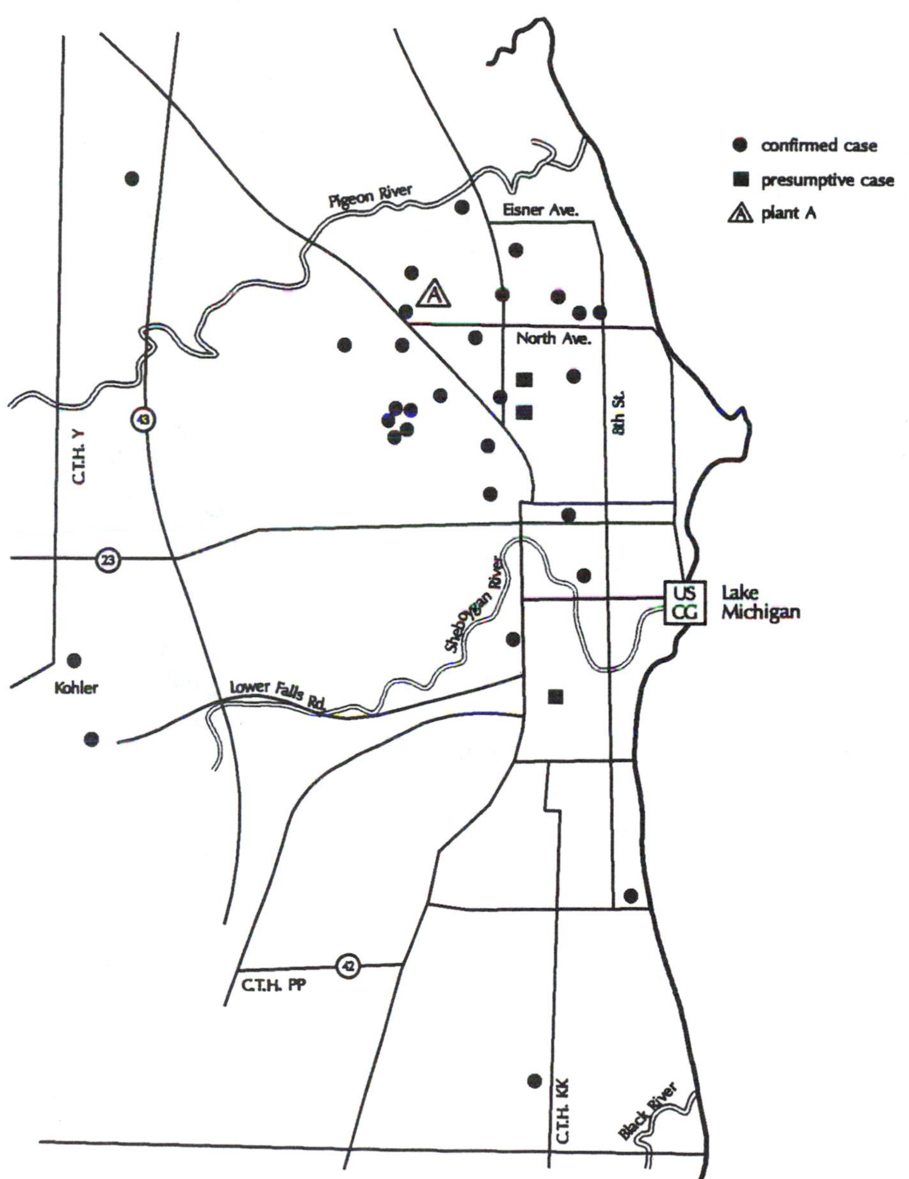

SOURCE: Addiss et al., 1989.

FIGURE 9.6 *Residence of patients with Legionnaires' disease, Sheboygan, Wisconsin, 1986*

On a spot map of a hospital, nursing home, or other such facility, clustering is consistent with either a focal source or person-to-person spread, while scattering of cases throughout the facility is more consistent with a widely disseminated vehicle or a source common to the residents that is not associated with room assignment, such as a common dining hall.

Although we often use spot maps to plot location of residence, place of work is sometimes more revealing. Certainly, place of work is important is assessing "sick building syndrome" and other disorders related to airflow patterns in buildings. In studying an outbreak of surgical wound infections in a hospital, we might plot cases by operating room, recovery room, and ward room to look for clustering. We can even use maps to plot recreational opportunities. For example, Figure 9.7 shows persons with shigellosis plotted by where they swam in the Mississippi River (Rosenberg et al., 1976).

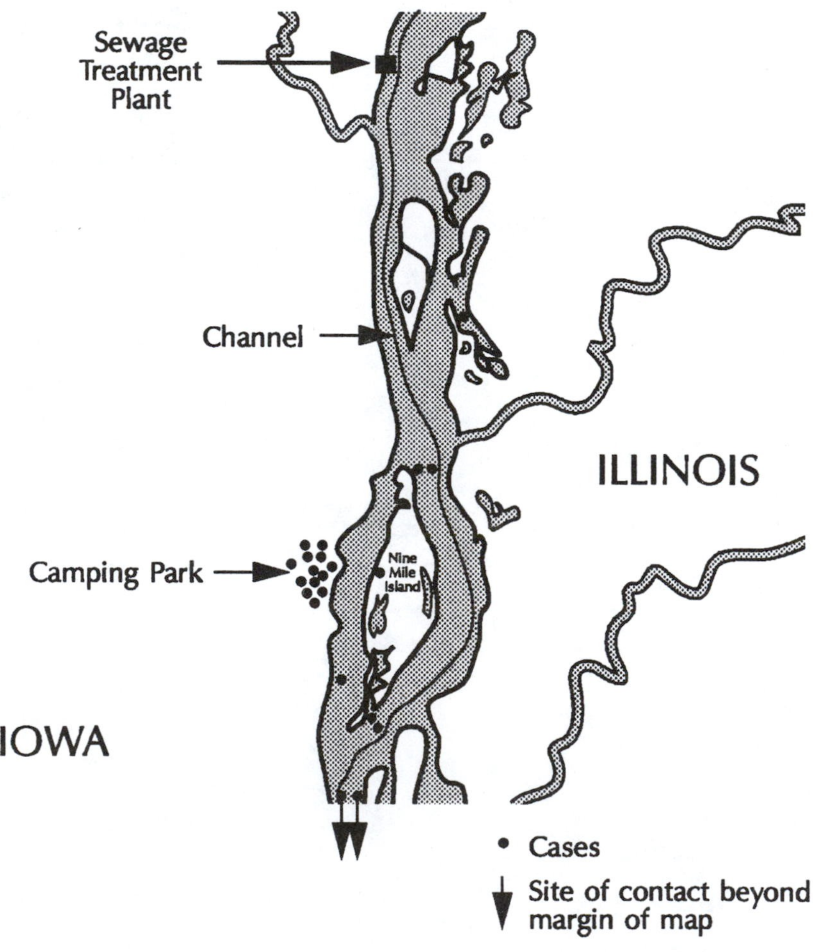

SOURCE: Rosenberg et al., 1976. Reprinted by permission; © 1976, American Medical Association.

FIGURE 9.7 *Mississippi River sites where 22 culture-positive cases swam within three days of onset of illness*

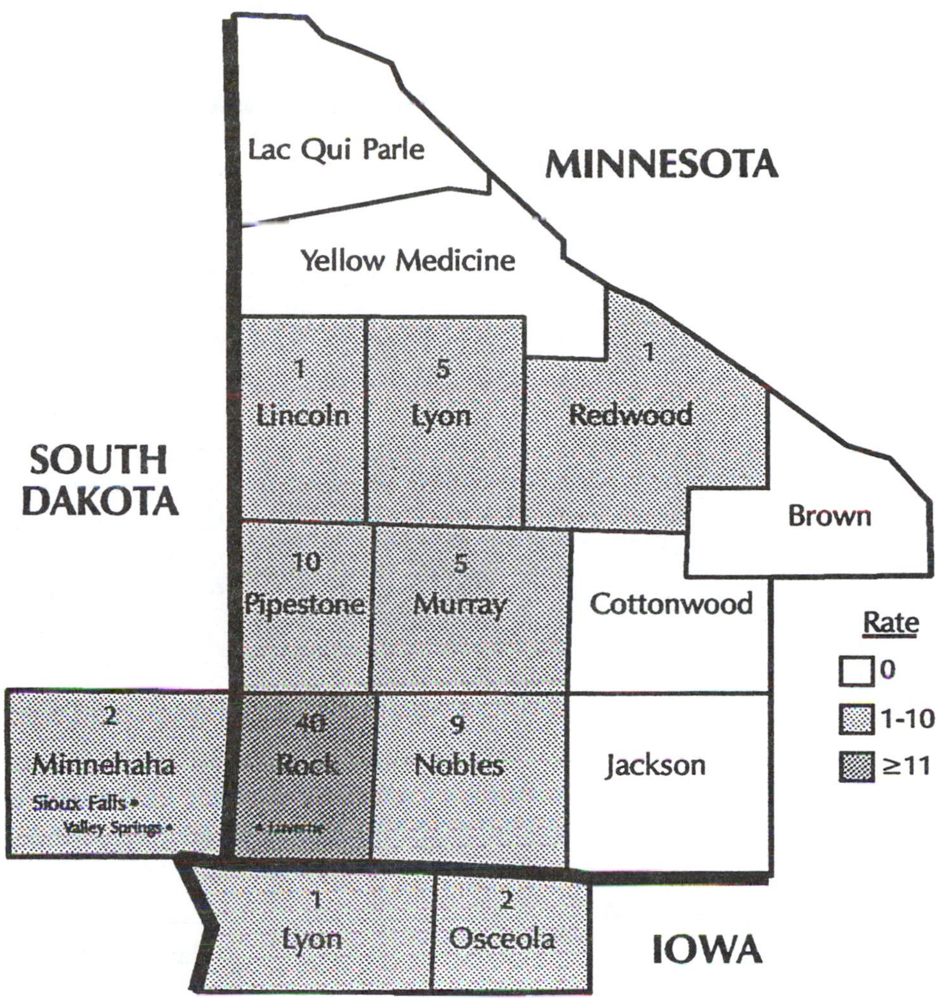

SOURCE: Hedberg et al., 1987.

FIGURE 9.8 *Rate per 10,000 persons of thyrotoxicosis by county, Minnesota, South Dakota, and Iowa, February 1984-August 1985*

If the size of the population varies between the areas you are comparing, a spot map—which shows *numbers of cases*—can be misleading. This is a weakness of spot maps. In such an instance, you should show area-specific attack rates with an area map. For example, Figure 9.8 is an area map that shows county-specific attack rates of thyrotoxicosis in 15 counties near the junction of Minnesota, South Dakota, and Iowa (Hedberg et al., 1987). If we had used a spot map to plot cases rather than rates, we might have misinterpreted the risk among Minnehaha residents. Seventeen residents of that county were affected, exceeded only by Rock County (43) and Nobles County (20). But because the population of Minnehaha is much larger than the population of the other counties, the risk was actually fairly low. Since this outbreak crosses state lines, it alerts us to maintain broad perspective and not restrict our thinking to artificial geopolitical boundaries.

Person

Characterizing an outbreak by person is how we determine what populations are at risk for the disease. We usually define such populations by host characteristics (age, race, sex, or medical status) or by exposures (occupation, leisure activities, use of medications, tobacco, drugs). Both of these influence susceptibility to disease and opportunities for exposure. As described in Chapter 2, we use rates to identify high-risk groups. In order to calculate rates, we must first have both numerators (numbers of cases) and denominators (number of people at risk).

Usually, age and sex are the two host factors we assess first, because they are often the person characteristics most strongly related to exposure and to the risk of disease. The categories used for age and sex in a frequency distribution should be appropriate for the particular disease and should match the available denominator data.

In many outbreaks, occupation is another important person characteristic. Although we like to calculate rates, it may be difficult to get denominator data for occupation. Nonetheless, the distribution of the cases themselves may suggest hypotheses worth pursuing.

Other person characteristics to analyze will be more specific to the disease under investigation and the setting of the outbreak. For example, if you were investigating an outbreak of hepatitis B, you should consider the usual high-risk exposures for that infection, such as intravenous drug use, sexual contacts, and health care employment. You might characterize an outbreak centered in a school by grade or classroom, and by student versus teacher or other staff.

Summarizing by Time, Place, and Person

After characterizing an outbreak by time, place, and person, it is useful to summarize what you know. For example, during an investigation of a different outbreak of Legionnaires' disease, this time in Louisiana, members of the investigative team discussed what they knew based on the descriptive epidemiology (CDC, 1989). Specifically, the epidemic curve indicated that the outbreak was basically over; no new case had been reported in the last two weeks. The affected population had a greater proportion of persons who were black, female, young, and less likely to smoke than persons in the usual Legionnaires' outbreak. There appeared to be no clustering by either residence or worksite, and no connection with exposure to the town's cooling towers. Thus the investigators were forced to develop new hypotheses about a source of Legionnaires' disease to explain this outbreak.

Step 6: Developing Hypotheses

The next conceptual step in an investigation is formulating hypotheses. However, in reality we usually begin to generate hypotheses with the first phone call. But at this point in an investigation, after talking with some case-patients and with local public health officials, and having characterized the outbreak by time, place, and person, our hypotheses will be sharpened and more accurately focused. The hypotheses should address the source of the agent, the mode (and vehicle or vector) of transmission, and the exposures that caused the disease. Also, the hypotheses should be testable, since evaluating hypotheses is one of the goals of the next step in an investigation.

You can generate hypotheses in a variety of ways. First, consider what you know about the disease itself: What is the agent's usual reservoir? How is it usually transmitted? What vehicles are commonly implicated? What are the known risk factors? In other words, simply by becoming familiar with the disease, you can, at the very least, "round up the usual suspects."

Another useful way you can generate hypotheses is to talk to a few of the case-patients, as discussed under "Step 3: Verifying the Diagnosis." Your conversations about possible exposures should be open-ended and wide-ranging, not necessarily confined to the known sources and vehicles. In some difficult investigations which yielded few clues, investigators have convened a meeting of several case-patients to search for common exposures. In addition, investigators have sometimes found it useful to visit the homes of case-patients and look through their refrigerators and shelves for clues.

Just as case-patients may have important insights into causes, so too may the local health department staff. The local staff know the people in the community and their practices, and often have hypotheses based on their knowledge.

The descriptive epidemiology often provides some hypotheses. If the epidemic curve points to a narrow period of exposure, what events occurred around that time? Why do the people living in a particular area have the highest attack rates? Why are some groups with particular age, sex, or other person characteristics at greater risk than other groups with different person characteristics? Such questions about the data should lead to hypotheses which can be tested by appropriate analytic techniques.

As noted earlier, outliers also can provide important clues. In the outbreak of thyrotoxicosis presented in Figure 9.8, most cases came from Luverne, Minnesota, and the surrounding areas. Only one case was identified in Sioux Falls, South Dakota, 60 miles away. Did this person ever go to Luverne? *Yes*. Was she a friend or acquaintance of any of the Luverne cases? *Not really*. What does she do when she goes to Luverne? *Visit my father and buy the locally produced ground beef that he sells in his store*. Aha! The hypothesis that the locally produced ground beef was the vehicle could easily be tested by asking cases and noncases whether they ate ground beef from the same source. Cases did, noncases didn't (Hedberg et al., 1987).

Step 7: Evaluating Hypotheses

The step after developing hypotheses to explain an outbreak is evaluating the credibility of those hypotheses. In a field investigation, you can evaluate hypotheses in one of two ways: either by comparing the hypotheses with the established facts, or by using analytic epidemiology to quantify relationships and explore the role of chance.

You would use the first method when the clinical, laboratory, environmental, and/or epidemilogic evidence so obviously supports the hypotheses that formal hypothesis testing is unnecessary. For example, in an outbreak of hypervitaminosis D that occurred in Massachusetts in 1991 it was found that all of the case-patients drank milk delivered to their homes by a local dairy. Therefore, investigators hypothesized that the dairy was the source and the milk was the vehicle. When they visited the dairy, they quickly recognized that the dairy was inadvertently adding far more than the recommended dose of vitamin D to the milk. No analytic epidemiology was really necessary to evaluate the basic hypotheses in this setting (CDC, unpublished data, 1991).

In many other settings, however, the circumstances are not as straightforward. In those instances, you should use **analytic epidemiology** to test your hypotheses. The key feature of analytic epidemiology is a comparison group. With a comparison group, you are able to quantify relationships between exposures and disease, and to test hypotheses about causal relationships. Careful analysis of the series of cases is insufficient for these purposes; a comparison group is essential. You can use comparison groups in two types of studies: cohort and case-control.

Cohort Studies

A cohort study is the best technique for an outbreak in a small, well-defined population. For example, you would use a cohort study if an outbreak of gastroenteritis occurred among persons who attended a wedding and a complete list of wedding guests was available.

In this situation, you would contact each attendee and ask a series of questions. You would determine not only whether the attendee had become ill (and met whatever case definition you had developed), but also what foods and drinks he/she had consumed. You might even try to quantify how much of each item he/she had consumed.

After collecting similar information from each attendee, you would be able to calculate an attack rate for those who ate a particular item and an attack rate for those who did not eat that item. Generally, you should look for three characteristics:

1. The attack rate is high among those exposed to the item
2. The attack rate is low among those not exposed, so the difference or ratio between attack rates is high
3. Most of the cases were exposed, so that the exposure could "explain" most, if not all, of the cases

You could, in addition, compute the ratio of these attack rates. Such a ratio is called a **relative risk**, and is a measure of the association between exposure (the food item) and disease. You could also compute a chi-square

TABLE 9.3 Attack rates by items served at the church supper, Oswego, New York, April 1940

	Number of Persons Who Ate Specified Item				Number of Persons Who Did Not Eat Specified Item			
	Ill	*Well*	*Total*	*Attack Rate (%)*	*Ill*	*Well*	*Total*	*Attack Rate (%)*
Baked ham	29	17	46	63	17	12	29	59
Spinach	26	17	43	60	20	12	32	62
Mashed potato*	23	14	37	62	23	14	37	62
Cabbage salad	18	10	28	64	28	19	47	60
Jello	16	7	23	70	30	22	52	58
Rolls	21	16	37	57	25	13	38	66
Brown bread	18	9	27	67	28	20	48	58
Milk	2	2	4	50	44	27	71	62
Coffee	19	12	31	61	27	17	44	61
Water	13	11	24	54	33	18	51	65
Cakes	27	13	40	67	19	16	35	54
Ice cream (van.)	43	11	54	80	3	18	21	14
Ice cream (choc.)*	25	22	47	53	20	7	27	74
Fruit salad	4	2	6	67	42	27	69	61

*Excludes 1 person with indefinite history of consumption of that food.

SOURCE: Gross, 1976

or other test of statistical significance to determine the likelihood of finding an association as large or larger on the basis of chance alone.

Table 9.3, which is based on a famous outbreak of gastroenteritis following a church supper in Oswego, New York in 1940, illustrates the use of a cohort study in an outbreak investigation (Gross, 1976). Of 80 persons who attended the supper, 75 were interviewed. Forty-six persons met the case definition. Attack rates for those who did and did not eat each of 14 items are presented in Table 9.3

Scan the column of attack rates among those who ate the specified items. Which item shows the highest attack rate? Were most of the 46 cases exposed to that food item? Is the attack rate low among persons not exposed to that item?

You should have identified vanilla ice cream as the implicated vehicle. The data for an individual item are often presented in a two-by-two table. The following two-by-two table shows the data on vanilla ice cream.

TABLE 9.4 Attack rate by consumption of vanilla ice cream, Oswego, New York, April 1940

		Ill	**Well**	**Total**	**Attack Rate (%)**
Ate vanilla ice cream?	Yes	43	11	54	79.6
	No	3	18	21	14.3
	Total	46	29	75	61.3

SOURCE: CDC, 1992.

The relative risk is calculated as 79.6/14.3, or 5.6. The relative risk indicates that persons who ate the vanilla ice cream were 5.6 times more likely to become ill than those who did not eat the vanilla ice cream. Sometimes, attack rate tables such as Table 9.3 include an additional column on the far right for relative risks.

Statistical Significance Testing We use tests of statistical significance to determine how likely it is that our results could have occurred by chance alone, if exposure was not actually related to disease.

The first step in testing for statistical significance is to assume that the exposure is not related to disease. This assumption is known as the **null hypothesis.** (The **alternative hypothesis,** which may be adopted if the null hypothesis proves to be implausible, is that exposure *is* associated with disease.) Next, you should compute a measure of association, such as a relative risk or odds ratio. Then, you calculate a chi-square or other statistical test. This test tells you the probability of finding an association as strong as, or stronger than, the one you have observed if the null hypothesis is really true. This probability is called the **p-value.** A very small p-value means that you are very unlikely to observe such an association if the null hypothesis is true. If you find a p-value smaller than some cutoff that you have decided on in advance, such as 5%, you may discard or reject the null hypothesis in favor of the alternative hypothesis.

Recall the notation of the two-by-two table described in Chapter 5.

TABLE 9.5 Standard notation of a two-by-two table

	Ill	Well	Total
Exposed	a	b	H1
Unexposed	c	d	H2
Total	V1	V2	T

SOURCE: CDC, 1992.

The most common statistical test in the outbreak setting is the chi-square test. For a two-by-two table, the chi-square formula is:

$$\text{Chi-square} = \frac{T[\,|\,ad - bc\,|\, - (T/2)]^2}{V1 \times V2 \times H1 \times H2}$$

Once you have a value for chi-square, you look up its corresponding p-value in a table of chi-squares, such as Table 9.6. Since a two-by-two table has 1 degree of freedom, a chi-square larger than 3.84 corresponds to a p-value smaller than 0.05. This means that if you have planned to reject the null hypothesis when the p-value is less than 0.05, you can do so if your value for chi-square is greater than 3.84.

TABLE 9.6 Table of chi-squares

	Probability						
Degree of Freedom	*.50*	*.20*	*.10*	*.05*	*.02*	*.01*	*.001*
1	.455	1.642	2.706	3.841	5.412	6.635	10.827
2	1.386	3.219	4.605	5.991	7.824	9.210	13.815
3	2.366	4.642	6.251	7.815	9.837	11.345	16.268
4	3.357	5.989	7.779	9.488	11.668	13.277	18.465
5	4.351	7.289	9.236	11.070	13.388	15.086	20.517
10	9.342	13.442	15.987	18.307	21.161	23.209	29.588
15	14.339	19.311	22.307	24.996	28.259	30.578	37.697
20	19.337	25.038	28.412	31.410	35.020	37.566	43.315
25	24.337	30.675	34.382	37.652	41.566	44.314	52.620
30	29.336	36.250	40.256	43.773	47.962	50.892	59.703

SOURCE: CDC, 1992.

The chi-square test works well if the number of people in the study is greater than about 30. For smaller studies, a test called the **Fisher Exact Test** may be more appropriate. Again, we refer you to any statistics book for further discussion of this topic.

Case-Control Studies

In many outbreak settings, the population is not well defined. Therefore, cohort studies are not feasible. However, since cases have been identified in an earlier step of the investigation, the case-control study is ideal. Indeed, case-control studies are more common than cohort studies in the investigation of an outbreak.

As we discussed in Chapter 3, in a case-control study you ask both case-patients and a comparison group of persons without disease ("controls") about their exposures. You then compute a measure of association—an **odds ratio** —to quantify the relationship between exposure and disease. Finally, as in a cohort study, you can compute a chi-square or other test of statistical significance to determine your likelihood of finding this relationship by chance alone.

This method, while not *proving* that a particular exposure caused disease, certainly has served epidemiologists well over time in implicating sources and vehicles associated with disease, and leading them to appropriate control and prevention measures.

Choosing controls When you design a case-control study, your first, and perhaps most important, decision is who the controls should be. Conceptually, the controls must not have the disease in question, but should represent the population that the cases come from. In other words, they should be similar to the cases except that they don't have the disease. If the null hypothesis were true, the controls would provide us with the level of exposure that you should expect to find among the cases. If exposure is much higher among the cases than the controls, you might choose to reject the null hypothesis in favor of a hypothesis that says exposure *is* associated with disease.

In practice, it is sometimes difficult to know who the controls should be. Precisely what is the population that the cases came from? In addition, we must consider practical matters, such as how to contact potential controls, gain their cooperation, ensure that they are free of disease, and get appropriate exposure data from them. In a community outbreak, a random sample of the healthy population may, in theory, be the best control group. In practice, however, persons in a random sample may be difficult to contact and enroll. Nonetheless, many investigators attempt to enroll such "population-based" controls through dialing of random telephone numbers in the community or through a household survey.

Other common control groups consist of:

- neighbors of cases
- patients from the same physician practice or hospital who do not have the disease in question
- friends of cases

While controls from these groups may be more likely to participate in the study than randomly identified population-based controls, they may not be as representative of the population. These **biases** in the control group can distort the data in either direction, masking an association between the exposure and disease, or producing a spurious association between an innocent exposure and disease.

In designing a case-control study, you must consider a variety of other issues about controls, including how many to use. Sample size formulas are widely available to help you make this decision. In general, the more subjects (cases and controls) you use in a study, the easier it will be to find an association.

Often, the number of cases you can use will be limited by the size of the outbreak. For example, in a hospital, 4 or 5 cases may constitute an outbreak. Fortunately, the number of potential controls will usually be more than you need. In an outbreak of 50 or more cases, 1 control per case will usually suffice. In smaller outbreaks you might use 2, 3, or 4 controls per case. More than 4 controls per case will rarely be worth your effort.

As an example, consider again the outbreak of Legionnaires' disease which occurred in Louisiana. Twenty-seven cases were enrolled in a case-control study. The investigators enrolled 2 controls per case, or a total of 54 controls. Using descriptive epidemiology, the investigators did not see any connection with the town's various cooling towers. Using analytic epidemiology, the investigators determined quantitatively that cases and controls were about equally exposed to cooling towers. However, cases were far more likely to shop at Grocery Store A, as shown in the two-by-two Table 9.7.

TABLE 9.7 Exposure to Grocery Store A among cases and controls, Legionellosis outbreak, Louisiana, 1990

		Cases	Controls	Total
Shopped at Grocery Store A?	Yes	25	28	53
	No	2	26	28
	Total	27	54	81

SOURCE: CDC, 1992.

In a case-control study, we are unable to calculate attack rates, since we do not know the total number of people in the community who did and did not shop at Grocery Store A. Since we cannot calculate attack rates, we cannot calculate a relative risk. The measure of association of choice in a case-control study is the **odds ratio.** Fortunately, for a rare disease such as legionellosis or most other diseases which cause occasional outbreaks, the odds ratio approximately equals the relative risk we would have found if we had been able to conduct a cohort study.

The odds ratio is calculated as ad / bc. The odds ratio for Grocery Store A is thus 25 × 26 / 28 × 2, or 11.6. These data indicate that persons exposed to Grocery Store A were 11.6 times more likely to develop Legionnaires' disease than persons not exposed to that store!

To test the statistical significance of this finding, we can compute a chi-square test using the following formula:

$$\text{Chi-square} = \frac{T[\,|\,ad - bc\,|\, - (T/2)]^2}{V1 \times V2 \times H1 \times H2}$$

For Grocery Store A, the chi-square becomes:

$$= \frac{81 \times [\,|\,25 \times 26 - 28 \times 2\,|\, - 81/2]^2}{27 \times 54 \times 53 \times 28}$$

$$= 24{,}815{,}342.25 \,/\, 2{,}163{,}672$$

$$= 11.47$$

Referring to Table 9.6, a chi-square of 11.47 corresponds to a p-value less than 0.001. A p-value this small indicates that the null hypothesis is highly improbable, and investigators rejected the null hypothesis.

Step 8: Refining Hypotheses and Executing Additional Studies

Epidemiologic Studies

Unfortunately, analytic studies sometimes are unrevealing. This is particularly true if the hypotheses were not well founded at the outset. It is an axiom of field epidemiology that if you cannot generate good hypotheses (by talking to some cases or local staff and examining the descriptive epidemiology and outliers), then proceeding to analytic epidemiology, such as a case-control study, is likely to be a waste of time.

When analytic epidemiology is unrevealing, you need to reconsider your hypotheses. This is the time to convene a meeting of the case-patients to look for common links and to visit their homes to look at the products on their shelves. Consider new vehicles or modes of transmission.

An investigation of an outbreak of *Salmonella muenchen* in Ohio illustrates how a reexamination of hypotheses can be productive. In that investigation, a case-control study failed to implicate any plausible food source as a common vehicle. Interestingly, *all* case-households, but only 41% of control households, included persons 15 to 35 years. The investigators thus began to consider vehicles of transmission to which young adults were commonly exposed. By asking about drug use in a second case-control study, the investigators implicated marijuana as the likely vehicle. Laboratory analysts subsequently isolated the outbreak strain of *S. muenchen* from several samples of marijuana provided by case-patients (Taylor et al., 1982).

Even when your analytic study identifies an association between an exposure and disease, you often will need to refine your hypotheses. Sometimes you will need to obtain more specific exposure histories. For example, in the investigation of Legionnaires' disease, what about Grocery Store A linked it to disease? The investigators asked cases and controls how much time they spent in the store, and where they went in the store. Using the epidemiologic data, the investigators were able to implicate the ultrasonic mist machine that sprayed the fruits and vegetables. This association was confirmed in the laboratory, where the outbreak subtype of the Legionnaires' disease bacillus was isolated from the water in the mist machine's reservoir (CDC, 1989).

Sometimes you will need a more specific control group to test a more specific hypothesis. For example, in many hospital outbreaks, investigators use an initial study to narrow their focus. They then conduct a second study, with more closely matched controls, to identify a more specific exposure or vehicle. In a large community outbreak of botulism in Illinois, investigators used three sequential case-control studies to identify the vehicle. In the first study, investigators compared exposures of cases and controls from the general public to implicate a restaurant. In a second study they compared restaurant exposures of cases and healthy restaurant patrons to identify a specific menu item, a meat and cheese sandwich. In a third study, investigators used radio broadcast appeals to identify healthy restaurant patrons who had eaten the implicated sandwich. Compared to cases who had also eaten the sandwich, controls were more likely to have avoided the onions that came with the sandwich. Type A *Clostridium botulinum* was then identified from a pan of leftover sauteed onions used only to make that particular sandwich (MacDonald et al., 1985).

Finally, recall that one reason to investigate outbreaks is research, that is, to expand our knowledge. An outbreak may provide an "experiment of nature," which would be unethical for us to set up deliberately, but which we can learn from when it occurs naturally. For example, in the previously described outbreak of hypervitaminosis D in Massachusetts, investigators quickly traced the source to a dairy that was adding too much vitamin D to its milk. After they had instituted the appropriate control measures, the investigators used the "experiment of nature" to characterize the spectrum of health effects caused by overexposure to vitamin D (CDC, unpublished data, 1991). Thus the investigation led to increased knowledge about an unusual problem as well as to prompt action to remove the source.

When an outbreak occurs, whether it is routine or unusual, consider what questions remain unanswered about that particular disease and what kind of study you might do in this setting to answer some of those questions. The circumstances may allow you to learn more about the disease, its modes of transmission, the characteristics of the agent, host factors, and the like. For example, an outbreak of mumps in a highly immunized population may be an opportunity to study vaccine efficacy and duration of protection.

Laboratory and Environmental Studies

While epidemiology can implicate vehicles and guide appropriate public health action, laboratory evidence can clinch the findings. The laboratory was essential in both the outbreak of salmonellosis linked to marijuana and in the Legionellosis outbreak traced to the grocery store mist machine. You may recall that the investigation of Legionnaires' disease in Philadelphia in 1976 was not considered complete until the new organism was isolated in the laboratory some 6 months later (Fraser et al., 1977).

Environmental studies are equally important in some settings. They are often helpful in explaining *why* an outbreak occurred. For example, in the investigation of the outbreak of shigellosis among swimmers in the Mississippi (Figure 9.7), the local sewage plant was identified as the cause of the outbreak (Rosenberg, 1976). In the study of thyrotoxicosis described earlier, a review of the procedures used in a slaughterhouse near Luverne, Minnesota, identified a practice that caused pieces of the animals' thyroid gland to be included with beef (Hedberg, 1987). Use a camera to photograph working conditions or environmental conditions. Bring back physical evidence to be analyzed in the laboratory, such as the slabs of beef from the slaughterhouse in the thyrotoxicosis study or the mist machine from the grocery store in the Legionellosis outbreak investigation.

Step 9: Implementing Control and Prevention Measures

In most outbreak investigations, your primary goal will be control and prevention. Indeed, although we are discussing them as Step 9, you should implement control measures as soon as possible, You can usually implement control measures early if you know the source of an outbreak. In general, you aim control measures at the weak link or links in the chain of infection. You might aim control measures at the specific agent, source, or reservoir. For example, an outbreak might be controlled by destroying contaminated foods, sterilizing contaminated water, or destroying mosquito breeding sites. Or an infectious food handler could be removed from the job and treated.

In other situations, you might direct control measures at interrupting transmission or exposure. You could have nursing home residents with a particular infection "cohorted," put together in a separate area to prevent transmission to others. You could instruct persons wishing to reduce their risk of acquiring Lyme disease to avoid wooded areas or to wear insect repellent and protective clothing.

Finally, in some outbreaks, you would direct control measures at reducing the susceptibility of the host. Two such examples are immunization against rubella and malaria chemoprophylaxis for travelers.

Step 10: Communicating the Findings

Your final task in an investigation is to communicate your findings. This communication usually takes two forms: (1) an oral briefing for local authorities and (2) a written report.

Your oral briefing should be attended by the local health authorities and persons responsible for implementing control and prevention measures. Usually these persons are not epidemiologists, so you must present your findings in clear and convincing fashion with appropriate and justifiable recommendations for action. This presentation is an opportunity for you to describe what you did, what you found, and what you think should be done about it. You should present your findings in scientifically objective fashion, and you should be able to defend your conclusions and recommendations.

You should also provide a written report that follows the usual scientific format of introduction, background, methods, results, discussion, and recommendations. By formally presenting recommendations, the report provides a blueprint for action. It also serves as a record of performance and a document for potential legal issues. It serves as a reference if the health department encounters a similar situation in the future. Finally, a report that finds its way into the public health literature serves the broader purpose of contributing to the knowledge base of epidemiology and public health.

REFERENCES

Addiss DG, Davis JP, LaVenture M, Wand PJ, Hutchinson MA, McKinney RM: Community-acquired Legionnaires' disease associated with a cooling tower: evidence for longer-distance transport of *Legionella pneumophila*. *American Journal of Epidemiology* 1989;130:557-568.

Bender AP, Williams AN, Johnson RA, Jagger HG: Appropriate public health responses to clusters: the art of being responsibly responsive. *American Journal of Epidemiology* 1990;132:S48-S52.

Benenson AS (ed): *Control of communicable diseases in man*. Fifteenth Edition. Washington, DC: American Public Health Association, 1990.

Caldwell GG: Twenty-two years of cancer cluster investigations at the Centers for Disease Control. *American Journal of Epidemiology* 1990;132:S43-S47.

Centers for Disease Control: Hepatitis—Alabama. *MMWR* 1972;21:439-444.

Centers for Disease Control: Legionnaires' disease outbreak associated with a grocery store mist machine—Louisiana, 1989. *MMWR* 1990;39:108-110.

Centers for Disease Control: Pertussis—Washington, 1984. *MMWR* 1985; 34:390-400.

Devier JR, Brownson RC, Bagby JR, Carlson GM, Crellin JR: A public health response to cancer clusters in Missouri. *American Journal of Epidemiology* 1990;132:S23-31.

Fiore BJ, Hanrahan LP, Anderson HA: State health department response to disease cluster reports: a protocol for investigation. *American Journal of Epidemiology* 1990;132:S14-22.

Fraser DW, Tsai TF, Orenstein W, et al.: Legionnaires' disease: Description of an epidemic of pneumonia. *New England Journal of Medicine* 1977;297: 1189-1197.

Goodman RA, Beuhler JW, Koplan JP: The epidemiologic field investigation: science and judgment in public health practice. *American Journal of Epidemiology* 1990;132:9-16.

Gross, M: Oswego County revisited. *Public Health Report* 1976;91:168-170.

Hedberg CW, Fishbein DB, Janssen RS, et al.: An outbreak of thyrotoxicosis caused by the consumption of bovine thyroid gland in ground beef. *New England Journal of Medicine* 1987;316:993-998.

Hertzman PA, Blevins WL, Mayer J, Greenfield B, Ting M, Gleich GJ: Association of the eosinophilia-myalgia syndrome with the ingestion of tryptophan. *New England Journal of Medicine* 1990;322:869-873.

Hopkins RS, Juranek DD: Acute giardiasis: an improved clinical case definition for epidemiologic studies. *American Journal of Epidemiology* 1991;133: 402-407.

Hutchins SS, Markowitz LE, Mead P, et al.: A school-based measles outbreak: the effect of a selective revaccination policy and risk factors for vaccine failure. *American Journal of Epidemiology* 1990;132:157-168.

MacDonald KL, Spengler RF, Hatheway CL, et al.: Type A botulism from sauteed onions. *Journal of the American Medical Association* 1985;253:1275-1278.

Neutra RR: Counterpoint from a cluster buster. *American Journal of Epidemiology* 1990;132:1-8.

Rimland D, Parkin WE, Miller GB, Schrack WD: Hepatitis B outbreak traced to an oral surgeon. *New England Journal of Medicine* 1977;296:953-958.

Rosenberg MD, Hazlet KK, Schaefer J, Wells JG, Pruneda RC: Shigellosis from swimming. *Journal of the American Medical Association* 1976;236: 1849-1852.

Ryan CA, Nickels MK, Hargett-Bean NT, et al.: Massive outbreak of antimicrobial-resistant salmonellosis traced to pasteurized milk. *Journal of the American Medical Association* 1987;258:3269-3274.

Schulte PA, Ehrenberg RL, Singal M: Investigation of occupational cancer clusters: theory and practice. *American Journal of Public Health* 1987;77:52-56.

Swygert LA, Maes EF, Sewell LE, Miller L, Falk H, Kilbourne EM: Eosinophilia-myalgia syndrome: results of national surveillance. *Journal of the American Medical Association* 1990;264:1698-1703.

Taylor DN, Wachsmuth IK, Shangkuan Y-H, et al.: Salmonellosis associated with marijuana: a multistate outbreak traced by plasmid fingerprinting. *New England Journal of Medicine* 1982;306:1249-1253.

PROBLEMS

1. During the previous year, nine residents of a community died from the same type of cancer. List some reasons that might justify an investigation.

2. For the month of August, 12 new cases of tuberculosis and 12 new cases of aseptic meningitis were reported to a county health department. Would you call either group of cases a cluster? Would you call either group of cases an outbreak? What additional information might be helpful in answering these questions?

3. Review the following six case report forms. Create a line listing based on this information.

STATE DISEASE REPORT FORM

NAME Ring, K. | AGE 29 | PHONE 555-3631
ADDRESS 52 Eufala Rd. | SEX M | RACE W
CITY, STATE Columbia | COUNTY Columbia
DISEASE Probable Trichinosis | DATE OF ONSET 7/23 | LAB CONFIRMED? Not Done
HOSPITAL ALERTED? No | HOSPITAL NAME | ADMISSION DATE | DISCHARGE DATA
LAB TEST RESULTS Eosinophil Count 24% of total WBC's
COMMENTS (Clinical description, immunization theory, etc.)
POSSIBLE EXPOSURE Cleveland-McKay Wedding
PHYSICIAN REPORTING Dr. Goodman | PHONE 555-3636 | DATE OF REPORT 8/14

STATE DISEASE REPORT FORM

NAME McDowell, D. | AGE 33 | PHONE 555-3707
ADDRESS 2020 Alabama | SEX M | RACE W
CITY, STATE Columbia | COUNTY Columbia
DISEASE Trichinosis | DATE OF ONSET 7/27 | LAB CONFIRMED? Muscle Biopsy
HOSPITAL ALERTED? Yes | HOSPITAL NAME Columbia General | ADMISSION DATE 7/27 | DISCHARGE DATA 7/30
LAB TEST RESULTS Eosinophilia = 2500
COMMENTS (Clinical description, immunization theory, etc.)
POSSIBLE EXPOSURE Cleveland-McKay Wedding
PHYSICIAN REPORTING Dr. Baker | PHONE 555-1900 | DATE OF REPORT 8/17

STATE DISEASE REPORT FORM

NAME Gordon, Jack | AGE 26 | PHONE 556-1213
ADDRESS 110 Clifton Street | SEX M | RACE W
CITY, STATE Columbia | COUNTY Columbia
DISEASE Probable Trichinosis | DATE OF ONSET 8/14 | LAB CONFIRMED? No
HOSPITAL ALERTED? No | HOSPITAL NAME | ADMISSION DATE | DISCHARGE DATA
LAB TEST RESULTS Eosinophils = 37%
COMMENTS (Clinical description, immunization theory, etc.)
POSSIBLE EXPOSURE Cleveland-McKay Wedding
PHYSICIAN REPORTING Dr. Gibbs | PHONE 555-3841 | DATE OF REPORT 8/14

STATE DISEASE REPORT FORM

NAME Dickens, R. | AGE 45 | PHONE 555-2662
ADDRESS 34 Winifred Ave. | SEX M | RACE
CITY, STATE Seattle, WA | COUNTY King
DISEASE Trichinosis | DATE OF ONSET 7/25 | LAB CONFIRMED? Serologic
HOSPITAL ALERTED? No | HOSPITAL NAME | ADMISSION DATE | DISCHARGE DATA
LAB TEST RESULTS Eosinophils = 4100
COMMENTS (Clinical description, immunization theory, etc.)
POSSIBLE EXPOSURE Cleveland-McKay Wedding
PHYSICIAN REPORTING Dr. Webster | PHONE 555-0511 | DATE OF REPORT 8/15

STATE DISEASE REPORT FORM

NAME Thomas, Nancy	AGE 27	PHONE 555-3761
ADDRESS	SEX F	RACE W
CITY, STATE	COUNTY Columbia	
DISEASE Trichinosis	DATE OF ONSET 8/4	LAB CONFIRMED? No
HOSPITAL ALERTED? No HOSPITAL NAME	ADMISSION DATE	DISCHARGE DATA
LAB TEST RESULTS 18% Eosinophilia		
COMMENTS (Clinical description, immunization theory, etc.)		
POSSIBLE EXPOSURE Cleveland-McKay Wedding		
PHYSICIAN REPORTING Dr. Stanley	PHONE 555-0400	DATE OF REPORT 8/15

STATE DISEASE REPORT FORM

NAME McKay, Alice	AGE 54	PHONE 555-6256
ADDRESS 406 Tugalo Lane	SEX F	RACE W
CITY, STATE Brighton	COUNTY Clayton	
DISEASE R/o Trichinosis	DATE OF ONSET 8/11	LAB CONFIRMED? Serology Pending
HOSPITAL ALERTED? Yes HOSPITAL NAME Columbia General	ADMISSION DATE 8/14	DISCHARGE DATA
LAB TEST RESULTS Eosinophils = 3600		
COMMENTS (Clinical description, immunization theory, etc.)		
POSSIBLE EXPOSURE Cleveland - McKay Wedding		
PHYSICIAN REPORTING Dr. Mason	PHONE 555-3291	DATE OF REPORT 8/15

4. Using the data from a hepatitis A outbreak in Table 9.8, draw an epidemic curve. From your epidemic curve and your knowledge of the average and minimum incubation periods for hepatitis A, identify the likely exposure period.

TABLE 9.8 Hepatitis A outbreak data

Case #	Age	Sex	Date of Onset	Case #	Age	Sex	Date of Onset
2	16	F	4-3	41	37	F	5-9
3	34	M	4-6	43	16	M	5-10
6	15	M	4-28	45	29	F	5-10
7	46	M	4-30	46	5	M	5-10
8	21	F	5-1	47	8	F	5-11
9	14	M	5-1	48	15	F	5-11
11	13	M	5-2	49	14	M	5-11
12	43	M	5-2	50	16	M	5-11
13	14	M	5-3	52	16	M	5-12
15	37	M	5-3	53	19	M	5-12
16	5	F	5-3	54	15	M	5-12
17	11	F	5-3	55	10	F	5-12
18	19	M	5-4	56	6	M	5-12
19	14	F	5-4	57	20	M	5-12
20	35	F	5-4	58	43	M	5-12
21	11	F	5-4	59	15	F	5-12
22	14	M	5-4	60	12	F	5-12
23	14	M	5-4	61	14	M	5-13
25	15	M	5-5	62	34	M	5-13
26	12	M	5-5	63	15	F	5-13
27	50	M	5-5	64	30	M	5-13
29	50	M	5-6	65	16	M	5-13
31	11	M	5-7	66	15	M	5-14
32	15	M	5-7	67	15	M	5-14
33	18	F	5-7	68	16	M	5-14
34	14	M	5-7	69	16	M	5-14
35	15	M	5-8	70	18	F	5-15
36	30	M	5-8	72	12	M	5-18
37	20	F	5-9	74	22	F	5-20
38	14	F	5-9	75	15	F	5-24
39	17	M	5-9	76	14	M	5-26
40	15	M	5-9				

5. You are called to help investigate a cluster of 17 men who developed leukemia in a community. Some of them worked as electrical repair men, and others were ham radio operators. Which study design would you choose to investigate a possible association between exposure to electromagnetic fields and leukemia?

6. To study rash illness among grocery store workers, investigators conducted a cohort study. The following table shows the data for exposure to celery. What is the appropriate measure of association? Calculate this measure and a chi-square test of statistical significance.

		Rash	No rash	Total	Attack rate
Exposed to celery?	Yes	25	31	56	44.64%
	No	5	65	70	7.14%
	Total	30	96	126	23.81%

How would you interpret your results?

ANSWERS

1. One reason to investigate is simply **to determine how many cases we would expect in the community.** In a large community, nine cases of a common cancer (for example, lung, breast, or colon cancer) would not be unusual. In a very small community, nines cases of even a common cancer may seem unusual. If the particular cancer is a rare type, then nine cases even in a large community may be unusual.

   If the number of cancer cases turns out to be high for that community, we might pursue the investigation further. We may have a **research** motive—perhaps we will identify a new risk factor (workers exposed to a particular chemical) or predisposition (persons with a particular genetic marker) for the cancer.

   Control and prevention may be a justification. If we find a risk factor, control/prevention measures could be developed. Alternatively, if the cancer is one which is generally treatable if found early, and a screening test is available, then we might investigate to determine not why these persons developed the disease, but why they died of it. If the cancer were cancer of the cervix, detectable by Pap smear and generally treatable if caught early, we might find (1) problems with access to health care, or (2) physicians not following the recommendations to screen women at the appropriate intervals, or (3) laboratory error in reading or reporting the test results. We could then develop measures to correct the problems we found (public screening clinics, education of physicians, or laboratory quality assurance.)

   If new staff need to gain experience on a cluster investigation, **training** may be a reason to investigate. More commonly, cancer clusters frequently generate **public concern**, which, in turn, may generate **political pressure.** Perhaps one of the affected persons is a member of the mayor's family. A health department must be responsive to such concerns, but does not usually need to conduct a full-blown investigation. Finally, **legal concerns** may prompt an investigation, especially if a particular site (manufacturer, houses built on an old dump site, etc.) is accused of causing the cancers.

2. Tuberculosis does not have a striking seasonal distribution. The number of cases during August could be compared with (a) the numbers reported during the preceding several months, and (b) the numbers reported during August of the preceding few years.

   Aseptic meningitis is a highly seasonal disease which peaks during August–September–October. As a result, the number of cases during August is expected to be higher than the numbers reported during the preceding several months.

   To determine whether the number of cases in August is greater than expected, we must look at the numbers reported during August of the preceding few years.

3. Which items to include in a line listing is somewhat arbitrary. The following categories of information are often included:

Identifying information

- Identification number or case number, usually in the leftmost column
- Names or initials as a cross-check

Information on diagnosis and clinical illness

- Physician diagnosis
- Was diagnosis confirmed? If so, how?
- Symptoms
- Laboratory results
- Was the patient hospitalized? Did the patient die?

Descriptive epidemiology—time

- Date of onset
- Time of onset

Descriptive epidemiology—person

- Age
- Sex
- Occupation, if relevant, or other seemingly relevant characteristics

Descriptive epidemiology—place

- Street, city, or county
- Worksite, school, day care center, etc., if relevant

Risk factors and possible causes

- Specific to disease and outbreak setting

An example of a line listing from the six case report forms is shown in Table 9.9.

TABLE 9.9 Example of a line listing

ID #	*Initials*	*Date of Onset*	*Diagnosis*	*How Confirmed*	*Age*	*Sex*	*County*	*Physician*	*Cleveland-McKay Wedding*
1	KR	7/23	Probable trichinosis	Not done	29	M	Columbia	Goodman	Yes
2	DM	7/27	Trichinosis	Biopsy	33	M	Columbia	Baker	Yes
3	JG	8/14	Probable trichinosis	Not done	26	M	Columbia	Gibbs	Yes
4	RD	7/25	Trichinosis	Serologic	45	M	King	Webster	Yes
5	NT	8/4	Trichinosis	Not done	27	F	Columbia	Stanley	Yes
6	AM	8/11	R/O trichinosis	Pending	54	F	Clayton	Mason	Yes

4. The epidemic curve shown in Figure 9.9 suggests a common source outbreak. We can estimate time of exposure by starting at the peak of the epidemic and going back the mean incubation period, or by starting at the rise of the epidemic and going back the minimum incubation period. Going back 30 days (mean incubation period for hepatitis A) from the epidemic peak on May 9 puts the estimated exposure on April 9. Assuming the minimum incubation period (15 days) for the April 28 case, exposure would have occurred on April 13. So, we can estimate that exposure

occurred between April 9 and April 13, give or take a few days on either side.

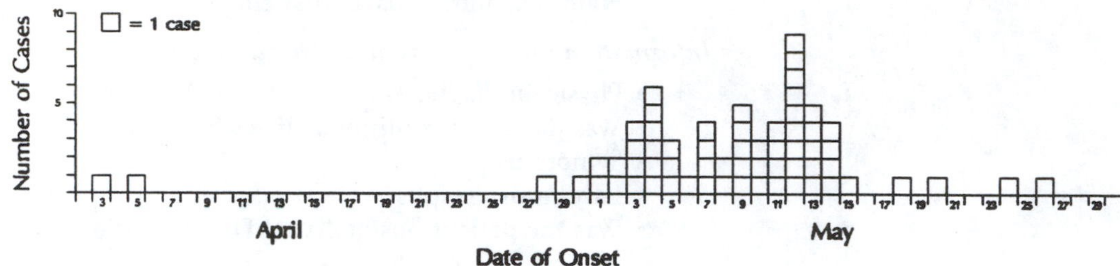

FIGURE 9.9 *Epidemic curve for Question 4: Hepatitis A by date of onset, April-May*

5. A case-control study is the design of choice, since 17 persons with the disease of interest have already been identified. We would need to enroll these 17 persons as the case group. We would also need to determine what group might serve as an appropriate comparison or control group. Neighbors might be used for the control group, for example. In our case-control study we would determine whether each case and each control was exposed to electromagnetic fields (however we defined that exposure). Finally, we would compare the exposure experience of cases and controls.

   The alternative to a case-control study is a cohort study. For a cohort study we would have to enroll a group of persons exposed to electromagnetic fields (however we defined that exposure), and a comparison group of persons not exposed. We would then have to determine how many in each group developed leukemia. Since leukemia is a relatively rare event, we would need rather large groups in order to have enough leukemia cases to make our study valid. Therefore, a cohort study is less practical than a case-control study in this setting.

6. The appropriate measure of association for a cohort study is the relative risk, calculated as the ratio of attack rates.

$$\text{Relative risk} = 44.64/7.14 = 6.2$$

$$\text{Chi-square} = \frac{T[\,|ad - bc| - (T/2)]^2}{V1 \times V2 \times H1 \times H2}$$

   For the table shown in Problem 6 on page 345, the chi-square becomes:

$$= \frac{126 \times [\,|25 \times 65 - 31 \times 5| - 126/2]^2}{30 \times 96 \times 56 \times 70}$$

$$= 249{,}435{,}774/11{,}289{,}600$$

$$= 22.09$$

A chi-square of 22.09 corresponds to a p-value of < 0.00001. A p-value this small indicates that the null hypothesis is highly improbable, and the investigators rejected the null hypothesis.

10 Now It's Your Turn: Evaluating Your Understanding

The purpose of this chapter is to help you evaluate your learning. The following problems are designed to assist you in this process. You can check your learning progress by referring to the answers and explanations for each problem located at the end of this chapter. We suggest you record your own responses before you check the answers. All problems are based on hypothetical data.

1. Suppose a highly effective new drug is discovered for treating a form of cancer that previously had been rapidly fatal. Which of the following rates will be *least* affected by the widespread use of the drug? (Check one.)

   a. _______ Five-year survival rate for this type of cancer.

   b. _______ Prevalence rate for this type of cancer.

   c. _______ Incidence rate for this type of cancer.

   d. _______ Mortality rate for this type of cancer.

2. In a study concerned with the possible effects of air pollution on the development of chronic bronchitis, the following data were obtained:

   A population of 9,000 men aged 45 years was examined in January 1985. Of these, 6,000 lived in areas that exposed them to air pollution and 3,000 did not. At this examination, 90 cases of chronic bronchitis were discovered, 60 among those exposed to air pollution.

   All the men initially examined who did not have chronic bronchitis were available for subsequent repeated examinations during the next five years. These examinations revealed 268 new cases of chronic bronchitis in the total group, including 30 among those not exposed to air pollution.

   The prevalence rates of chronic bronchitis in January 1985 were:

	Numerator	Denominator		Prevalence Rate per 1,000
a.	________	__________	Among those exposed to air pollution	__________
b.	________	__________	Among those not exposed to air pollution	__________

The incidence rates of chronic bronchitis for the five years were:

	Numerator	Denominator		Prevalence Rate per 1,000
c.	________	__________	Among those exposed to air pollution	__________
d.	________	__________	Among those not exposed to air pollution	__________
e.	________	__________	In the total sample	__________

f. Which of the following conclusions can be drawn from the *prevalence* data? (Check one.)

_______ (1) Air pollution is associated with chronic bronchitis.

_______ (2) Air pollution is not associated with chronic bronchitis.

g. Which of the following conclusions can be drawn from the *incidence* data? (Check one.)

_______ (1) Air pollution is associated with chronic bronchitis.

_______ (2) Air pollution is not associated with chronic bronchitis.

To determine whether air pollution is causally related to chronic bronchitis, one must consider the possibility that the conclusions, drawn from either the prevalence or the incidence data, may be artifactual (spurious). Three common sources of spurious conclusions are: selective survival, selective migration, and secondary association (due to confounding variables). For each source of spurious conclusions, indicate whether it is more likely to apply to the prevalence data, to the incidence data, or equally to both sets of data. (Check the one best answer for each.)

h. Selective survival is:

_______ (1) More likely to have influenced the conclusions drawn from the prevalence data than from the incidence data.

_______ (2) More likely to have influenced the conclusions drawn from the incidence data than from the prevalence data.

_______ (3) Equally likely to have influenced the conclusions drawn from the prevalence or the incidence data.

i. Selective migration is:

_______ (1) More likely to have influenced the conclusions drawn from the prevalence data than from the incidence data.

_______ (2) More likely to have influenced the conclusions drawn from the incidence data than from the prevalence data.

_______ (3) Equally likely to have influenced the conclusions drawn from the prevalence or the incidence data.

j. Secondary (artifactual) associations are:

_______ (1) More likely to have influenced the conclusions drawn from the prevalence data than from the incidence data.

_______ (2) More likely to have influenced the conclusions drawn from the incidence data than from the prevalence data.

_______ (3) Equally likely to have influenced the conclusions drawn from the prevalence or the incidence data.

3. Death rates from all causes are reported to be lower in professional and managerial occupations than in unskilled occupations. You would suspect this association between occupational status and death to be secondary (due to confounding variables) if you knew the following facts. (Check as many as would make you suspect a secondary association.)

   a. _______ People in unskilled occupations are older than those in professional and managerial occupations.

   b. _______ People in professional and managerial occupations are older than those in unskilled occupations.

   c. _______ Professional and managerial occupations contain a greater proportion of women than do unskilled occupations.

   d. _______ There are more people in unskilled occupations than there are in professional and managerial occupations.

4. A health agency was concerned with two problems: the high rate of recurrence of rheumatic heart disease in children with rheumatic fever and the high rate of complications occurring in children with diabetes. The consequences (in terms of subsequent disability and death) of rheumatic fever recurrences and diabetic complications are equally serious. Furthermore, the prevalence of diabetes and rheumatic heart disease were the same in the population for which the agency was responsible.

The high rate of recurrence of rheumatic heart disease was due to the failure of many children with rheumatic fever to take penicillin regularly. The high rate of diabetic complications was due to the failure of diabetic children to take insulin regularly. To reduce these problems, the agency wished to try two approaches: first, sending a postcard each month to the families to remind them the patient must have penicillin or insulin regularly, and second, a regular home visit by a nurse. The agency drew a random sample of their rheumatic fever patients and a similar sample of their diabetic patients. One third of each sample received no intervention, one third received a regular postcard, and one third a home visit.

Tables 10.1 and 10.2, compiled one year after the trials started, show that sending a postcard had little effect, but home visits were highly effective for both rheumatic fever and diabetes.

TABLE 10.1 Recurrence of rheumatic heart disease in children with rheumatic fever

Method of Intervention	*Recurrences of Rheumatic Heart Disease per 1,000*
No intervention	15.7
Regular postcard	15.5
Home visits	5.0

TABLE 10.2 Occurrences of diabetic complications in diabetic children

Method of Intervention	*Diabetic Complications per 1,000*
No intervention	4.5
Regular postcard	4.2
Home visits	0.5

As a result of this information, home visiting became a routine program of the agency. Because of a shortage of personnel, however, home visits could be made either to all rheumatic fever patients or to all diabetic patients (but *not* to both). On the basis of the data presented in Tables 10.1 and 10.2, which condition should receive home visits? (Check one.)

a. _______ Children with rheumatic fever.

b. _______ Children with diabetes.

Indicate the data from which you drew your conclusions.

5. A study was undertaken to evaluate the effectiveness of a prenatal program. An objective of this program was to reduce the perinatal mortality rate (rate of deaths of infants during the first seven days of life).

Two populations were studied: (1) all primigravidae (women with a first pregnancy) aged 20 to 24 who attended the clinic for prenatal care during a particular year and (2) a representative sample of primigravidae who were pregnant during this same period and who received no prenatal care. This sample was from the community served by the clinic and was of the same age and ethnic group as the attenders.

The results are as shown in Tables 10.3 and 10.4.

TABLE 10.3 Perinatal mortality rates in women receiving and not receiving prenatal care

Prenatal Care at Clinic	*Number of Women*	*Perinatal Deaths*	*Perinatal Mortality Rate per 1,000*
Receiving prenatal care	200	5	25.0
No prenatal care	150	10	66.7
Total	350	15	42.9

TABLE 10.4 Perinatal mortality rates by educational level of women

Education	*Number of Women*	*Perinatal Deaths*	*Perinatal Mortality Rate per 1,000*
High school graduates	190	6	31.6
Non-high school graduates	160	9	56.3
Total	350	15	42.9

If you knew that 110 of the women who had received prenatal care were high school graduates and that two of them had infants that died in the perinatal period (assuming all the results are statistically significant), what would you conclude from these data? (Check as many as are correct.)

a. ______ That primigravidae aged 20 to 24 who received prenatal care had a reduced perinatal mortality rate compared to those receiving no prenatal care.

b. ______ That the prenatal program had *not* been effective. The reduction in perinatal mortality rate was not due to the program but due to the higher educational level of the woman using the program.

c. ______ That prenatal care was beneficial for more educated mothers but did not help less educated mothers in this country.

d. ______ That in this country the higher rates of perinatal mortality in less educated as compared with more educated women were due to other factors besides the lack of prenatal care.

Present the complete table from which you drew your conclusions.

6. To determine whether a newly invented birth control pill increased the risk of stroke, a cohort study was started. A random sample of women of child-bearing age was selected and examined to make sure that none had any evidence of stroke; 9,920 individuals were identified as being eligible

for study. Of these, 1,000 were taking the new birth control pill regularly and the remainder were not taking it at all. The entire sample was followed for ten years with the results shown in Table 10.5. From these data, which of the following conclusions can be drawn? (Check the one best answer.)

TABLE 10.5 New cases of stroke during ten-year time period, by pill-taking status

	New Cases of Stroke during Ten Years	*Free of Stroke during Ten Years*	*Total*
Women taking pill	10	990	1,000
Women not taking pill	10	8,910	8,920
Total	20	9,900	9,920

a. ______ Taking the pill *does* increase the risk of stroke and the degree of this risk is shown by the fact that 10/1,000 (1%) of those taking the pill developed a stroke, but only 10/8,920 (0.1%) of those not taking the pill developed a stroke.

b. ______ Taking the pill *does not* increase the risk of stroke because 50% (10/20) of stroke cases were taking the pill and 50% (10/20) of stroke cases were not taking the pill.

c. ______ Taking the pill *does not* increase the risk of stroke because although 10/1,000 (1%) of those taking the pill did develop a stroke, 990/9,900 (10%) of those also taking the pill did not develop a stroke.

d. ______ Taking the pill *does* increase the risk of stroke and the degree of this risk is shown by the fact that 10/20 (50%) of the stroke cases were taking the pill, but only 990/9,900 (10%) of those free of stroke were taking the pill.

7. In order to determine whether exposure to various industrial pollutants increased the risk of lung cancer, the average annual death rates for lung cancer over a ten-year period were analyzed for male employees in five different sorts of industries. These industries are labeled A-E in Table 10.6. (Because lung cancer is almost always fatal and there is a short interval between diagnosis and death, death rates are good approximations of incidence.)

   The death rates in industries A and B were higher than those in C, D, and E. (The differences were statistically significant.) Both the age distribution and cigarette-smoking patterns differed in industries A and B. Because both age and cigarette smoking increase the risk of lung cancer, it was necessary to control for these before concluding that some factor in industries A and B was responsible for an increased risk of lung cancer. To control for them, a standardized mortality ratio (SMR) for age and cigarette smoking was computed. The results are shown in Table 10.7.

TABLE 10.6 Average annual death rates for lung cancer for male employees, by industry, 1980-1989

Industry	*Death Rate per 100,000 Employees*
A	72
B	71
C	50
D	49
E	49

TABLE 10.7 Standardized mortality ratios for lung cancer for male employees, by industry

Industry	*SMR*
A	180.6
B	101.1
C	210.2
D	98.9
E	101.3

From these data, which of the following conclusions can be drawn? (Check as many as may be true.)

a. _______ Some factors in industries A and C probably increased the risk of lung cancer.

b. _______ These data show that neither cigarette smoking nor age was related to lung cancer in industries B, D, and E.

c. _______ Industry B must have had either more cigarette smokers and/or older employees than industry C.

8. For a particular county, all mothers giving birth to a first child during a particular year were classified by place of residence (urban or rural) and by social class. The *mean birthweights* of the babies were tabulated as shown in Table 10.8.

If these data were available, and a new investigation were being planned to search for the causes of low birthweight, what is the most logical way to start this search? (Check the one best answer.)

a. _______ By attempting to identify the relevant factors in a rural way of living contrasted to an urban way of life.

b. _______ By attempting to identify the relevant factors in the way of life of lower-class people as compared with those for higher-class people.

TABLE 10.8 Mean birthweights in grams, by maternal place of residence and social class

	Place of Residence		
Social Class	*Rural*	*Urban*	*All Places*
Low	3,300	3,309	3,303
High	3,672	3,669	3,671
All classes	3,364	3,592	3,475

c. ______ By attempting to identify the relevant factors that distinguish rural people from urban people *and* low social class from high social class.

d. ______ To ignore both place of residence and social class status because neither of these is associated with birthweight.

9. Sensitivity and specificity are useful indices in the evaluation of a newly developed screening test. Table 10.9 represents the evaluation of a screening test for a particular disease compared with a well-established method of diagnosing that disease. A, B, C, and D represent frequencies.

TABLE 10.9 Presence and absence of disease, by screening test and by established method

	According to Well-established Method	
According to Screening Test	*Disease Present*	*Disease Absent*
Disease present	A	B
Disease absent	C	D

a. The *sensitivity* of the screening test may be defined as (check one):

______ (1) C/(C + D)

______ (2) C/(A + C)

______ (3) A/(A + C)

______ (4) A/(A + B)

b. The *specificity* of the screening test may be defined as (check one):

______ (1) D/(C + D)

______ (2) D/(A + D)

______ (3) D/(B + D)

______ (4) None of the above.

c. The frequency that represents the *false positives* of the screening test is (check one):

_______ (1) A

_______ (2) B

_______ (3) C

_______ (4) D

10. The data in Table 10.10 were available for one particular county for a disease known to be spread by food and water. Assuming that the data in the table are accurate and complete, which of the following do these data suggest? (Check one.)

TABLE 10.10 Number of new cases, all cases, and deaths from disease, by year

Year	*Population of County*	*New Cases*	*All Cases*	*Deaths*
1980	50,000	100	200	5
1985	75,000	150	225	5
1990	100,000	200	250	5

a. _______ A successful environmental health program; that is, improvement in the sanitary quality of food and water.

b. _______ Improvement in the treatment of the disease.

c. _______ A successful environmental health program *and* improvement in treatment.

d. _______ None of the above.

11. For each statement, check one numbered heading that is most closely related to the statement.

a. Evaluation of a newly developed procedure compared with a standard procedure.

_______ (1) Validity

_______ (2) Reliability

_______ (3) Both

_______ (4) Neither

b. Comparisons of responses obtained one month apart for a newly developed questionnaire.

_______ (1) Validity

_______ (2) Reliability

_______ (3) Both

_______ (4) Neither

c. Expressed as sensitivity and specificity.

_______ (1) Validity

_______ (2) Reliability

_______ (3) Both

_______ (4) Neither

12. For each of the circumstances listed below, check which study method applies.

a. A study concerned with a rare disease.

_______ (1) Case-control

_______ (2) Cohort

b. A study that attempted to determine whether a high absenteeism rate for school children led to poor grades or whether poor grades led to high absenteeism.

_______ (1) Case-control

_______ (2) Cohort

c. A study in which selective survival could seriously bias the results.

_______ (1) Case-control

_______ (2) Cohort

d. A study in which it was important to quantify the attributable risk of the characteristic.

_______ (1) Case-control

_______ (2) Cohort

e. A study in which the latent or determination period between exposure to the characteristic and the onset of the condition (or determination) might be as long as 20 years.

_______ (1) Case-control

_______ (2) Cohort

13. Which of the following explanations could account for the phenomenon in Figure 10.1? (Check as many as are correct.)

a. _______ Improvements in treatment between 1937 and 1955 may have benefited the younger age groups more than the older ones.

b. _______ A bias in diagnosing the causes of deaths at different ages.

c. _______ Selective migration to Europe in 1945 of younger couples with low risk of death from appendicitis.

d. _______ Changes in the numbers of people of different ages in the population at the two points in time.

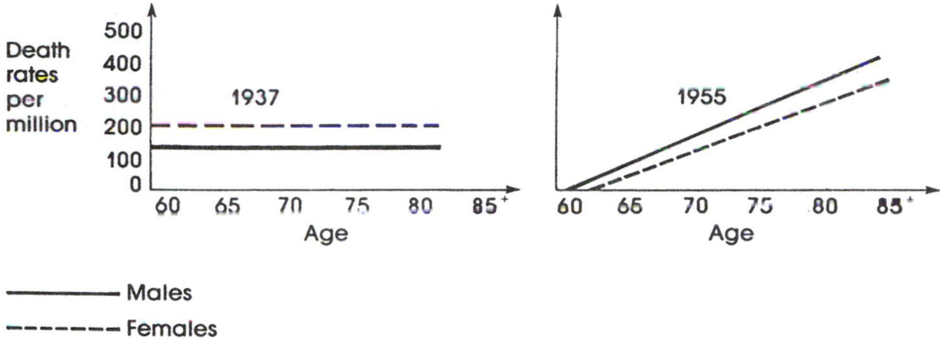

FIGURE 10.1 *Death rate from appendicitis by age and sex in the United States, 1937 and 1955*

14. In two hypothetical cohort studies—one in Boise, Idaho, and another in Jamaica—the methods used in each study were identical and standardized criteria for diagnoses were used. There was minimal (and approximately equal) attrition in both studies over the course of time the studies were conducted. No known cure for coronary heart disease exists. The results are shown in Table 10.11.

TABLE 10.11 Prevalence and incidence of coronary heart disease in men aged 60-64, Boise and Jamaica, 1980-1989

	Prevalence per 1,000 (1989)	*Average Incidence per 100,000 (1980-1989)*
Boise	37.4	27.0
Jamaica	15.5	5.2

From these data would you infer that the death rate from coronary heart disease in men of this age was (check one):

a. ______ Higher in Boise than in Jamaica.

b. ______ Higher in Jamaica than Boise.

c. ______ Equal in Boise and Jamaica.

15. In the continuing controversy over the role of cigarette smoking as a cause of lung cancer, an investigator makes the following statement:

> There are certain well-known data that refute the hypothesis that cigarette smoking is a cause of lung cancer. For example, in Great Britain the *per capita* consumption of cigarettes is half as much as in the United States, but the incidence of lung cancer is twice as much. In Australia the *per capita* consumption of cigarettes is about the same as in Great Britain, yet Australians have half as much lung cancer. In Holland the *per capita* consumption of cigarettes is lower than the United States but there is 33% more lung cancer.

What reasoning would lead you to agree or disagree with the investigator that these data refute the hypothesis that cigarette smoking causes lung cancer? (Check the one best answer.)

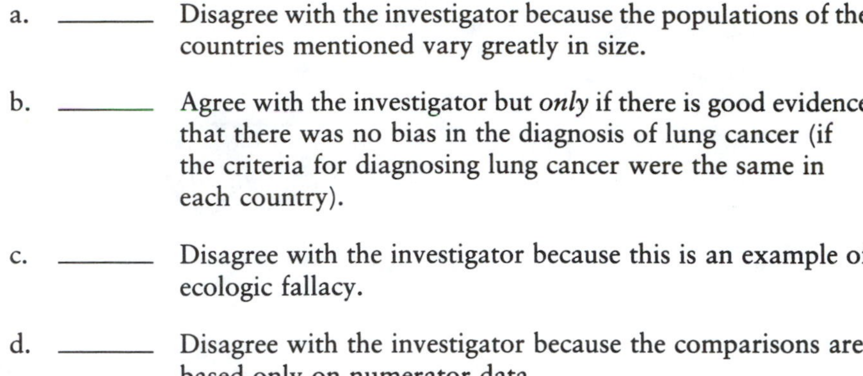

a. ______ Disagree with the investigator because the populations of the countries mentioned vary greatly in size.

b. ______ Agree with the investigator but *only* if there is good evidence that there was no bias in the diagnosis of lung cancer (if the criteria for diagnosing lung cancer were the same in each country).

c. ______ Disagree with the investigator because this is an example of ecologic fallacy.

d. ______ Disagree with the investigator because the comparisons are based only on numerator data.

16. In a study of broken appointments by patients attending a clinic, the effect of distance from the clinic was examined. Part of the results are shown in Table 10.12.

TABLE 10.12 Rate of broken appointments, by distance which patients live from clinic, for women aged 45-49

Miles from Clinic	*% Broken Appointments*
10 or greater	53
5-9	47
1-4	39
less than one	29

These differences were statistically significant. It was suspected, however, that the social class composition of the patients living at different distances from the clinic varied, which may have affected the number of broken appointments. Accordingly, to control for social class, each patient was given a social class score, and a *social class adjusted* rate of broken appointments was computed, as shown in Table 10.13. The adjusted rates were not statistically significantly different from each other.

TABLE 10.13 Rate of broken appointments, adjusted for social class, by distance which patients live from clinic, for women aged 45-49

Miles from Clinic	*% Broken Appointments*
10 or greater	42
5-9	44
1-4	40
less than one	41

From these data, which of the following conclusions can be drawn (in each case the conclusions are restricted to females aged 45 to 49)? (Check as many as are correct.)

a. _______ The social class adjusted results decrease the likelihood that distance from the clinic was related causally to broken appointments.

b. _______ The social class adjusted results decrease the likelihood that social class was related to broken appointments.

c. _______ The data confirm that the *social class distribution* of patients living at different distances from the clinic does vary.

d. _______ The data increase the likelihood that *both distance from the clinic* and *social class* of the patients are related to broken appointments.

17. As an administrator of a chronic disease control program, you have two screening tests available for the early detection of a particular disease. Screening test A has a sensitivity of 95% and a specificity of 70%. Screening test B has a sensitivity of 60% and a specificity of 90%. Given the following circumstances, which test would you choose? (Check A or B for each circumstance.)

    a. If the disease were one whose presence caused a high level of anxiety, to avoid needless emotional suffering you wanted to reduce the probability that healthy people would be told that they had the disease. _______ A _______ B
    b. If the most important concern were to not overburden the health care system with unnecessary referrals for further diagnostic workups after the screening. _______ A _______ B
    c. If this were a treatable disease in its early stages, but fatal if not detected early. _______ A _______ B
    d. If this were a highly infectious disease in its early stages, but less infectious in later stages and you had to protect the public from contact with the infectious stage of the disease. _______ A _______ B

18. Two observers examined the same 100 subjects independently. Each observer reported the prevalence of diabetes as 25% in the sample. Construct a table demonstrating how it is possible for observer 1 and observer 2 to have inter-observer reliability of only 50%, despite their identical estimates of prevalence.

19. As part of a cancer control program, a state's Department of Human Services started a program in 1960 to reduce the exposure of the population to x-rays. To evaluate the effectiveness of the program, a statewide cancer register was developed to record all newly diagnosed cases of cancer. The data in Table 10.14 refer to a specific, incurable form of cancer in children (aged 0 to 4); exposure to x-rays is thought to be an important part of the cause.

    Assume that the reporting of new cases was reasonably complete and that there had been minimal in- or out-migration from the state during

TABLE 10.14 Total number of children aged 0 to 4, number of new cases, and number of cases on register, by year

Year	*Children Aged 0 to 4*	*Newly Diagnosed Cases of Cancer*	*Cancer Cases in Register*
1980	100,000	100	200
1985	150,000	120	350
1990	200,000	130	550

the ten-year period. Assume, also, that in the neighboring states that had not had such a program, none of the cancer rates (for this particular form of cancer in this age group) had changed in the ten-year period. What would you regard these data as suggesting for this particular cancer in this age group? (Check the <u>one best</u> answer.)

a. ______ The program to prevent cancer was *not* successful, but there had been an improvement in the ability to treat cancer during this period.

b. ______ The program to prevent cancer was successful but there had been no improvement in the ability to treat cancer.

c. ______ The program was successful in preventing cancer *and* there had been an improvement in the ability to treat cancer.

d. ______ Neither the program to prevent cancer was successful *nor* had there been any improvement in treatment.

20. Suppose you read an article about a study of lead poisoning in 136 children. All of the children reported by hospitals in Mytown, Colorado between 1987 and 1993 with lead poisoning were included in the study. The data in Tables 10.15 and 10.16 present the results of the study.

TABLE 10.15 Distribution of lead poisoning in children, by age, 1987-1993

Age in Months	*Cases of Lead Poisoning*
9 and under	0
10-12	3
13-18	25
19-24	39
25-30	30
31-36	17
37-42	13
43-48	4
49 and over	4
Unknown	1
Total	136

TABLE 10.16 Month of first admission of 136 lead-poisoned children in Mytown, Colorado, 1987-1993

Month	*Cases Admitted*
January	3
February	5
March	2
April	5
May	12
June	19
July	32
August	28
September	15
October	9
November	4
December	2
Total	136

On the basis of these data, the authors concluded that: (1) The most vulnerable age for lead poisoning was between 1 and 3.5 years (12-42 months). (2) More hospital admissions for lead poisoning occur during the summer months than at any other time. For each conclusion, check the one best answer.

Conclusion 1 (The most vulnerable age is between 1 and 3.5 years.)

a. ______ Disagree with the conclusion because this is an example of ecologic fallacy.

b. ______ Disagree with the conclusion because it is based on numerator data only.

c. ______ Agree with the conclusion, but only if there has been no bias in the diagnosis of lead poisoning.

d. ______ Disagree with the conclusion because the antecedent-consequent relationship cannot be determined from this study design.

Conclusion 2 (More hospital admissions occur during the summer months.)

a. ______ Disagree with the conclusion because this is an example of ecologic fallacy.

b. ______ Disagree with the conclusion because it is based on numerator data only.

c. ______ Agree with the conclusion, but only if there has been no bias in the diagnosis of lead poisoning.

d. ______ Disagree with the conclusion because the antecedent-consequent relationship cannot be determined from this study design.

21. The data in Table 10.17 were reported from a cohort study conducted on professional male workers. The results indicate (check *as many* as are correct and show the figures on which you based your conclusions):

TABLE 10.17 Age-adjusted mortality rates from lung cancer and coronary heart disease, for heavy cigarette smokers and nonsmokers

	Annual Age-adjusted Death Rate per 100,000 Men	
	Lung Cancer	*CHD*
Heavy smokers	160	599
Nonsmokers	7	422

a. ______ More workers would be saved from lung cancer than from coronary disease if no one smoked.

b. ______ More workers would be saved from coronary heart disease than from lung cancer if no one smoked.

c. ______ Heavy smoking carries a higher relative risk for lung cancer than for CHD.

d. ______ Heavy smoking carries a higher relative risk for CHD than for lung cancer.

22. From the data of a well-conducted cohort study concerned with the incidence of stroke in rural and urban men, Tables 10.18 and 10.19 were constructed. Diagnostic criteria were well standardized (no bias), the samples were representative, and there was minimal attrition (no selection). Differences were statistically significant. From these data, what would be the most appropriate conclusion? (Check the one best answer.)

TABLE 10.18 Incidence of stroke in rural and urban men

	Rural Men	*Urban Men*
Population at risk	529	937
Cases of stroke	24	41
Incidence rate per 1,000	45.3	43.8

a. ______ In this sample, the higher incidence rates in rural men indicate some increased risk (other than age) associated with rural living.

b. ______ In this sample, there is an increased risk (other than age) associated with urban living because at each age the urban incidence rates are higher than the rural.

TABLE 10.19 Incidence of stroke in rural and urban men

	Rural			*Urban*		
Age	*PAR*	*Cases of Stroke*	*Incidence Rate per 1,000*	*PAR*	*Cases of Stroke*	*Incidence Rate per 1,000*
35-44	147	1	6.8	436	6	13.8
45-54	87	3	4.5	188	7	37.2
55-64	133	4	30.1	195	13	66.7
65-74	160	16	100.0	103	15	145.6
Unknown	2	0	—	15	0	—
Total	529	24		937	41	

c. ______ No comparison of urban versus rural rates can be made from these tables because there are nearly twice as many urban as rural men at risk.

d. ______ Some error in assigning ages must have been made in this study because although the total rates (Table 10.18) are higher in rural men, when the two populations are broken into age groups (Table 10.19), the urban rates are always higher than the rural rates for each age group.

23. In an attempt to determine the effect of driver education on automobile accidents, a case-control study was undertaken. One hundred fifty individuals between the ages of 16 and 25 who had been responsible for an automobile accident were suitably matched with 300 controls who had had no accident. The "exposure" (number of miles driven) was the same in the two groups. The analyses were performed separately for females and males. Differences were statistically significant. On the basis of the data in Table 10.20, the investigators drew the following conclusions. *For females*: "There is an association between lack of driver education and accidents because the majority of the accident cases did not have driver education." *For males*: "In males, however, the opposite association exists because the majority of the accident cases *did* have driver education."

TABLE 10.20 Driver education and automobile accidents in cases and controls

	Females		*Males*	
Driver Education	*Accident Cases*	*No Accident*	*Accident Cases*	*No Accident*
Had driver education	10	50	60	120
Did not have driver education	40	50	40	280
Total	50	100	100	400

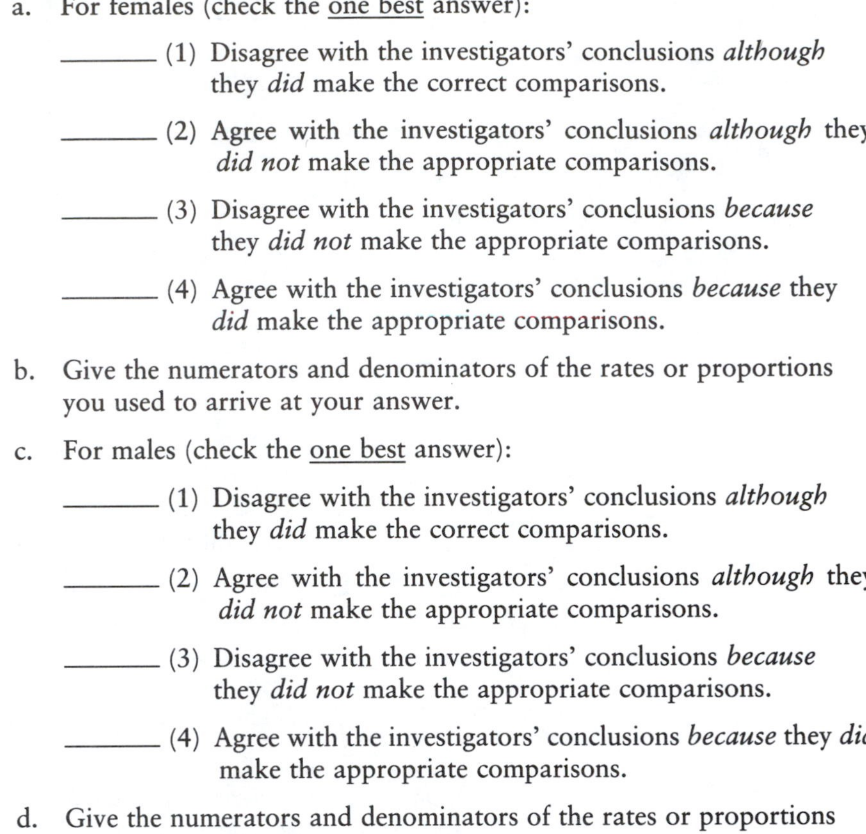

a. For females (check the one best answer):

_______ (1) Disagree with the investigators' conclusions *although* they *did* make the correct comparisons.

_______ (2) Agree with the investigators' conclusions *although* they *did not* make the appropriate comparisons.

_______ (3) Disagree with the investigators' conclusions *because* they *did not* make the appropriate comparisons.

_______ (4) Agree with the investigators' conclusions *because* they *did* make the appropriate comparisons.

b. Give the numerators and denominators of the rates or proportions you used to arrive at your answer.

c. For males (check the one best answer):

_______ (1) Disagree with the investigators' conclusions *although* they *did* make the correct comparisons.

_______ (2) Agree with the investigators' conclusions *although* they *did not* make the appropriate comparisons.

_______ (3) Disagree with the investigators' conclusions *because* they *did not* make the appropriate comparisons.

_______ (4) Agree with the investigators' conclusions *because* they *did* make the appropriate comparisons.

d. Give the numerators and denominators of the rates or proportions you used to arrive at your answer.

24. In a study to determine the relationship between physical activity and coronary heart disease, men of similar age and of the same ethnic group in three different occupations were compared. The occupations were classified as physically active, moderately active, and sedentary. The findings are shown in Table 10.21. Questions (a) and (b) are true-false questions relating to the data in Table 10.21.

TABLE 10.21 Coronary heart disease, by occupational type

Occupational Type	*Number of Men*	*Cases of CHD*	*Rate per 1,000*
Active	6,000	20	3.3
Moderate	3,000	30	10.0
Sedentary	1,000	20	20.0
Total	10,000	70	7.0

a. If the data shown in Table 10.21 are from a *cross-sectional study* (prevalence data) and the differences are statistically significant, indicate whether *each* of the following statements is true or false.

True _______
False _______
(1) The associations shown in Table 10.21 could have occurred if physical activity was protective against coronary heart disease.

True ______ (2) The associations could be entirely a result of men with CHD changing occupations from active to more sedentary jobs.
False ______

True ______ (3) The associations could be entirely a result of a higher case-fatality rate in men in active jobs as compared with those in sedentary jobs.
False ______

b. If the data shown in Table 10.21 were from a *cohort study* (incidence data) and the differences were statistically significant, indicate whether *each* of the following statements would be true or false.

True ______ (1) The associations shown in Table 10.21 could have occurred if physical activity was protective against coronary heart disease.
False ______

True ______ (2) The associations could be entirely a result of men with CHD changing occupations from active to more sedentary jobs.
False ______

True ______ (3) The associations could be entirely a result of a higher case-fatality rate in men in active jobs as compared with those in sedentary jobs.
False ______

REVIEW EXERCISE—INVESTIGATING AN OUTBREAK

This review exercise[1] is a case study of an outbreak of enteritis during a pilgrimage to Mecca. After reading this case study and answering all 16 embedded questions, a student will be able to do the following:

- Define an epidemic, an outbreak, and a cluster
- Create and understand the uses of a case definition
- Draw an epidemic curve
- Calculate food-specific attack rates
- List the steps in investigating an acute outbreak

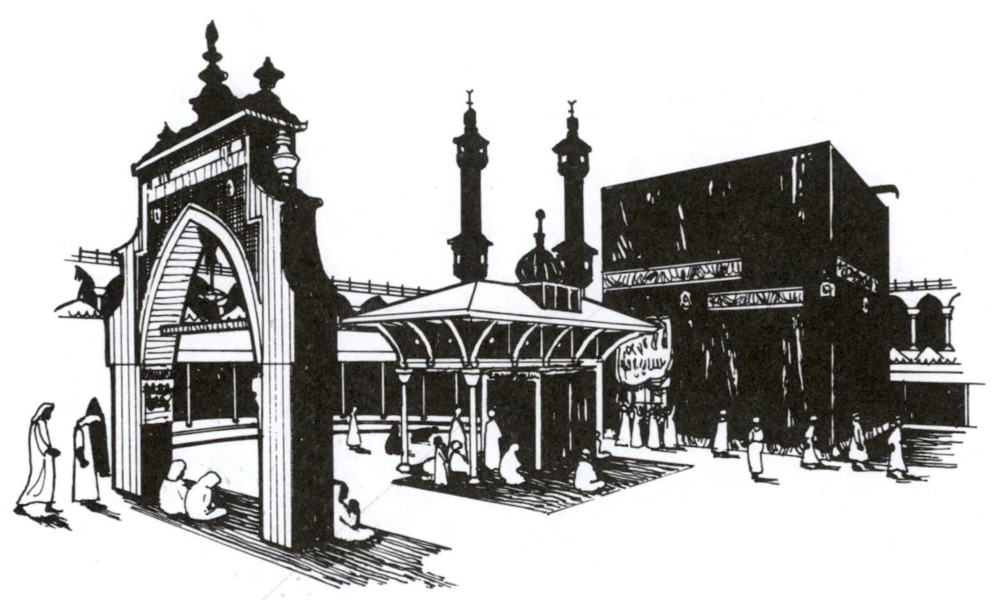

FIGURE 10.2 *Illustration of the Kaaba in Mecca*

AN OUTBREAK OF ENTERITIS DURING A PILGRIMAGE TO MECCA

Part I

On the morning of November 1, 1979, during a pilgrimage to Mecca, the epidemiologist assigned to the Kuwaiti medical mission experienced acute onset of abdominal cramps and diarrhea at the holy mosque before the walk around the Kaaba. He subsequently learned that other members of the mission had developed similar symptoms. When he returned that evening to Muna, he initiated an investigation.

[1]Taken from Centers for Disease Control and Prevention: *Principles of epidemiology: An introduction to applied epidemiology and biostatistics* (pp. 387-413). Atlanta, GA: 1992.

Question 1. What information do you need to decide if this is an epidemic?

The epidemiologist interviewed several ill members of the mission to better characterize the illness. On the basis of these interviews, the epidemiologist quickly prepared a questionnaire and conducted interviews with the 112 members of the Kuwaiti medical mission.

A total of 66 cases of illness were identified; 2 had onset in Kuwait prior to the beginning of the pilgrimage and 64 had onset of symptoms beginning late in the afternoon on October 31.

Question 2. Is this an epidemic? Explain your answer.

Description of the Pilgrimage

The Kuwaiti medical mission, consisting of 112 members, traveled by automobile from Kuwait to Mecca. On October 30 all members of the mission slept in Muna. At sunrise on October 31 they traveled to Arafat, where at 8:00 A.M. they had tea with or without milk for breakfast. The milk was prepared immediately before consumption by mixing powdered milk with boiled water. The remainder of the day was devoted to religious services. At 2:00 P.M., a lunch was served for all members of the mission who wished to partake. It was a typical Kuwaiti meal consisting of three dishes: rice, meat, and tomato sauce. Most individuals consumed all three dishes. The lunch had been prepared in Muna on October 30 and transported to Arafat by truck early on October 31. At sunset on October 31 the mission members returned to Muna.

Clinical Description

The investigator identified a total of 66 cases of gastroenteritis. The onset of all cases was acute, characterized chiefly by diarrhea and abdominal pain. Nausea, vomiting, and blood in the stool occurred infrequently. No case-patient reported fever. All recovered within 12 to 24 hours. Approximately 20% of the ill individuals sought medical advice. The investigator did not obtain any fecal specimens for examination.

Question 3. Develop a preliminary case definition.

Question 4. List the broad categories of diseases that must be considered in the differential diagnosis of an outbreak of gastrointestinal illness.

Note: These concepts have not been covered in this course. If you are not familiar with disease agents, review the answer to this question.

Question 5. What clinical and epidemiologic information might be helpful in determining the etiologic agent(s)?

Question 6. The Kuwaiti investigators distributed a questionnaire to all members of the mission. What information would you solicit on this questionnaire?

Part II

Investigators determined that of the 64 cases with onset during the pilgrimage, all had eaten lunch in Arafat at 2:00 P.M. on October 31. Fifteen members of the mission did not eat lunch; none became ill.

Question 7. Calculate the attack rate for those who ate lunch and those who did not. What do you conclude?

Table 10.22 on pages 374-375 presents some of the information collected by the investigators. The two members who developed illness prior to October 31 have been excluded. The 15 members of the mission who did not eat lunch are not included in Table 10.22.

Question 8. Using appropriate time periods, draw an epidemic curve.

Question 9. Are there any cases for which the time of onset seems inconsistent? How might they be explained?

Question 10. Modify the graph you have drawn (Question 8) to illustrate the distribution of incubation periods.

Question 11. Determine or calculate the minimum, maximum, mean, median, mode, range, and standard deviation of the incubation periods.

Question 12a. Calculate the frequency of each clinical symptom among the cases.

Question 12b. How does the information on the symptoms and incubation periods help you to narrow the differential diagnosis? (You may refer to the attached "Abbreviated Compendium of Acute Foodborne Gastrointestinal Diseases" in Appendix D.)

Question 13a. Using the food consumption histories in Table 10.22, complete item 7 of the "Investigation of a Foodborne Outbreak" report form in Appendix E.

Question 13b. Do these calculations help you to determine which food(s) served at the lunch may have been responsible for the outbreak?

Question 14. Outline further investigations which should be pursued. List one or more factors that could have led to the contamination of the implicated food.

TABLE 10.22 Selected characteristics of Kuwaiti medical mission members who ate lunch at Arafat, Saudi Arabia, October 31, 1979

			Onset of Illness		*Foods*			*Signs/Symptoms**				
ID#	*Age*	*Sex*	*Date*	*Hour*	*Rice*	*Meat*	*TS**	*D*	*C*	*BS*	*N*	*V*	*F*
31	36	M	Oct. 31	5 P.M.	X	X	X	D	C	BS			
77	28	M	Oct. 31	5 P.M.	X	X		D	C				
81	33	M	Oct. 31	10 P.M.	X	X	X	D	C				
86	29	M	Oct. 31	10 P.M.	X	X	X	D	C				
15	38	M	Oct. 31	10 P.M.		X		D		BS	N		
17	48	M	Oct. 31	10 P.M.	X	X		D	C				
18	35	M	Oct. 31	10 P.M.	X	X	X	D	C				
35	30	M	Oct. 31	11 P.M.	X	X	X	D	C				
88	27	M	Oct. 31	11 P.M.	X	X	X	D	C				
76	29	M	Oct. 31	11 P.M.	X	X	X	D	C	BS			
71	50	M	Oct. 31	12 MN	X	X	X	D					
1	39	F	Nov. 1	1 A.M.	X	X	X	D	C			V	
27	36	M	Nov. 1	1 A.M.	X	X	X	D	C		N		
28	44	M	Nov. 1	1 A.M.	X	X	X	D	C				
29	48	M	Nov. 1	1 A.M.	X	X	X	D	C	BS			
30	35	M	Nov. 1	2 A.M.	X	X	X	D	C				
50	29	M	Nov. 1	2 A.M.	X	X	X	D	C				
59	51	M	Nov. 1	2 A.M.	X	X	X	D	C				
67	40	M	Nov. 1	2 A.M.	X	X		D					
72	58	M	Nov. 1	2 A.M.	X	X	X	D	C				
73	28	M	Nov. 1	3 A.M.	X	X	X	D	C				
60	31	M	Nov. 1	3 A.M.	X	X	X	D	C				
61	38	M	Nov. 1	3 A.M.	X	X	X	D		BS			
51	32	M	Nov. 1	3 A.M.	X	X	X	D	C			V	
52	37	M	Nov. 1	3 A.M.	X	X		D					
58	30	M	Nov. 1	3 A.M.	X	X	X	D	C				
22	35	M	Nov. 1	3 A.M.	X	X	X	D	C				
25	30	M	Nov. 1	3 A.M.	X	X		D	C				
32	50	M	Nov. 1	3 A.M.	X	X	X	D	C				
38	26	M	Nov. 1	3 A.M.	X	X	X	D	C				
79	29	M	Nov. 1	3 A.M.	X	X	X	D	C				
80	28	M	Nov. 1	3 A.M.	X	X	X	D	C				
37	30	M	Nov. 1	4 A.M.	X	X	X	D					
65	34	M	Nov. 1	4 A.M.	X	X		D		BS			
66	45	M	Nov. 1	4 A.M.	X	X		D	C				
87	41	M	Nov. 1	4 A.M.	X	X	X	D	C				
89	43	M	Nov. 1	4 A.M.	X	X	X	D	C				
90	43	M	Nov. 1	4 A.M.	X	X	X	D	C				
91	38	M	Nov. 1	4 A.M.	X	X	X	D	C				
92	37	M	Nov. 1	4 A.M.	X	X	X	D	C				
70	31	M	Nov. 1	5 A.M.	X	X	X	D	C				
2	34	F	Nov. 1	5 A.M.	X	X	X	D	C				
21	38	M	Nov. 1	5 A.M.	X	X	X	D	C				
40	38	M	Nov. 1	5 A.M.	X	X	X	D					
78	27	M	Nov. 1	5 A.M.	X	X	X	D	C				
82	39	M	Nov. 1	5 A.M.	X	X	X	D	C				
83	40	M	Nov. 1	5 A.M.	X	X	X	D	C				
84	34	M	Nov. 1	5 A.M.	X	X		D	C				

Continued

TABLE 10.22 *Continued*

			Onset of Illness		*Foods*			*Signs/Symptoms**					
ID#	*Age*	*Sex*	*Date*	*Hour*	*Rice*	*Meat*	*TS**	*D*	*C*	*BS*	*N*	*V*	*F*
14	52	M	Nov. 1	6 A.M.	X	X	X	D					
16	40	M	Nov. 1	6 A.M.	X	X	X	D		BS			
93	30	M	Nov. 1	6 A.M.	X	X	X	D	C				
94	39	M	Nov. 1	6 A.M.	X	X	X	D	C				
33	55	M	Nov. 1	7 A.M.	X	X	X	D	C				
34	28	M	Nov. 1	7 A.M.	X	X	X	D	C				
85	38	M	Nov. 1	7 A.M.	X	X		D	C				
43	38	M	Nov. 1	9 A.M.	X	X		D	C				
69	30	M	Nov. 1	9 A.M.	X	X	X	D	C				
4	30	F	Nov. 1	10 A.M.	X			D	C				
5	45	F	Nov. 1	10 A.M.		X			C				
3	29	F	Nov. 1	1 P.M.	X	X		D	C				
12	22	F	Nov. 1	2 P.M.	X	X	X		C				
74	44	M	Nov. 1	2 P.M.	X	X	X	D					
75	45	M	Nov. 1	5 P.M.	X	X	X	D		BS			
95	40	M	Nov. 1	11 P.M.	X	X	X	D	C				
6	38	F	WELL		X	X							
7	52	F	WELL		X	X	X						
8	35	F	WELL		X		X						
9	27	F	WELL		X	X	X						
10	40	F	WELL		X	X	X						
11	40	F	WELL		X	X	X						
13	50	M	WELL		X	X	X						
19	38	M	WELL		X	X	X						
20	38	M	WELL		X	X	X						
23	29	M	WELL		X	X	X						
24	27	M	WELL		X	X	X						
26	47	M	WELL		X	X	X						
36	60	M	WELL		X								
39	27	M	WELL		X	X	X						
41	30	M	WELL		X	X	X						
42	38	M	WELL		X	X	X						
44	50	M	WELL		X	X	X						
45	27	M	WELL		X	X	X						
46	31	M	WELL		X	X	X						
47	46	M	WELL		X	X	X						
48	38	M	WELL		X	X							
49	36	M	WELL		X		X						
53	36	M	WELL		X	X	X						
54	27	M	WELL		X	X	X						
55	40	M	WELL		X	X	X						
56	30	M	WELL		X	X	X						
57	25	M	WELL		X	X	X						
62	50	M	WELL		X								
63	44	M	WELL		X								
64	47	M	WELL		X		X						
68	31	M	WELL		X	X	X						

*TS = Tomato sauce; D = diarrhea, C = cramps, BS = blood in stool, N = nausea, V = vomiting, F = fever

SOURCE: CDC, 1992.

Part III

The lunch which was served in Arafat at 2:00 P.M. on October 31 was prepared at 10:00 P.M. the night before in Muna. It consisted of boiled rice, chunks of lamb fried in oil, and tomato sauce prepared from fresh tomatoes which were sectioned and stewed. The cooked rice was placed in two large pots and the lamb was divided evenly on top. The tomato sauce was kept in a third pot.

These pots were covered with metal tops and placed in an open spot among some rocks near the kitchen and allowed to stand overnight. They were presumably not touched by anyone during this period. Early in the morning on October 31, the pots were transported by truck from Muna to Arafat where they stood in the truck until 2:00 P.M. The temperature in Arafat at noon that day was 35°C. The food was not refrigerated from the time of preparation to the time of consumption.

Cooks and all other individuals who helped in preparing the meal were intensively interviewed regarding any illness present before or at the time of preparation. All individuals interviewed denied having any illness and knew of no illness among other members of the group responsible for meal preparation. No specimens were obtained from any of the cooks for laboratory examination.

The following is quoted verbatim from the report prepared by the epidemiologist who investigated the outbreak:

> This clinical picture probably suggests an infection by *Clostridium perfringens*. This organism could be detected in the food elements consumed as well as in the patient's stool. However, no laboratory diagnostic procedures were possible in the outbreak site. All the investigations conducted were based entirely on epidemiologic grounds.
>
> The incubation period as well as other data extrapolated from epidemiological analysis suggests that *Clostridium perfringens* is the causative agent. This organism is widely distributed in nature especially in soil and dust. So there is ample opportunity for contamination of the food. If cooked meat is allowed to cool slowly under suitable anaerobic conditions, spores which might have survived cooking or have subsequently come from dust may germinate and within a few hours produce large numbers of vegetative bacilli. In fact, the pilgrimage camp in Muna lacks sanitary cooking facilities. The food is usually prepared in a dusty place open to the blowing winds creating an ideal situation for *Clostridium perfringens* contamination.
>
> The type of the organism, the type of food dish it usually contaminates, its mode of spread and the differences in the attack rates for those who consumed meat and those who did not points to the meat as the probable source of infection in this outbreak.
>
> *Conclusion*: The acute illness of enteritis in Arafat affected many persons in an epidemic form. It was a common-source outbreak, the source being the meat consumed at the Arafat lunch. The incubation period was about 13 hours. The illness was characterized by colicky abdominal pain and diarrhea with no elevation of temperature. The

responsible agent for this outbreak is most probably *Clostridium perfringens*. The lunch at Arafat should have been prepared in the same day of consumption, or kept refrigerated if it had to be prepared the day before. Although kitchens could not be fully equipped to fulfill the essential safety measures in a place like Muna, they should be supplied by essential measures to protect food from contamination. The remaining food in Arafat should have been condemned after the investigation, but none remained at that time.

The epidemiological investigations carried out in this epidemic could explore the nature of this epidemic and answer most of the questions raised. The laboratory investigation, although helpful to detect the causative organisms, should not replace the more efficient epidemiological methods in the exploration of such epidemics. The lack of the necessary laboratory facilities to detect the causative organisms in foodborne outbreaks should not discourage the investigative epidemiologist and make him doubtful and lose confidence in his epidemiological tools.

Question 15. In the context of this outbreak, what control measures would you recommend?

Question 16. Was it important to work up this outbreak?

ANSWERS

1. The rate *least* affected is the incidence rate, so (c) is the correct answer because treatment cannot affect the development of new cases (the incidence).
2. Prevalence rates in January 1985:

   a. Among those exposed to air pollution = 60/6,000 = 10 per 1,000.
   b. Among those *not* exposed to air pollution = 30/3,000 = 10 per 1,000.

   Incidence rates for the five years:

   c. Among those exposed to air pollution = 238/5,940 = 40.1 per 1,000 (note that the 60 cases prevalent in this group in 1985 are *not* at risk in the incidence rates and so are excluded from the denominator).
   d. Among those *not* exposed to air pollution = 30/2,970 = 10.1 per 1,000 (denominator reduced because 30 cases prevalent in 1985 are not at risk in incidence).
   e. In total sample = 268/8,910 (this is simple addition; do not add the rates and divide by 2).
   f. Correct answer is (2). There is no difference in prevalence rates of exposed and nonexposed groups.
   g. Correct answer is (1). Incidence rate among the exposed is four times the rate among the nonexposed.
   h. Correct answer is (1). Selective survival should not influence conclusions from the cohort study (which provides incidence data) because all subjects of the cohort are followed (even to death). Thus (2) and (3) are incorrect.
   i. Correct answer is (1) for the same reasons as in (h).
   j. Correct answer is (3). Secondary associations due to confounding variables can be found in all study methods.

3. a. Correct answer is (a). Age is associated with death, and the fact that people in unskilled occupations are older makes age a possible confounder.
   b. Statement (b) is incorrect. It says people in professional and managerial occupations are *older*; they are the group with the lower rates, so age is unlikely as a confounder.
   c. Statement (c) is correct because women have lower death rates; here sex is the suspected confounder.
   d. Statement (d) is irrelevant because rates are compared.

4. Correct answer is (a). This is shown by calculating the relative risk of occurrence with no home visits and the attributable risk with no home visits, for each disease in Table 10.23 on page 379.

   With home visits, rheumatic heart disease is less likely (3.1 compared to 9) to recur than diabetes complications. However, home visits have a greater effect on preventing complications of rheumatic fever than they do on diabetes (10.7 per 1,000 compared to 4 per 1,000).

5. a. Statement (a) is correct. The perinatal mortality rate is lower in those who received prenatal care.

TABLE 10.23 Relative risk and attributable risk of complications in children with rheumatic fever or diabetes

	Relative Risk with No Home Visits	*Attributable Risk with No Home Visits*
Rheumatic fever recurrence	15.7/5.0 = 3.1	15.7 − 5.0 = 10.7 per 1,000
Diabetic complications	4.5/0.5 = 9.0	4.5 − 0.5 = 4 per 1,000

b. Statement (b) is incorrect. The difference in rates for those who received care and those who did not receive care is found in both less educated and more educated women (the table controls for education levels).
c. Statement (c) is incorrect. The difference in rates for those who received care and those who did not receive care is also found among less educated women.
d. Statement (d) is correct. Among those receiving care, the rate is higher among less educated women.

Your table should resemble Table 10.24. (For clarity the numerators and denominators were included; they all can be derived from the data given.)

Although the perinatal mortality rate is lower for those women who received prenatal care, it is not certain that prenatal care *caused* reduced mortality. For example, if the women chose to attend prenatal care, healthier women may have selected such care. If the women were randomly assigned to either prenatal or no prenatal care, the cause-effect relationship could be argued with more persuasion.

TABLE 10.24 Perinatal death rates per 1,000, by education and prenatal care, primigravidae 20-24 years old

	High School Graduate	*Non-High School Graduate*	*Total*
Prenatal care	2/100 = 18.2	3/90 = 33.3	5/200 = 25.0
No prenatal care	4/80 = 50.0	6/70 = 85.7	10/150 = 66.7
Total	6/190 = 31.6	9/160 = 56.3	15/350 = 42.9

6. We compare the incidence rates of stroke in pill takers and non-pill takers. These are 10/1,000 in pill takers and 10/8,920 in non-pill takers.

a. The only correct answer is statement (a).
b. This comparison is incorrect and deals only with stroke victims (numerator data only).
c. The rate of non-pill takers developing stroke must be compared (not 990/1,000, which is the pill takers' rate of *not* developing stroke).
d. The decision is right about risk, but the comparisons made to support the decision are incorrect in a cohort study.

7. Correct answers are (a) and (c).

   The age and cigarette-smoking SMRs adjust for age and smoking differences between the industries' employees, using the indirect adjustment method.

   Because industries A and C shows SMRs much higher than 100 (the baseline standard for SMRs), factors other than smoking and age are operative.

   Although the average annual death rate in B is high (71 per 100,000), adjustment for confounders of age and cigarette smoking shows its risk equal to that of industry E and nearly the same as that of industry D. Thus, cigarette smoking and age are related to lung cancer in B, which makes answer (b) incorrect.

8. Correct answer is (b). In the control table, there are differences in birthweights by social class position in both rural and urban residents, but little difference by places of residence for the two social classes. When residence is controlled, only social class is associated with birthweight.

9. a. The correct answer is (3). Sensitivity is A/(A + C).
   b. The correct answer is (3). Specificity is D/(B + D).
   c. The correct answer is (2). Frequency of false positives is B.

10. If (a) is correct, you would find a decline in incidence rates; if (b) is correct, you would find a decline in case-fatality ratios, suggesting improved treatment (see Table 10.25).

TABLE 10.25 Incidence rates and case-fatality ratios of disease, by year

	Incidence Rate	*Case-Fatality Ratio*
1980	100/(50,000 − 100) = 2 per 1,000	5/200 = 25 per 1,000
1985	150/(75,000 − 75) = 2 per 1,000	5/225 = 22 per 1,000
1990	200/(100,000 − 50) = 2 per 1,000	5/250 = 20 per 1,000

   In calculating incidence rates, deduct cases that are *not* incidence cases from denominators for each year. These cases may be from previous years and therefore cannot be *new*. Because there is no secular change in incidence rates but a decline in case-fatality ratios, (b) is the correct answer.

11. a. The correct answer is (1).
    b. The correct answer is (2).
    c. The correct answer is (3).

12. a. The correct answer is (1). Rare diseases are not easily studied in cohort style because we would need a large population to ascertain enough cases.
    b. The correct answer is (2). This needs a strategy to establish which factor is the cause. The best way is to use a cohort study.
    c. The correct answer is (1), case-control; both the cases studied and the controls are survivors; this may be selective. Selective survival does *not* bias the results of cohort studies, because we gather data from all members of the cohort regardless of whether they survive.

d. The correct answer is (2). The best quantification of attributable risk comes from cohort studies. Case-control studies only *estimate* relative risk.
e. The correct answer is (1), case-control. Cohort studies lasting 20 years have occurred, but the logistics are very difficult and there are low success rates for continued participation and follow-up of participants. An historical cohort study is more advisable, but that was not given as an option.

13. The differences in rates between 1937 and 1955 are explained by the fact that in 1937 there was no association with age for the death rates; in 1955, there was a possible association. There were no changes in the association with gender; at all ages males had higher rates than females.

    a. Statement (a) is correct. The improvement of treatment over time for younger people explains the positive association with age in 1955.
    b. Statement (b) is correct. In 1955 doctors may have started labeling appendicitis deaths in younger people as something else; for example, as alcoholic enteritis, which would artifactually reduce the rates in younger people; or doctors may have increased labeling deaths as appendicitis among older people in 1955. This would be a change in diagnostic custom.
    c. Statement (c) is incorrect. Migration would have to be of young couples with *high* risk of death from appendicitis.
    d. Statement (d) is incorrect. We are dealing with rates; they are comparable.

14. Statement (a) is correct. The prevalence of CHD in 1989 is about twice as high in Boise than in Jamaica. The incidence rate is five times higher in Boise than in Jamaica in the ten-year period preceding 1989. Thus, if the death rates were the same in the two areas, one would expect the prevalence rate in Boise to be about five times higher than that in Jamaica. Since it is only 2.4 times higher, the death rate in Boise must be higher than in Jamaica. Immigration and cure are not factors.

15. a. Statement (a) is incorrect. It is not relevant because indices are per capita or a proportion (a rate).
    b. Statement (b) is an unlikely explanation.
    c. Statement (c) is correct. The investigator is using ecologic (group) indices and assuming association, or lack thereof, between group indices.
    d. Statement (d) is not correct. All comparisons are population-based.

16. Table 10.12 shows a positive association of distance and broken appointments. In Table 10.13 the effect of social class has been nullified in the rates. The association found in Table 10.12 is not seen in Table 10.13. Therefore, social class must be associated with distance; the social class with the greatest percentage of broken appointments is also living farther away.

    a. Statement (a) is correct. Because there is no association in Table 10.13, the effect in Table 10.12 must be dependent on social class.

b. Statement (b) is incorrect. See (a).
c. Statement (c) is correct. See (a).
d. Statement (d) is incorrect. Table 10.13 would show both associations if this statement were true.

17. Sensitivity addresses the likelihood of correctly identifying cases. Specificity addresses the likelihood of correctly identifying noncases.

    a. B is the correct choice. This statement concerns having a low rate of good specificity.
    b. B is the correct choice. A high rate of false positives (labeling people as cases whey they are not) overburdens the health care system. Test B will produce good specificity.
    c. A is the correct choice. Test A will produce good sensitivity.
    d. A is the correct choice. Test A will produce good sensitivity.

18. **TABLE 10.26** Results of two observers' independent examinations for diabetes (N = 100)

	Observer A		
Observer B	*Diabetics*	*Nondiabetics*	*Total*
Diabetics	0	25	25
Nondiabetics	25	50	75
Total	25	75	100

19. The correct answer is (c). By examining the new cases shown in Table 10.14, you find that the incidence rate declines and the prevalence rate increases. Therefore, the preventive program is effective and treatment improving because prevalence is increasing.

TABLE 10.27 Incidence and prevalence rates of cancer in children aged 0 to 4, 1980-1990

Year	*Incidence Rates*	*Prevalence Rates*
1980	100/100,000 = 1/1,000	200/100,000 = 2/1,000
1985	120/150,000 = 0.8/1,000	350/150,000 = 2.3/1,000
1990	130/200,000 = 0.65/1,000	550/200,000 = 2.75/1,000

20. Data in Table 10.15 represents only 136 cases of lead poisoning; there are no denominators.

    Conclusion 1: Answer (b) is correct.

    Conclusion 2: Answer (c) is correct. Admissions do occur more among summer months. Bias due to seasonal variation in diagnostic custom can produce artifactual seasonal variations.

21. We conclude that nonsmoking saves more workers from one disease than the other if attributable risks of death among smokers are different for the two diseases.

Attributable risk for lung cancer = 160 − 7 = 153/100,000
Attributable risk for CHD = 599 − 422 = 177/100,000

Therefore, (a) is incorrect; (b) is correct.

Relative risk for lung cancer = 160/7 = 23.7
Relative risk for CHD = 599/422 = 1.4

Therefore, (c) is correct; (d) is incorrect.

22. a. Statement (a) is incorrect. Age-specific rates in Table 10.19 are *lower* for rural men, so different age distribution explains the higher total rate for rural men.
 b. Statement (b) is correct.
 c. Statement (c) is incorrect; rates are compared.
 d. Statement (d) is incorrect; no bias was present.

23. For females, 80% of cases and 50% of controls (no accident) did not have driver education. For males, the rates are 40% and 40%, respectively. Therefore:

 a. Statement (1) is incorrect, but the investigators' conclusions are correct.
 Statement (2) is correct. You can agree with the investigators' conclusions, but the comparison should have been 80% with 50%; a "majority" of cases is not a comparison. Noncases need to be compared, where an equal "majority" may be found.
 Statement (3) is incorrect. The investigators' conclusions are correct.
 Statement (4) is incorrect. The investigators did not make appropriate comparisons.
 b. 40/50 and 50/100.
 c. Statement (1) is incorrect. You should disagree with the investigators' conclusions; incorrect comparisons were made.
 Statement (2) is incorrect. You should disagree with the investigators' conclusions.
 Statement (3) is correct.
 Statement (4) is incorrect. You should disagree with the investigators' conclusions.
 d. 40/100 and 80/200.

24. a. *If the data are from a cross-sectional study*:
 Statement (1) is true. The associations could have occurred.
 Statement (2) is true.
 Statement (3) is true. A higher case-fatality rate in active men means fewer cases in that group.
 b. *If the data are from a cohort study*:
 Statement (1) is true.
 Statement (2) is false. Persons were classified by activity before the occurrence of CHD.
 Statement (3) is false. Case-fatality ratio does not affect incidence rates.

ANSWERS—REVIEW EXERCISE

An Outbreak of Enteritis During a Pilgrimage to Mecca

Question 1. What information do you need to decide if this is an epidemic?

Answer 1.

- Is the number of cases more than the number expected?
- Therefore, we need to know background rate.

Question 2. Is this an epidemic?

Answer 2. Yes. An epidemic can be defined as the occurrence of more cases in a place and time than expected in the population being studied. Of the 110 members without signs and symptoms of gastroenteritis prior to the pilgrimage, 64 (58%) developed such signs and symptoms during this trip. This is clearly above the expected or background rate of gastroenteritis in most populations. Gastroenteritis prevalence rates from recent surveys are approximately 5% and are consistent with this population (2/112 had such signs and symptoms at the time of the pilgrimage).

One could survey other groups of pilgrims originating from the same country to determine their rates of diarrheal illness if the existence of an outbreak was uncertain. Practically speaking, however, an attack rate of 58% is an epidemic until proven otherwise.

The term "outbreak" and "epidemic" are used interchangeably by most epidemiologists. The term "outbreak" is sometimes preferred, particularly when talking to the press or public, because it is not as frightening as "epidemic." The term "cluster" may be defined as the occurrence of a group of cases in a circumscribed place and time. In a cluster, the number of cases may or may not be greater than expected.

Question 3. Develop a preliminary case definition.

Answer 3. Points to consider:

- As a general rule, during the initial phase of an investigation, the case definition should be broad.
- The case definition should include four components: **time, place, person,** and **diagnosis** (or signs, symptoms). Depending on the frequency of the symptoms observed and the probable etiologic agent, a more precise case definition can be developed later.

Case definition:

Clinical: acute onset of abdominal cramps and/or diarrhea
Time: onset after noon on October 31 and before November 2
Place/Person: member of the Kuwaiti medical mission en route to Mecca

Note: The Kuwaiti investigators had already decided that lunch on October 31 was the responsible meal and defined an outbreak-associated case of enteritis as a person in the Kuwaiti mission who ate lunch at Arafat at 2:00 P.M. on October 31 and subsequently developed abdominal pain and/or diarrhea prior to November 2, 1979.

However, at this point in your consideration of the outbreak you have not implicated the lunch, and it would probably be premature to limit your case definition to those who ate lunch.

Question 4. List the broad categories of diseases that must be considered in the differential diagnosis of an outbreak of gastrointestinal illness.

Answer 4.

Broad categories:
- Bacterial
- Viral
- Parasitic
- Toxins

More specifically:

Differential diagnosis of acute foodborne enteric illness

Bacteria and bacterial toxins	Viruses
*Bacillus cereus**	Norwalk-like agents (i.e., 27 nm viruses)
Campylobacter *jejuni*	Rotavirus*
Clostridium botulinum (initial symptoms)	**Toxins**
*Clostridium perfringens**	Heavy metals (especially cadmium, copper, tin, zinc)
*Escherichia coli**	Mushrooms
Salmonella, non-typhoid	Fish and shellfish (e.g., scombroid, ciguatera)
Salmonella typhi	Insecticides
Shigella	**Parasites**
Staphylococcus aureus	*Cryptosporidium*
Vibrio cholerae O1	*Entamoeba histolytica*
Vibrio cholerae non-O1	*Giardia lamblia*
Vibrio parahemolyticus	
Yersinia enterocolitica	

*These agents are most compatible with the following characteristics of this outbreak:
- acute onset
- lower GI signs and symptoms
- no fever
- appreciable proportion seeking medical advice
- no mention of non-enteric (dermatologic, neurologic) manifestations

However, you have not yet reached the point in your investigation to consider the most likely etiologic possibilities for the illness.

Question 5. What clinical and epidemiologic information might be helpful in determining the etiologic agent(s)?

Answer 5.

- Incubation period
- Symptom complex
- Duration of symptoms
- Severity of symptoms
- Seasonality
- Geographic location
- Biologic plausibility of pathogens

Question 6. The Kuwaiti investigators distributed a questionnaire to the persons who ate the implicated lunch. What information would you solicit on this questionnaire?

Answer 6.

- Identifying information
- Demographics (age, sex, race)
- Clinical information
  –Symptoms
  –Date and time of onset of symptoms
  –Duration of symptoms
  –Medical intervention, if required
- Information on possible causes
  –Exposure information regarding foods consumed, including amounts
  –Other potential exposures
  –Other factors that may modify risk of diarrhea (e.g., antacids, antibiotics)

Question 7. Calculate the attack rate for those who ate lunch and those who did not. What do you conclude?

Answer 7.

112 members of the mission
− 15 members who didn't eat lunch
− **2 members sick before pilgrimage**
95 at risk of developing illness

64 became ill among those who ate lunch
0 became ill among those who didn't eat lunch

Attack rate for those who ate lunch: 64 ill/95 at risk = 67%

Attack rate for those not eating lunch: 0 ill/15 at risk = 0%

Conclusion: Lunch is strongly associated with disease.

Question 8. Using appropriate time periods, draw an epidemic curve.

Answer 8.

Points for consideration about epi curves:

1. The epi curve is a basic tool of epidemiologists to
   a. establish existence of epidemic vs. endemic illness
   b. delineate time course and magnitude of an epidemic
   c. develop inferences about transmission (e.g., common source, person to person, intermittent exposure). Note that changing the interval on the x-axis can significantly alter the shape of an epi curve.
   d. predict future course of an epidemic: when it will end, that a second wave is underway, that secondary cases are occurring, etc.
2. With common source outbreaks, the width of the curve is determined by the incubation period, varying doses, and host susceptibility.
3. Often a few cases don't fit into the body of an epi curve. Such exceptions may be quite important—as index cases or other special situations.
4. *A rule of thumb*: When the incubation period is known, the maximum time period on the x-axis should not usually exceed 1/4 to 1/3 of the incubation period.

Summary of the temporal distribution (see Figure 10.3).

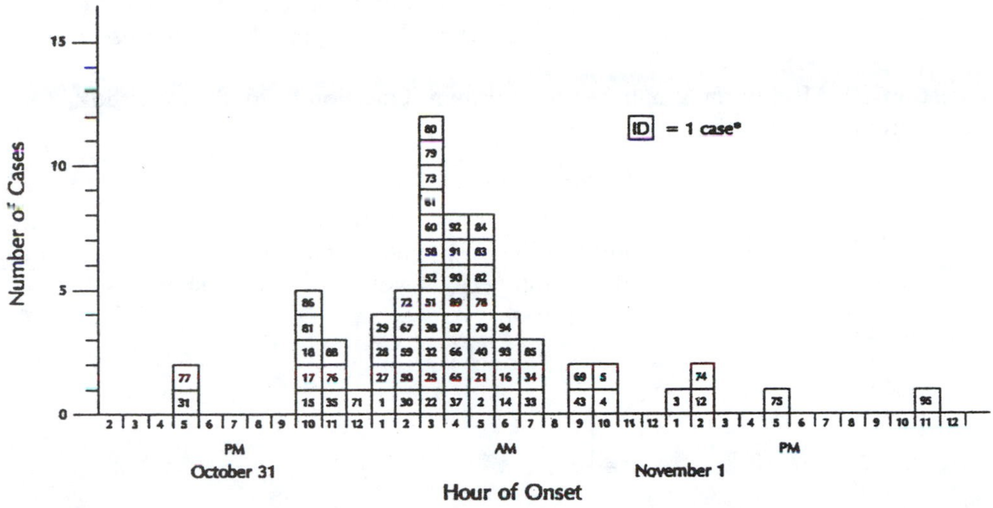

*ID# included for reference only.

FIGURE 10.3 *Outbreak-associated cases of enteritis by hour of onset of illness, Kuwaiti Mission, Arafat, Saudi Arabia, October 31–November 1, 1979*

a. Onsets of cases occurred over a period of 31 hours extending from 5 P.M. on October 31 to 11 P.M. on November 1.
b. Onsets of 53 (82.8%) of the cases occurred throughout the 10-hour interval from 10 P.M. on October 31 through 7 A.M. on November 1.
c. The peak (12 cases) occurred at 3 A.M. on November 1.
d. The median hour of onset = 3:30 A.M. November 1 (actual middle rank = 32.5 which falls between the 3 and 4 A.M. measurement intervals).
e. It is likely that the way the questionnaire was designed forced the interviewees to give a rounded time for onset of symptoms.

Question 9. Are there any cases for which the times of onset seem inconsistent? How might they be explained?

Answer 9.

1. The two cases (#31 and 77) with onsets at 5 P.M. on October 31
   a. Illnesses unrelated to the outbreak?
   b. Earlier exposures to food items? Cooks?
   c. Short incubation periods? Large doses? Enhanced susceptibility?
   d. Times of onset incorrect?

2. The two cases (#75 and 95) occurring late on November 1
   a. Illnesses unrelated to the outbreak?
   b. Foods eaten at later time?
   c. Secondary cases?

d. Times of onset incorrect?
e. Long incubation periods? Small doses? Enhanced resistance?

Question 10. Modify the graph you have drawn (Question 8) to illustrate the distribution of incubation periods.

Answer 10.

Since all meal participants were served at 2:00 P.M. the distribution of onsets and incubation periods is the same. Therefore, to illustrate the distribution of incubation periods, you need only to show a second label for the *x-axis*, as in Figure 10.4.

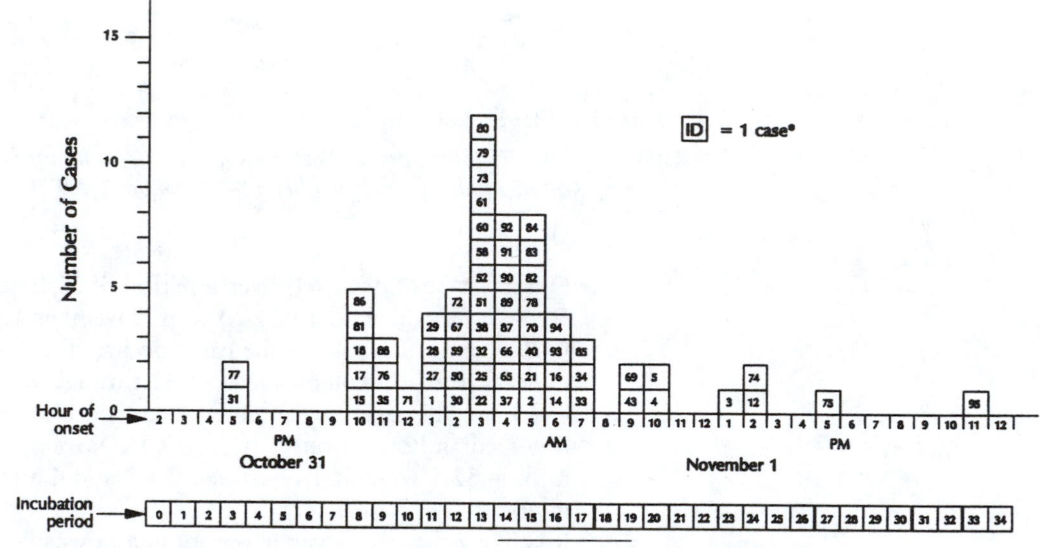

*ID# included for reference only.

FIGURE 10.4 *Outbreak-associated cases of enteritis by hour of onset of illness and incubation period, Kuwaiti Mission, Arafat, Saudi Arabia, October 31–November 1, 1979*

Question 11. Determine or calculate the minimum, maximum, mean, median, mode, range, and standard deviation of the incubation periods.

Answer 11.

Minimum = 3 hours

Maximum = 33 hours

Mean = 14 hours

Median = 13.5 hours (middle rank = 64 + 1)/2 = 32.5, which falls between the intervals for 13 and 14 hours)

Mode = 13 hours

Range = maximum − minimum = 30 hours

Standard deviation = 5 hours

Note: The range in which roughly 95% of the observations fall = $\overline{x} \pm 1.96$ (rounded to 2) standard deviations = 4 to 24 hours.

Comment

The incubation period (though not necessarily the clinical features) is about right for *Clostridium perfringens*, *Salmonella*, *Vibrio parahemolyticus*, and *Bacillus cereus*. The incubation period is a bit short for enterotoxigenic *E. coli* and *Vibrio cholerae* non-O1, and too long for staph enterotoxin, heavy metals, chemicals, and most toxins produced by fish, shellfish, and mushrooms. Illnesses that have upper GI signs and symptoms, such as nausea and vomiting, and intoxications due to chemicals, metals, etc., usually have short incubation periods, while illnesses with predominately lower GI signs and symptoms, such as diarrhea, have longer incubation periods.

Question 12a. Calculate the frequency of each clinical symptom among the cases.

Answer 12a.

The distribution of signs and symptoms are given in Table 10.28. Diarrhea occurred among all but two of the cases, with 78.1% experiencing both diarrhea and abdominal pain. Blood in the stool was reported by 8 (12.5%) of the cases. Symptoms of upper GI distress occurred among 4 (6.3%) of the cases (2 persons experienced nausea while two others reported vomiting). No temperature elevations were recorded.

TABLE 10.28 Frequency distribution of signs and symptoms among outbreak-associated cases of enteritis, Kuwaiti Mission, Arafat, Saudi Arabia, October 31-November 1, 1979 (n=64)

Sign or Symptom	*Number of Cases*	*Percent*
Diarrhea	62	96.9
Abdominal pain	52	81.3
(Diarrhea + abdominal pain)	(50)	(78.1)
Blood in stool	8	12.5
(Diarrhea + blood in stool)	(5)	(7.8)
(Diarrhea + abdominal pain + blood in stool)	(3)	(4.7)
Nausea	2	3.1
Vomiting	2	3.1
Fever	0	0

Question 12b. How does the information on the symptoms and incubation period help you to narrow the differential diagnosis? (You may refer to the attached compendium in Appendix D, which describes a number of acute foodborne gastrointestinal diseases.)

Answer 12b.

The clinical findings, including an apparent absence of malaise, myalgias, chills, and fever, are more consistent with an intoxication resulting from the presence of toxin in the lower GI tract than with an invasive infectious agent. The recovery of all cases within 24 hours is also consistent with such an intoxication. The absence of dermatologic and neurologic signs and symptoms in conjunction with the incubation period (the median was 13.5 hours and the mean was 14 hours) would lessen the likelihood of heavy metals, organic and inorganic chemicals, and toxins produced by fish, shellfish, and mushrooms. The incubation period and clinical features help narrow the list to the following: *Clostridium perfringens*, *Bacillus cereus*, *Vibrio parahemolyticus*, and, less likely, *Vibrio cholerae* non-O1, and enterotoxin producing *E. coli*.

Question 13a. Using the food consumption histories in Table 10.22, complete item 7 of the "Investigation of a Foodborne Outbreak" report form in Appendix E.

Answer 13a.

	# Persons Who ATE Specified Food				*# Who DID NOT EAT Specified Food*			
	Ill	*Well*	*Total*	*Attack Rate*	*Ill*	*Well*	*Total*	*Attack Rate*
Rice	62	31	93	66.7%	2	0	2	100.0%
Meat	63	25	88	71.6%	1	6	7	14.3%
T.S.	50	26	76	65.8%	14	5	19	73.7%

You may analyze these data with 2 × 2 tables:

Exposed?		ILL	WELL	TOTAL	Attack Rate	
	Yes	a	b	a+b	AR1 = a/a+b	RR = AR1/AR2
	No	c	d	c+d	AR2 = c/c+d	
		a+c	b+d	T=a+b+c+d		

Ate Rice		ILL	WELL	TOTAL	Attack Rate	
	Yes	62	31	93	62/93 = 66.7%	RR = 66.7/100
	No	2	0	2	2/2 = 100.0%	= 0.67
		64	31			

Ate Meat		ILL	WELL	TOTAL	Attack Rate	
	Yes	63	25	88	63/88 = 71.6%	RR = 72.6/14.3
	No	1	6	7	1/7 = 14.3%	= 5.0
		64	31			

Ate Tomato Sauce		ILL	WELL	TOTAL	Attack Rate	
	Yes	50	26	76	50/76 = 65.8%	RR = 65.8/73.7
	No	14	5	19	14/19 = 73.7%	= 0.89
		64	31			

Question 13b. Do these calculations help you to determine which food(s) served at the lunch may have been responsible for the outbreak?

Answer 13b.

Attack rates were high for those who ate rice, meat, and tomato sauce. However, meat is the likely culprit because it was the only food associated with a high attack rate among those who ate it, but a low attack rate among those who did not. Almost all (63/64) who ate meat also ate the other items, which probably accounts for the high attack rates for those items, too.

One of the cases did not admit to eating meat and could be explained in any number of ways:

- Unrelated illness
- Cross-contamination, e.g., common server, spoon, dish, counter, etc., or from meat to rice
- Reporting error (e.g., forgot or purposely denied eating meat)
- Transcription error (e.g., misrecorded response)

Note: Epidemiologic evidence shows an association between exposure and subsequent disease but **does not prove causal relationship.**

Question 14. Outline further investigations which should be pursued. List one or more factors that could have led to the contamination of the implicated food.

Answer 14.

A. Detailed review of ingredients, preparation, and storage of incriminated food. For bacterial food poisoning need:

   1) initial combination (point of origin vs. point of consumption)
   2) improper time-temperature relationships with respect to preparation, cooking, serving, and storage

B. Specific things about which one might inquire:

   1) Origin of the meat—some sources may be at higher risk than others. Animal meats are often contaminated at time of slaughter. This aspect is usually quite difficult to control.
   2) Storage of meat to time of cooking (should be kept frozen or refrigerated). This usually doesn't pose problems and since most meat is *not* eaten raw, subsequent cooking would considerably lessen the risk of disease.
   3) Cooking procedures—often difficult to control both in public/private sectors. Temperatures attained and duration of optimum cooking temperatures poorly monitored. Failure to reach adequate cooking temperatures associated with diseases other than *C. perfringens* for the most part.
   4) Cross-contamination—a factor difficult to control since knives, counter space, cutting boards, and pots or pans are often used for both raw foods and cooked foods without interim cleansing.
   5) Inadequate refrigeration of cooked foods—common in *C. perfringens* outbreaks. Cooked foods essentially allowed to incubate for several hours during cooling process. Not easy to correct as may involve expenditures for additional refrigeration appliances and use of shallow pans.

6) Inadequate reheating of cooked foods—as with 3).
7) Improper holding temperatures while serving—Here again, difficult to control, but commonly associated with disease outbreaks including *C. perfringens*. The food was essentially held at temperatures that permitted the growth of contaminating organisms rather than at 140°F or above which would have prevented their multiplication.

Question 15. In the context of this outbreak, what control measures would you recommend?

Answer 15.

1. After collecting appropriate specimens for laboratory analysis, destroy remaining foods to prevent their consumption.
2. Prevent recurrence of similar event in the future.
   a. Educate food handlers in proper techniques, stressing importance of time–temperature relationships.
   b. Acquire necessary equipment for properly cooking, cooling, serving, and storing foods.
   c. When applicable, eliminate sources of contaminated food.
3. Basic principles in prevention of *C. perfringens*.
   a. Cook all foods to minimum internal temperature of 165°F.
   b. Serve immediately or hold at >140°F.
   c. Any leftovers should be discarded or immediately chilled and held at <40°F using shallow pans.
   d. All leftovers should be reheated and held at temperatures given above for cooked foods.

Question 16. Was it important to work up this outbreak?

Answer 16.

Reasons why it was important:

1. To identify factors associated with its occurrence in order to institute the necessary measures to prevent future recurrences.
2. To provide reassurance that a deliberate act of poisoning was not involved.
3. To demonstrate that public health officials can react promptly to a problem and identify causative factors utilizing epidemiologic methods.

Appendix A

Glossary

Absolute difference. The difference in the prevalence for a risk factor between two groups.

Active immunity. The development of protective antibodies in a potential host through response to infection or immunization. See **Passive immunity**.

Adjusted rate. A rate that has been statistically adjusted to "remove" any effects a given variable may have in relation to the comparisons being made.

Agent. A necessary but not always sufficient cause of disease. An agent must be present for disease to occur but its presence is not always sufficient to produce the disease. Recently, the concept of agent has been broadened from infectious microorganisms to include chemical and physical causes of disease. See **Epidemiologic triangle**.

Age-specific rate. The rate of an outcome calculated for a certain age group. Only people in the designated age brackets are included in the numerator and denominator.

Airborne transmission. Transmission of an infectious disease agent by particles that are suspended in air. See **Dust** and **Droplet nuclei**.

Alpha. The probability of rejecting a null hypothesis when it is true (Type I error).

Alternate hypothesis. A statistical statement that expresses a relationship between two (or more) variables.

Analytic epidemiology. The aspect of epidemiology concerned with the search for health-related causes and effects.

Artifactual. See **Spurious**.

Association. As one variable changes, a concomitant or resultant change in the quantity or quality of another variable.

At risk. Capable of experiencing the health state under study.

Asymptomatic carrier. Carrier who never shows symptoms of disease while infected.

Attributable risk. A figure that quantifies the amount of risk due to a certain characteristic. It is obtained by subtracting the incidence rate for the group without the characteristic from the rate for the groups with the characteristic.

Behavioral epidemiology. The application of epidemiological methods to the study of behaviors related to health and well-being. Thus, behavioral epidemiology is the study of the distribution and determinants of health behaviors.

Berkson's fallacy. Nonrepresentativeness of cases; those cases who seek care are selectively different from those who do not.

Beta. The probability of not rejecting a null hypothesis when it is false (Type II error).

Bias. A conscious or unconscious tendency to mislabel observations in a nonrandom (systematic) manner.

Bimodal distribution. A frequency distribution with two peaks (modes).

Biological variability. The differences in assessment or test results due to the natural changeability of individual subjects over time.

Biologic transmission. When an agent of disease undergoes changes within the vector (animate intermediary), the vector is serving as both an intermediate host and a mode of transmission. See **Vector** and **Indirect transmission.**

Biostatistics. The mathematical science of quantifying observed phenomena to describe and analyze epidemiological comparisons.

Box plot. A visual display that summarizes data using a "box and whiskers" format to show the minimum and maximum values (ends of the whiskers), interquartile range (length of the box), and median (line through the box).

Carrier. A person without apparent disease who is nonetheless capable of transmitting the agent to others.

Case-control method. A method of study that can support and test hypotheses about supposed causes. The data collection is retrospective, that is, the past characteristics and events are analyzed for cases and noncases.

Case (incident) control method. A case-control study in which only new cases are studied or the time of manifestation of the effect is known—for example, from clinical records. This avoids selective survival.

Case definition. A set of standard criteria for deciding whether a person has a particular disease or other health-related condition.

Case-fatality rate. The proportion of persons with a particular condition (cases) who die from that condition. The denominator is the number of incident cases; the numerator is the number of cause-specific deaths among those cases.

Case follow-up study. The descriptive epidemiology of the natural history of diseases, including recuperation.

Case-series study. A study of cases only, with no control group for comparison.

Categorical data or variables. Variable created by collapsing a larger number of values into a few categories, or that by its nature is not suited to a long continuum of possible values.

Causal. Inferring from findings that an antecedent leads to the health state under study.

Chain of infection. A model of how disease transmission occurs. Transmission occurs when the agent leaves its reservoir or host through a portal of exit, is conveyed by some mode of transmission, and enters through an appropriate portal of entry to infect a susceptible host.

Chi-square test. A statistical test applied to nominal or categorical data.

Chronic carrier. A person who continues to harbor an infectious agent for an extended period of time (months or years) following the initial infection.

Clinical epidemiology. The application of the science of epidemiology and biostatistics to clinical practice.

Clinical hunch. An idea that arises during clinical care that can be a valuable source of epidemiological hypothesis.

Clinical trial. An experimental study to test the efficacy and potential side effects of an intervention such as a drug, vaccine, or medical device.

Cluster. An aggregation of cases of a disease or other health-related condition, particularly cancer and birth defects, which are closely grouped in time and place. The number of cases may or may not exceed the expected number; frequently the expected number is not known.

Cohort. A group of persons who have characteristics in common and are studied prospectively.

Cohort effect. A special age group going through life with a high or low rate of a condition and carrying this characteristic with them into successive age categories over time.

Cohort study. A study design that looks forward in time from baseline data. Health status and related characteristics are assessed and later reassessed to determine which characteristics preceded or caused newly developed health outcomes. This design best allows for estimates of the probability or risk of developing the outcome.

Common source outbreak. Outbreak which occurs when a group of persons is exposed to a common noxious influence, such as an infectious agent or toxin. See **Point source outbreak** and **Propagated outbreak.**

Confidence interval. A range of values used within which a true value is expected to fall 95% of the time.

Contingency table. A two-variable table with cross-tabulated data.

Confounding variable. A health-state related variable that is distributed differently in different groups causing confusion (introduces artifactual estimates of effect) in comparing the rates of health states in the groups.

Construct validity. The degree to which a measure correlates with the characteristics one would expect, and so it is probably valid. See **Validity.**

Control table. Presentation of data relating two or more variables while showing or controlling for the effect of other variables.

Controlling for. Examining the effect of one variable on the health outcome while taking into account the effect of another; for example, looking at death rates by sex within specific age groups.

Convalescent carrier. Someone who is capable of transmitting an infectious disease after they are clinically ill (during convalescence).

Correlation. A statistical measure of an association. See **Association.**

Cross-sectional method. A study design that shows concurrently existing characteristics and health outcomes. Like a picture of the situation at a specific time, it cannot answer questions about cause and effect (whether the characteristics preceded the outcome).

Crude death (mortality) rate. The death (mortality) rate from all causes of death for a population. See **Crude rate.**

Crude rate. The rate of an outcome calculated without any restrictions (such as age, race, or sex) for who is counted in the numerator or denominator.

Cumulative incidence (rate). An incidence rate that covers a specified time period—for example, one year or five years—and for which all subjects are followed over the same period of time.

Death registration states. States registering deaths in a uniform manner and contributing to the national vital statistics system.

Death-to-case ratio. The number of deaths attributed to a particular disease during a specified time period divided by the number of new cases of that disease identified during the same time period.

Degrees of freedom (df). For chi-square tests, the number of cells in the table whose expected number of subjects does not depend on the expected number of subjects in other cells.

Denominator. The lower portion of a fraction used to calculate a rate or ratio. In a rate, the denominator is usually the population (or population experience, as in person-years, etc.) at risk. See **Numerator** and **Rate.**

Dependent variable. Usually the health outcome under study where the aim is to determine to what extent the health outcome is dependent on, or a result of, other variables.

Descriptive epidemiology. Explanation of the frequency and relative distributions of health and disease in populations.

Descriptive statistics. Statistical methods of organizing and summarizing information.

Direct contact. Transmission of an infectious agent through kissing, skin-to-skin contact, and sexual intercourse.

Direct method of age adjustment. Application of age-specific rates of the populations being compared to determine the expected number of events in a standard population.

Direct transmission. Immediate transfer of an agent from a reservoir to a susceptible host by direct contact or droplet spread. See **Direct contact** and **Droplet spread.**

Discrete quantitative variable. A quantitative variable that can assume only a limited set of values no matter how precise the measurement techniques are.

Dose-response relationship. As the amount of exposure to a risk factor increases, the rate of the effect of exposure increases.

Droplet nuclei. Residue of dried droplets that are less than 5 microns in size and may remain suspended in the air for long periods, may be blown over great distances, and are easily inhaled into the lungs and exhaled. An important means of transmission for some diseases.

Droplet spread. The spray produced by sneezing, coughing, or talking which produces relatively large, short-range aerosols that are capable of transmitting disease.

Dust. Particles blown from the soil by the wind as well as material that has settled on surfaces and become resuspended by air currents. Airborne transmission of disease includes transmission by dust particles. See **Airborne transmission.**

Ecologic fallacy. In interpreting associations between ecologic indices, an error committed by mistakenly assuming that, because the majority of a group has a characteristic, the characteristic is related to a health state common in the group.

Ecologic index. A system of classification that applies the majority characteristic of an entire group to all individuals within the group, irrespective of individual characteristics.

Effectiveness. The ability of a program to produce results in the field. See **Efficacy** and **Efficiency.**

Effect modifier. A variable that modifies or influences the effect (for instance, disease or outcome). It is often part of the causative network, in an interactive sense.

Efficacy. The ability of a program to produce results under ideal conditions. See **Effectiveness** and **Efficiency.**

Efficiency. The ability of a program to produce intended results with a minimum expenditure of time and resources. See **Effectiveness** and **Efficacy.**

Endemic level. A persistent level of disease occurrence with a low to moderate disease level. See **Hyperendemic, Epidemic, Pandemic.**

Epidemic. The occurrence of higher rate of a health state than would be expected, based on past experience. See **Endemic, Hyperendemic, Pandemic, Outbreak.**

Epidemiologic triangle. The traditional model of infectious disease causation. It consists of three components: an external agent, a susceptible host, and an environment that brings the host and the agent together. Also known as the epidemiologic triad.

Epidemiologic variables. Time, place, and person factors. See **Descriptive epidemiology.**

Epidemiology. A science concerned with the distribution and determinants of health events (health, disease, and health behavior) in human populations. It is both a body of knowledge and a method.

Etiologic fraction. See **population attributable risk percent.**

Exhaustive categories. Enough categories in a classification scheme so that all subjects are classifiable in some category for the variable.

Experimental epidemiology. Introducing a suspected cause and measuring its subsequent effect in populations. Used to evaluate the efficacy of an intervention procedure.

Extrapolation. Making numerical predictions for the future based on past and current rates or quantities.

Face validity. When a measure appears so logical to the study population that it can be accepted at face value as valid. See **Validity.**

False negatives. In tests of validity, labeling cases or the presence of a characteristic incorrectly; that is, categorizing cases as noncases or failing to identify the characteristic when it is actually present.

False positives. In tests of validity, labeling noncases or the absence of a characteristic incorrectly; that is, categorizing noncases as cases or identifying a characteristic when it is actually not present.

Fisher's Exact Test for 2 × 2 tables. A statistical test of significance that can be used in place of a chi-square test when the expected number of subjects in some cells is less than five.

Flow diagram. A diagram that shows progressive division of the original population into the groups from which inferences flow.

Herd immunity. The concept that in order to prevent or abort a disease outbreak, a certain high proportion of individuals in a population must be resistant to an infectious disease agent.

High-risk groups. Groups in a community with an elevated risk of disease or other health-related event.

Historical cohort study. A cohort study done on a cohort defined in the past.

Host. A person in whom infection may or may not occur.

Hybrid study. A combination of the case-incident-control method and cohort method in one study.

Hyperendemic level. A persistently high level of disease occurrence. See **Endemic, Epidemic, Pandemic.**

Hypothesis. A statistically testable statement. See **Null hypothesis.**

Incidence. The occurrence of new cases during a specified period of time.

Incidence density (rate). A rate in which the numerator is person-years instead of the number of people because all subjects have *not* been followed for the same period of time.

Incidence study. See **Cohort study.**

Incubation period. The period of time from exposure to the onset of symptoms. See **Natural history of disease** and **Latency period.**

Incubatory carrier. A person who is capable of transmitting disease before being clinically ill (during the incubation period).

Independent association. A relationship between two variables that holds when controlling or adjusting for other variables.

Independent variable. A characteristic or situation being considered for its relation (possibly causative) to a health outcome.

Indirect association. A dependent relationship between two variables, which appears to exist only because of the confounding influence of a third variable, and disappears when the third variable is controlled. See **Secondary association.**

Indirect transmission. Transfer of an agent from a reservoir to a susceptible host by suspended air particles or by animate intermediaries. See **Vector** and **Direct transmission.**

Indirect method of age adjustment. Standard rates applied to populations being compared in order to calculate the expected number of events, and then compared with the observed number of events.

Infant mortality rate. A ratio expressing the number of deaths among children under one year of age reported during a given time period divided by the number of births reported during the same time period. The infant mortality rate is usually expressed per 1,000 live births.

Infectivity. The proportion of exposed persons who become infected.

Inferential statistics. Statistical techniques which allow one to analyze information and generalize about a population on the basis of information obtained from a sample of a population. See **Descriptive statistics.**

Information bias. See **Bias.**

Inter-observer reliability. The degree to which two (or more) different observers classify consistently among themselves observations on a group of subjects.

Interval data or variables. Data that is measured in standard units where any given difference between two numerical values has the same meaning.

Intra-observer reliability. The degree to which one observer classifies observations the same at two different points in time.

Latency period. In chronic diseases, the period of time from exposure to the onset of symptoms. See **Incubation period** and **Natural history of disease.**

Life-table analysis. A method of including people in a cohort study for different durations during the overall study period.

Linear relationship. When two variables are considered together, the first increases as the second increases (or decreases), so that, when plotted graphically, a straight line results.

Matching. A technique for controlling for variables that are actual or potential confounders.

Mixed epidemic. An epidemic which has features of both common source and propagated epidemics, such as a common source outbreak followed by secondary person-to-person spread. See **Common source outbreak** and **Propagated outbreak.**

Mode of transmission. The means by which an infectious agent is conveyed from a reservoir to a host.

Morbidity rate. Rates used to express the incidence of disease or prevalence of disease. See **Incidence rate** and **Prevalence rate.**

Mortality rate (death rate). The probability of death occurring within a specified time period multiplied by a constant.

Mutually exclusive and exhaustive categories. Each subject is classifiable into only one category.

Natural history of disease. The description of what happens following the development of disease, including complications, cure, death, symptom change, remissions, and so forth. Systematic prospective study can quantify the probability of these events for a group of cases.

Negative (inverse) association. As the amount of the characteristic increases, the rate of the health state decreases.

Neonatal mortality rate. A ratio expressing the number of deaths among children from birth to (but not including) 28 days of age divided by the number of live births reported during the same time period. The neonatal mortality rate is usually expressed per 1,000 live births.

Nominal data or variables. The data from these variables label things; they do not measure or quantify amounts. Also called qualitative variables.

Nonparametric statistics. Statistical techniques that can be used on nominal or ordinal data.

Normal curve. A bell-shaped curve that results when a normal distribution is graphed.

Normal distribution. The symmetrical clustering of values around a central location.

Null hypothesis. A statement expressing no relationship or no difference between two (or more) variables.

Numerator. The upper portion of a fraction. See **Denominator** and **Rate.**

Odds ratio. A technique for estimating relative risk from case-control studies. See **Relative odds ratio.**

Ordinal variable. A variable having values that can be meaningfully ordered or ranked (for example, from less to more, from small to large).

Outbreak. A term meaning the same as epidemic; often used by public health officials because it is less alarming to the public than the term epidemic. See **Epidemic.**

Pandemic. An epidemic which spreads over several countries or continents and affects a large number of people. See **Epidemic.**

Parameter. The true value of a population's health attribute.

Passive immunity. Protection against a particular disease by acquiring antibodies either from one's mother or by the receipt of injections of antitoxins or immune globulin. See **Active immunity**.

Pathogenicity. The proportion of infected persons who develop clinical disease.

Period prevalence. The rate of cases of a disease or people with a health condition over a specified period of time. See **Prevalence rate** and **Point prevalence.**

Person-years. Sometimes used in the denominator of incidence rates. It is the accumulated period of time each person is in a study. Person-years is sometimes used in the denominator instead of the number of people. See **Incidence density rate.**

Placebo. In an experimental study a nontreatment or pseudo-treatment which is believed to be effective by the subject.

Point prevalence. The prevalence of a disease or health condition at a particular point-in-time (i.e., the number or rate of individuals with a specific health outcome at the time period when the count is taken). See **Prevalence rate** and **Period prevalence.**

Point prevalence study. See **Cross-sectional method.**

Point source outbreak. When a group of people is exposed to a common noxious influence for a brief period of time, and everyone who becomes ill develops disease at the end of one incubation period. This is a classification of a common source outbreak. See **Common source outbreak.**

Population. The whole group of individuals, objects, or measurements having some common observable characteristic. See **Sample.**

Population at risk (PAR). Those individuals capable of developing a specified health state; they become the denominator for calculating the rate of the health state.

Population attributable risk percent (PARP) or proportion. A measure of the benefit derived by modifying a risk factor.

Portal of entry. The path by which an agent enters to infect a susceptible host.

Portal of exit. The place where an agent leaves its reservoir or host.

Positive association. As the amount of the characteristic increases, the rate of the health state increases.

Postneonatal mortality rate. A ratio expressing the number of deaths among children 28 days to (but not including) 1 year of age during a given time period divided by the number of live births reported during the same time period. The postneonatal mortality rate is usually expressed per 1,000 live births.

Practical significance. This exists if the findings have important implications within the conceptual context of the study.

Predictive validity. The degree to which a measure forecasts the outcome of interest. See **Validity.**

Prevalence. The number or rate of cases that exist (prevail) at a specified time.

Prevalence rate. Rates that express in a given population the proportion of persons who have a particular disease or attribute at a specified point in time.

Prevalence ratio. The prevalence for a risk factor for one group divided by that for another group.

Probability. An estimate of the frequency or likelihood of the occurrence of an event.

Propagated outbreak. A disease outbreak which does not have a common source, but instead spreads gradually from person to person. See **Common source outbreak.**

Proportionate mortality. The proportion of deaths attributable to different causes in a specified population over a period of time. Each cause is expressed as a percentage of all deaths, and the sum of the causes must add to 100%. These proportions are not mortality rates, since the denominator is all deaths, not the population in which the deaths occurred.

Prospective method. See **Prospective study** and **Cohort study.**

Prospective study. See **Cohort study.**

Public health surveillance. The systematic collection, analysis, interpretation, and dissemination of health data on an ongoing basis.

P-value. The probability of obtaining a difference between sample estimates as large as the observed difference if the null hypothesis is true.

Qualitative variables. Variables that name or classify but do not indicate measurement. Also called nominal variables.

Quantitative data or variables. Variables that indicate measurement.

Quasi-experimental. Research designs in which the investigator does not have as much control as in an experimental design.

Randomization. Assigning people to treatment and control groups in an unbiased manner so as to produce groups similar in characteristics not controlled by other methods. Sometimes called random assignment of subjects to groups, or random allocation.

Randomized clinical trial. A clinical trial in which subjects have been randomly assigned to the various groups in the study.

Random sample. A selection of some members of a population such that each member is independently chosen and has a known non-zero probability of being selected.

Range. In a set of numbers or observations, the range is the largest observation minus the smallest.

Rate. A numerical statement of the frequency of an event obtained by dividing the number of individuals experiencing the event (the numerator) by the total number capable of experiencing the event (the denominator or the population at risk) and multiplying by a constant such as 100 or 1,000.

Ratio scale. Data that have a true zero point that represents total absence of the variable.

Relationship. See **Association.**

Relative odds (or odds ratio). Percentages of cases that were exposed to a presumed antecedent divided by the percentage of controls that were similarly exposed. It is sometimes used in case-control studies as an estimate of relative risk.

Relative risk. A ratio obtained by dividing the incidence rate of one group by the incidence rate of another group. If the rates are equal, the resulting relative risk is one.

Reliability (reproducibility). The degree to which observations are repeatedly classified the same.

Reproducibility. See **Reliability.**

Reservoir. The habitat in which an infectious agent normally lives, grows, and multiplies.

Retrospective. Looking back. A retrospective study is a case-control study.

Risk. The probability or likelihood of a health-related event or outcome.

Risk factor. A characteristic, behavior, or experience that increases the probability of (causes) disease or other health-related event or condition. See **High-risk group.**

Sample. A group of subjects chosen for study to represent a larger population.

Sample size. The number of subjects chosen for study to represent a larger population.

Sampling variability. The differences between findings for all possible samples from the same or equivalent populations. It is possible to draw many different samples from any one population, and each one would provide somewhat different findings.

Secondary association. Association produced by confounding variables. See **Indirect association.**

Secular trend. Refers to a trend over time.

Selection. Factors that affect the composition of the populations studied so as to confuse comparisons between groups, that is, produce artifactual findings.

Selection bias. Bias that is introduced into a study when study participants (subjects) are not representative of the population to which inferences are to be made. See **Selection.**

Selective survival. The result of differences between those who die and those who live; those who survive may have characteristics related to maintaining life that confound retrospective studies of the health outcome causing mortality.

Sensitize. See **Sensitivity.**

Sensitivity. In tests of validity, the percentage of all true cases identified correctly. See **Specificity.**

Simple attributable risk. See **Attributable risk.**

Specific. See **Specificity.**

Specificity. In tests of validity, the percentage of all true noncases identified correctly. See **Sensitivity.**

Sporadic level. An irregular pattern of disease occurrence, with occasional cases occurring at irregular intervals. See **Endemic, Hyperendemic, Epidemic, Pandemic.**

Spurious (artifactual). When applied to associations, false relationships produced by methodological errors or confounding variables.

Standardized Mortality Ratios (SMR). The ratio of observed events to events expected if standard rates are applied to the study populations. It is usually the figure used in indirect adjustments.

Standard error. The square root of the variance divided by the sample size. Describes how widely values are dispersed around the mean.

Standard population. As arbitrary distribution of a characteristic (for example, age) used as a common standard for two groups when comparing their rates.

Standardized rate. See **Adjusted rate.**

Statistical tests of significance. Methods of determining the likelihood that estimates of population parameters are different solely because of sampling variability.

Tables. A way to present and summarize numerical data in an organized fashion.

Table shells. A table that is complete except for the data.

Target population. The group a researcher wishes to study. Also known as a study population. See **Random sample.**

True negatives. In tests of validity, labeling noncases or the absence of characteristics correctly.

True positives. In tests of validity, labeling cases or characteristics correctly.

Type I error. Rejection of a null hypothesis that is actually true. See **Alpha.**

Type II error. Failure to reject a null hypothesis that is actually false. See **Beta.**

Universal variables (effect modifiers). Characteristics that in nature generally modify many health events and need to be considered when comparing groups.

Unweighted average. An equal weight to each component of the average.

Validity. The correctness of labeling; the ability of a criterion or tool to measure what it claims to measure, or the correctness of participants' reports.

Variance. A number that expresses the spread of individual data points around the mean for a sample.

Vector. Refers to an animate intermediary in disease transmission. Most vectors are arthropods such as mosquitoes, fleas, or ticks.

Vehicle. Objects such as food, water, biologic products (e.g., blood), and fomites (inanimate objects) that may indirectly transmit an infectious agent from a reservoir to a host.

Virulence. Refers to the proportion of persons with clinical disease who become severely ill or die.

Weighted average. Different weights to each component of the average.

Years of potential life lost (YPLL). A measure of the impact of premature mortality on a population, calculated as the sum of the differences between some predetermined minimum or desired life span and the age of death for individuals who died earlier than that predetermined age.

Zoonoses. Infectious diseases that are transmissible under normal conditions from animals to humans.

Z-statistic. A statistic computed to test the statistical difference between two numbers.

Appendix B

A Sample of Epidemiology and Biostatistics Resource Books

Abrahamson JH: *Making sense of data: A self-instruction manual on the interpretation of epidemiological data*. New York: Oxford University Press, 1988.

Aday LA: *Designing and conducting health surveys*. San Francisco: Jossey-Bass, 1989.

Austin DF, Werner SB: *Epidemiology for the health sciences: A primer on epidemiologic concepts and their uses*. Charles C Thomas, 1982.

Badura B, Kickbusch I: *Health promotion research: Towards a new social epidemiology*. Copenhagen, Denmark: WHO Regional Office for Europe, 1991.

Bernier RH, Mason VM: *EPISOURCE: A guide to resources in epidemiology*. Roswell, GA: The Epidemiology Monitor, 1991.

Brookmeyer R, Gail MH: *AIDS epidemiology: A quantitative approach*. New York: Oxford, 1994.

Brownson RC, Remington PL, Davis JR: *Chronic disease epidemiology and control*. Washington, DC: American Public Health Association, 1993.

Buck C, Llopis A, Najera E, Terris M: *The challenge of epidemiology: Issues and selected readings*. Washington, DC: Pan American Health Organization, 1988.

Checkoway H, Pearce N, Crawford-Brown DJ: *Research methods in occupational epidemiology*. New York: Oxford University Press, 1989.

Clayton D, Hills M: *Statistical models in epidemiology*. New York: Oxford, 1993.

Cook TD, Campbell DT: *Quasi-experimentation: Design and analysis issues for field settings*. Boston: Houghton Mifflin, 1979.

Cox DR, Oakes D: *Analysis of survival data*. New York: Chapman and Hall Ltd, 1984.

Dever GF: *Epidemiology in health services management*. Rockville, MD: Aspen Systems, 1984.

Duncan DF: *Epidemiology: Basis for disease prevention and health promotion*. New York: Macmillan, 1988.

Duncan RC, Knapp RG, Miller MC: *Introductory biostatistics for the health sciences*, 2d ed. New York: John Wiley and Sons, 1983.

Evans AS: *Viral infections in humans: Epidemiology and control*. New York: Plenum, 1989.

Eylenbosch WJ, Noah ND: *Surveillance in health and disease*. New York: Oxford University Press, 1988.

Feinstein AR: *Clinical Epidemiology: The architecture of clinical research*. Philadelphia: W. B. Saunders, 1985.

Fink A, Kosecoff J: *How to conduct surveys*. Newbury Park, CA: Sage, 1985.

Fleiss JL: *Statistical methods for rates and proportions*, 2d ed. New York: John Wiley and Sons, 1981.

Friedman GD: *Primer of epidemiology*, 3d ed. New York: McGraw-Hill, 1987.

Goldsmith JR: *Environmental epidemiology: Epidemiological investigation*. Boca Raton, FL: CRC Press, 1986.

Gordis L: *Epidemiology and health risk assessment*. New York: Oxford University Press, 1988.

Morton RF, Hebel JR, McCarter RJ: *A study guide to epidemiology and biostatistics*. Rockville, MD: Aspen Systems, 1990.

Hennekens C, Buring J: *Epidemiology in medicine*. Boston: Little, Brown, 1987.

Hosmer DW, Lemeshow S: *Applied logistic regression*. New York: John Wiley and Sons, 1989.

Hulka BS, Wilcosky TC, Griffith JD: *Biological markers in epidemiology*. New York: Oxford University Press, 1990.

Ibrahim MA: *Epidemiology and health policy*. Rockville, MD: Aspen Systems, 1985.

Ingelfinger JA, Mosteller F, Thibodeau LA, Ware JH: *Biostatistics in clinical medicine*, 2d ed. New York: Collier MacMillan, 1987.

Kahn HA: *An introduction to epidemiologic methods*. New York: Oxford University Press, 1983.

Kahn HA, Sempos CT: *Statistical methods in epidemiology*. New York: Oxford University Press, 1989.

Kaplan RM, Criqui MJ: *Behavioral epidemiology and disease prevention*. New York: Plenum, 1985.

Kelsey JL, Thompson WD, Evans AS: *Methods in observational epidemiology*. New York: Oxford University Press, 1986.

Kleinbaum DG, Kupper LL: *Applied regression analysis and other multivariable methods*. Boston: Duxbury Press, 1978.

Kleinbaum DG, Kupper LL, Morgenstern H: *Epidemiologic research: Principles and quantitative methods*. New York: Van Nostrand Reinhold, 1982.

Kopler FC, Craun G: *Environmental epidemiology*. Boca Raton, FL: Lewis, 1986.

Kramer MS: *Clinical epidemiology and biostatistics*. New York: Springer-Verlag, 1988.

Kraemer HC, Thiemann S: *How many subjects*. Newbury Park, CA: Sage, 1987.

Kelsey JL, Thompson WD, Evans AS: *Methods in observational epidemiology*. New York: Oxford University Press, 1986.

Kuzma JW: *Basic statistics for the health sciences*. Palo Alto, CA: Mayfield, 1984.

Last JM: *A dictionary of epidemiology*, 2d ed. New York: Oxford University Press, 1988.

Levy PS, Lemeshow S: *Sampling for health professionals*. Belmont, CA: Life Time Learning, 1981.

Lilienfeld AM, Lilienfeld DE: *Foundations of epidemiology*, 2d ed. New York: Oxford University Press, 1980.

Margetts BM, Nelson M: *Design concepts in nutritional epidemiology*. New York: Oxford University Press, 1991.

MacMahon B, Pugh T: *Epidemiology: Principles and methods*. Boston: Little, Brown, 1970.

Mausner JS, Kramer S. *Epidemiology: An introductory text*. Philadelphia: W. B. Saunders, 1985.

McDowell I, Newell C: *Measuring health: A guide to rating scales and questionnaires*. New York: Oxford University Press, 1987.

Meinert CL, Tonascia S: *Clinical trials: Design, conduct, and analysis*. New York: Oxford University Press, 1986.

Miettinen OS: *Theoretical epidemiology: Principles of occurrence research in medicine*. New York: John Wiley and Sons, 1985.

Monson RR: *Occupational epidemiology*, 2d ed. Boca Raton, FL: CRC Press, 1990.

Morrison AS: *Screening in chronic disease*. New York: Oxford University Press, 1985.

National Medical Series for Independent Study: *Epidemiology and public health*. New York: John Wiley and Sons, 1987.

Neter J, Wasserman W, Kutner MH: *Applied linear regression models*, 2d ed. Boston: Irwin, 1989.

Oakes M: *Statistical inference: A commentary for the social and behavioral sciences*. New York: John Wiley and Sons, 1986.

Olsen J, Merletti F, Snashall D, Vuylsteek K: *Searching for causes of work-related diseases: An introduction to epidemiology at the work site*. New York: Oxford University Press, 1991.

Phillips DS: *Basic statistics for health science students*. New York: W. H. Freeman, 1978.

Puri ML, Vilaplana JP, Wertz W: *New perspectives in theoretical and applied statistics*. New York: John Wiley and Sons, 1987.

Rappaport SM, Smith TJ: *Exposure assessment for epidemiology and hazard control*. Boca Raton: FL: Lewis, 1990.

Rothman KJ: *Causal inference*. Chestnut Hill, MA: Epidemiology Resources Institute, 1988.

Rothman KJ: *Modern epidemiology*. Boston: Little, Brown, 1986.

Rubinson L, Neutens JJ: *Research techniques for the health sciences*. New York: Macmillan, 1987.

Schefler WC: *Statistics for health professionals*. Reading: Addison-Wesley, 1984.

Schlesselman JJ, Stolley PD: *Case control studies: Design, conduct, analysis*. New York: Oxford University Press, 1982.

Selvin S: *Statistical analysis of epidemiologic data*. New York: Oxford University Press, 1991.

Streiner DL, Norman GR, Blum HM: *PDQ epidemiology*. Philadelphia: Decker, 1989.

Susser M: *Epidemiology, health, and society*. New York: Oxford University Press, 1987.

Walker AM: *Observation and inference: An introduction to the methods of epidemiology*. Chestnut Hill, MA: Epidemiology Resources Institute, 1991.

Wassertheil-Smoller S: *Biostatistics and epidemiology: A primer for health professionals*. New York: Springer-Verlag, 1990.

Weiss NS: *Clinical epidemiology: The study of the outcome of illness*. New York: Oxford University Press, 1986.

Willett W: *Nutritional epidemiology*. New York: Oxford University Press, 1990.

Appendix C

Graph Paper and Maps

SQUARE 10 X 10 TO THE HALF INCH

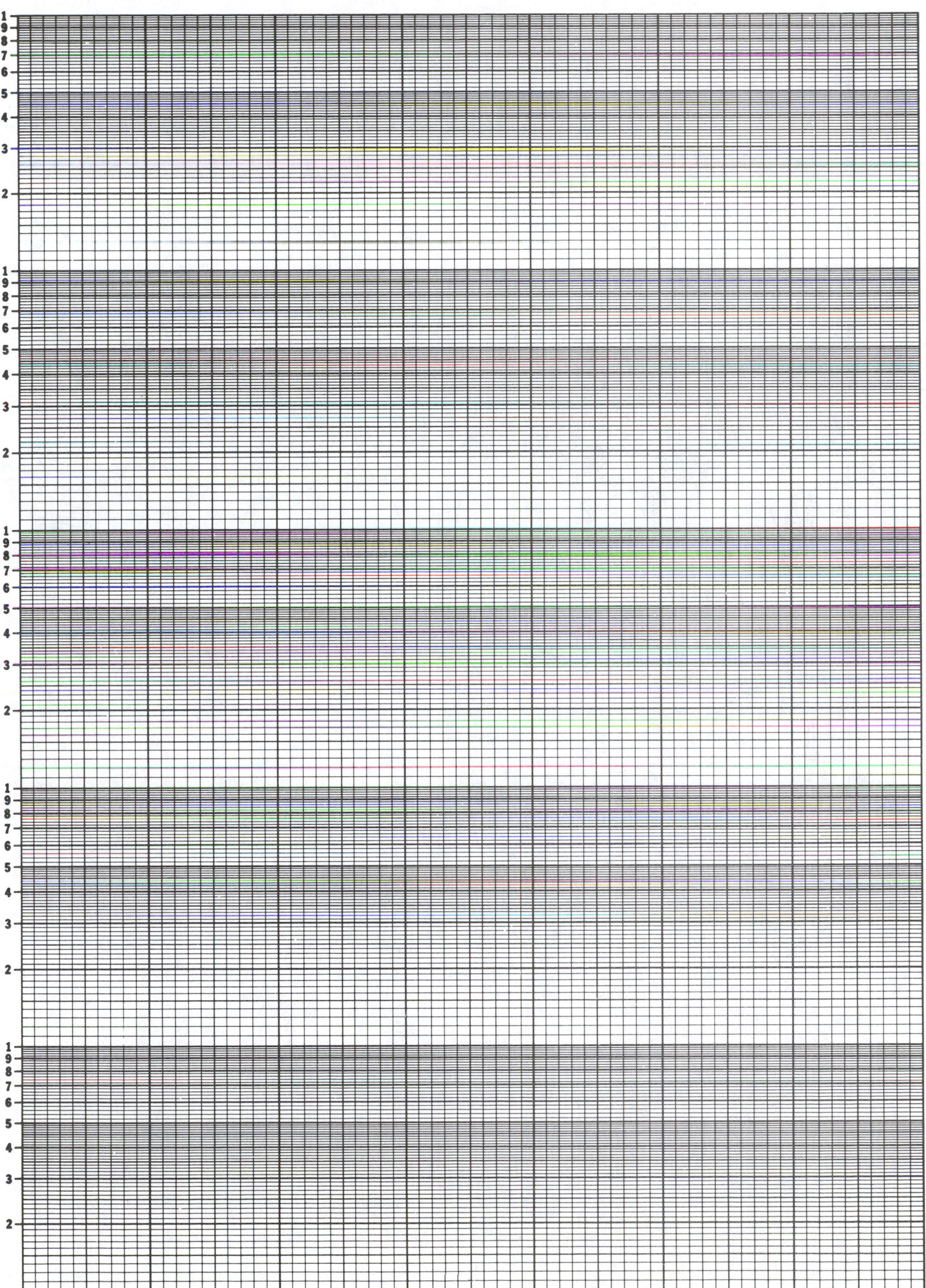

1
9
8
7
6
5
4
3
2
1
9
8
7
6
5
4
3
2
1
9
8
7
6
5
4
3
2
1
9
8
7
6
5
4
3
2
1
9
8
7
6
5
4
3
2
1

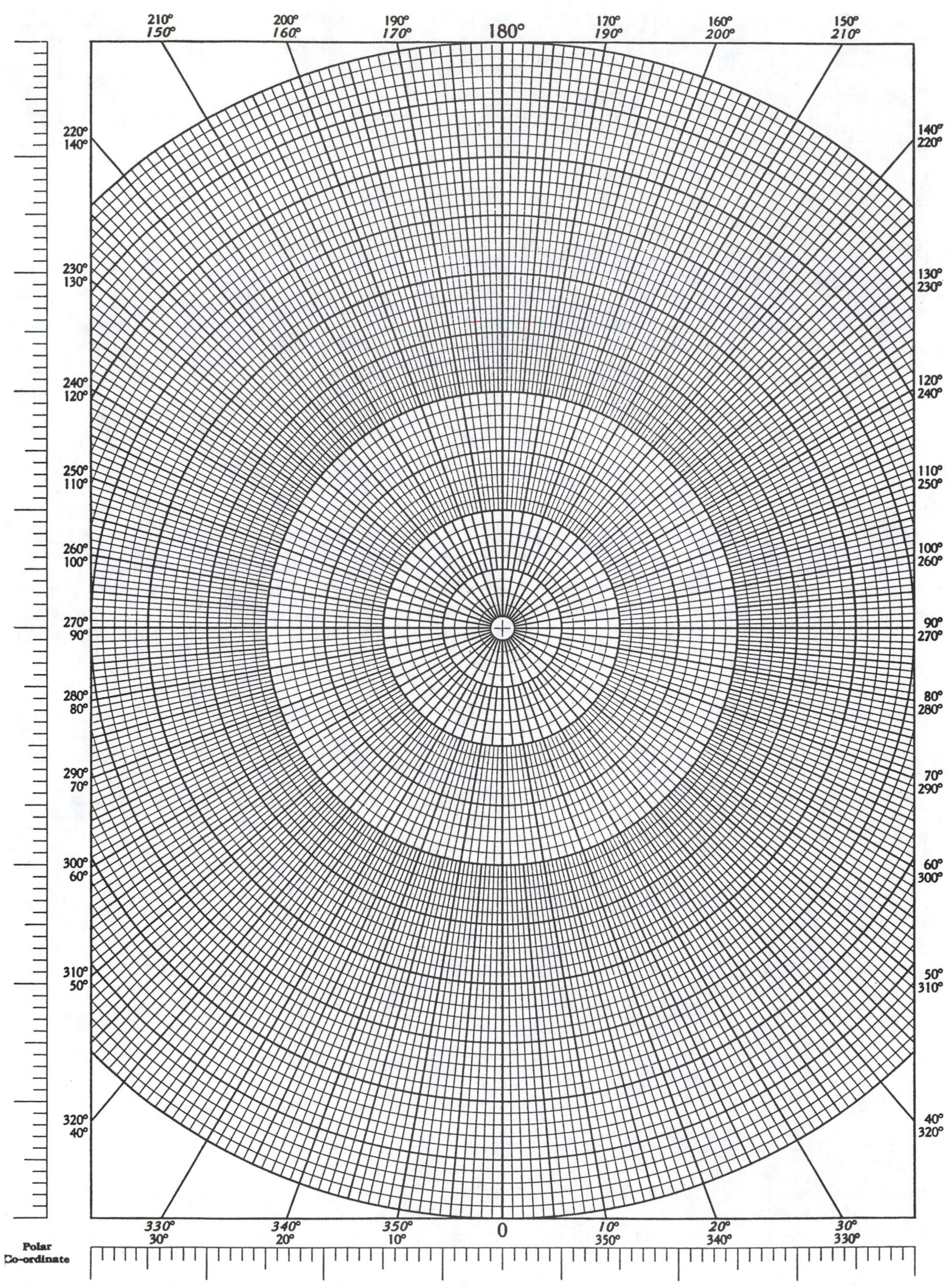

180°
210° 150°
200° 160°
190° 170°
170° 190°
160° 200°
150° 210°
220° 140°
230° 130°
240° 120°
250° 110°
260° 100°
270° 90°
280° 80°
290° 70°
300° 60°
310° 50°
320° 40°
140° 220°
130° 230°
120° 240°
110° 250°
100° 260°
90° 270°
80° 280°
70° 290°
60° 300°
50° 310°
40° 320°
330° 30°
340° 20°
350° 10°
0
10° 350°
20° 340°
30° 330°
Polar
Co-ordinate

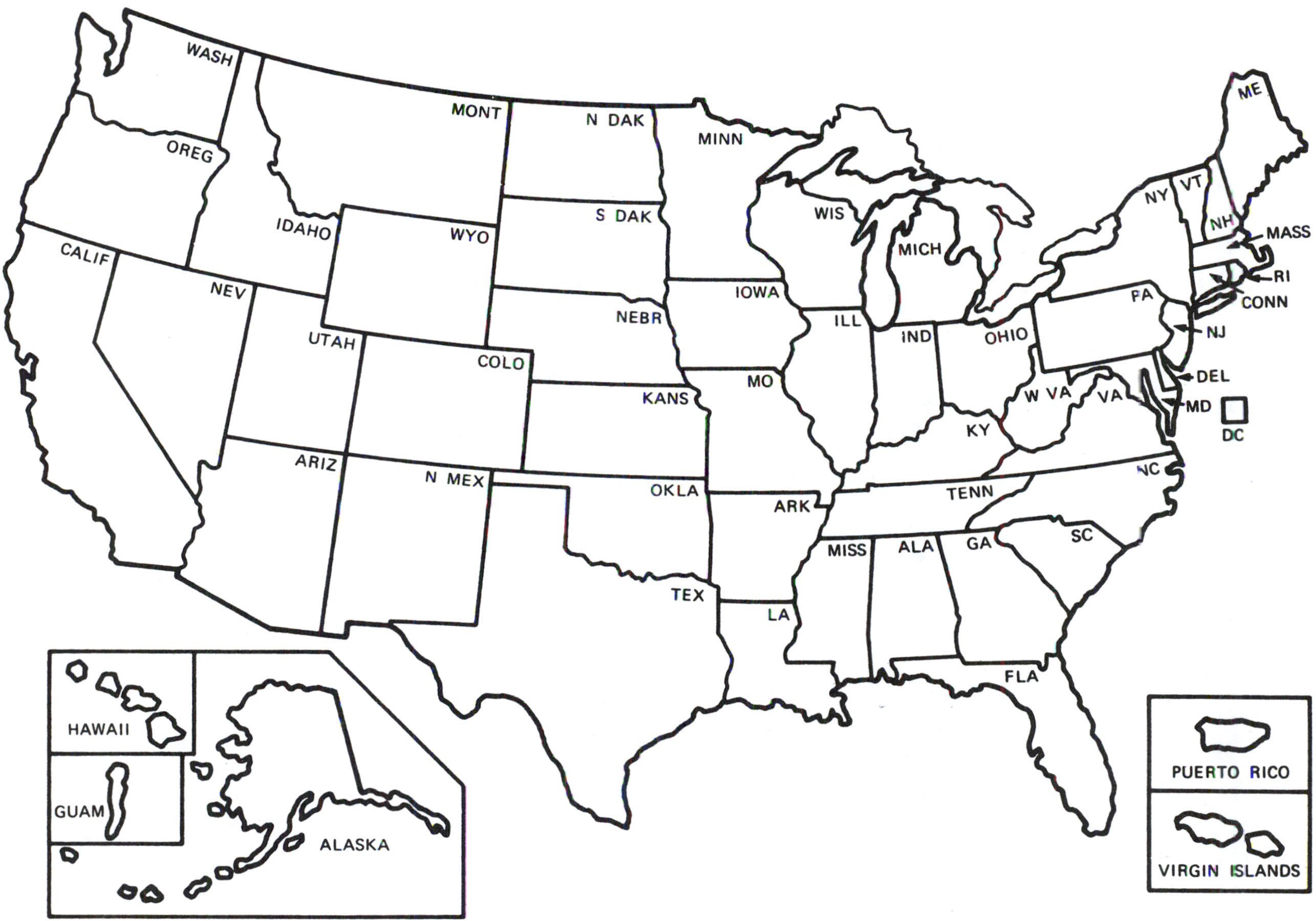
WASH
MONT
N DAK
MINN
ME
OREG
NY
VT
NH
MASS
IDAHO
WYO
S DAK
WIS
MICH
CALIF
RI
IOWA
PA
CONN
NEV
NEBR
ILL
IND
OHIO
NJ
UTAH
COLO
MO
DEL
KANS
W VA
VA
MD
DC
KY
ARIZ
N MEX
NC
OKLA
TENN
ARK
MISS
ALA
GA
SC
TEX
LA
FLA
HAWAII
GUAM
ALASKA
PUERTO RICO
VIRGIN ISLANDS

Appendix D

Abbreviated Compendium of Acute Foodborne Gastrointestinal Disease

NOTE: This is from *Principles of epidemiology: An introduction to applied epidemiology and biostatistics*. Atlanta, GA: Centers for Disease Control and Prevention, 1992.

I. Diseases typified by vomiting after a short incubation period with little or no fever

Agent	Incubation period Usual (and Range)	Symptoms* (Partial list)	Pathophysiology	Characteristic foods	Specimens
A. *Staphyloccocus aureus*	2–4 hours (1–6 hours)	N, C, V; D, F may be present	preformed enterotoxin	sliced/chopped ham and meats, custards, cream fillings	**Food:** enterotoxin assay (FDA), culture for quantitation and phage typing of staph, gram stain **Handlers:** culture nares, skin, skin lesions, and phage type staph **Cases:** culture stool and vomitus, phage type staph
B. *Bacillus cereus*	2–4 hours (1–6 hours)	N, V, D	? preformed enterotoxin	fried rice	**Food:** culture for quantitation **Cases:** stool culture
C. Heavy Metals 1. cadmium 2. copper 3. tin 4. zinc	5–15 minutes (1–60 minutes)	N, V, C, D		foods and beverages prepared/stored/cooked in containers coated/lined/contaminated with offending metal	Toxicologic analysis of food container, vomitus, stomach contents, urine, blood, feces

II. Diseases typified by diarrhea after a moderate to long incubation period, often with fever

Agent	Incubation period Usual (and Range)	Symptoms* (Partial list)	Pathophysiology	Characteristic foods	Specimens
A. *Clostridium perfringens*	12 hours (8–16 hours)	C, D (V, F rare)	enterotoxin formed *in vivo*	meat, poultry	**Food:** enterotoxin assay done as research procedure by FDA, culture for quantitation and serotyping **Cases:** culture feces for quantitation and serotyping of *C. perfringens*; test for enterotoxin in stool **Controls:** culture feces for quantitation and serotyping of *C. perfringens*
B. *Salmonella* (non-typhoid)	12–36 hours (6–72 hours)	D, C, F, V, H septicemia or enteric fever	tissue invasion	poultry, eggs, raw milk, meat (cross-contamination important)	**Food:** culture with serotyping **Cases:** stool culture with serotyping **Handlers:** stool culture with serotyping as a secondary consideration
C. *Vibrio parahaemolyticus*	12 hours (2–48 hours)	C, D N, V, F, H, B	tissue invasion, ? enterotoxin	seafood	**Food:** culture on TCBS, serotype, Kanagawa test **Cases:** stool cultures on TCBS, serotype, Kanagawa test

*B=bloody stools, C=cramps, D=diarrhea, F=fever, H=headache, N=nausea, V=vomiting, EM=electron microscopy, ELISA=enzyme-linked immunosorbent assay

II. Diseases typified by diarrhea after a moderate to long incubation period, often with fever, continued

Agent	Incubation period Usual (and Range)	Symptoms* (Partial list)	Pathophysiology	Characteristic foods	Specimens
D. *Escherichia coli* enterotoxigenic	16–48 hours	D, C	enterotoxin	uncooked vegetables, salads, water, cheese	**Food:** culture and serotype **Cases:** stool cultures; serotype and enterotoxin production, invasiveness assay
Escherichia coli enteroinvasive	16–48 hours	C, D, F, H	tissue invasion	same	**Controls**: stool cultures; serotype & enterotoxin production. Look for common serotype in food & cases not found in controls; DNA probes
Escherichia coli enterohemorrhagic (*E. coli* O157:H7 and others)	48–96 hours	B, C, D, H, F infrequent	cytotoxin	beef, raw milk, water	stool cultures on MacConkeys sorbitol; serotype
E. *Bacillus cereus*	8-16 hours	C, D	? enterotoxin	custards, cereals, puddings, sauces, meat loaf	**Food:** culture **Cases:** stool cultures
F. *Shigella*	24-48 hours	C, F, D B, H, N, V	tissue invasion	foods contaminated by infected foodhandler; usually not foodborne	**Food:** culture and serotype **Cases:** stool culture & serotype **Handlers**: stool culture & serotype
G. *Yersinia enterocolitica*	3 to 5 days (usual) range unclear	F, D, C, V, H	tissue invasion, ? enterotoxin	pork products, foods contaminated by infected human or animal	**Food:** culture **Cases:** stool, blood cultures, serology **Handlers:** stool cultures

II. continued

H. *Vibrio cholerae* O1	24–72 hours	D, V	enterotoxin formed *in vivo*	shellfish, water or foods contaminated by infected person or obtained from contaminated environmental source	**Food:** culture on TCBS, serotype **Cases:** stool cultures on TCBS, serotype Send all isolates to CDC for confirmation and toxin assay.
I. *Vibrio cholerae* non-O1	16–72 hours	D, V	enterotoxin formed *in vivo*? tissue invasion	shellfish	**Food:** culture on TCBS, serotype **Cases:** stool cultures on TCBS, serotype
J. *Campylobacter jejuni*	3–5 days	C, D, B, F	unknown	raw milk, poultry, water	**Food:** culture on selective media (5%0_2, 42°C) **Cases:** culture on selective media (5%0_2, 42°C), serology
K. Parvovirus-like agents (Norwalk, Hawaii, Colorado, cockle agents)	16–48 hours	N, V, C, D	unknown	shellfish, water	Stool for immune EM and serology by special arrangement
L. Rotavirus	16–48 hours	N, V, C, D	unknown	foodborne transmission not well documented	**Cases:** stool examination by EM or ELISA; serology

*B=bloody stools, C=cramps, D=diarrhea, F=fever, H=headache, N=nausea, V=vomiting, EM=electron microscopy, ELISA=enzyme-linked immunosorbent assay

III. Botulism

Agent	Incubation period Usual (and Range)	Symptoms* (Partial list)	Pathophysiology	Characteristic foods	Specimens
Clostridium botulinum	12–72 hours	V, D Descending paralysis	preformed toxin	improperly canned or preserved foods that provide anaerobic conditions	**Food:** toxin assay **Cases:** serum and feces for toxin assay by CDC or State Lab; stool culture for *C. botulinum*

IV. Diseases most readily diagnosed from the history of eating a particular type of food

Agent	Incubation period Usual (and Range)	Symptoms* (Partial list)	Pathophysiology	Characteristic foods	Specimens
A. Poisonous mushrooms	Variable	Variable		Wild mushrooms	**Food:** speciation by mycetologist
B. Other poisonous plants	Variable	Variable		Wild plant	**Cases:** vomitus, blood, urine **Food:** speciation by botanist; feces may sometimes be helpful in confirmation
C. Scombroid fish poisoning	5 minutes–1 hour	N, C, D, H, flushing, urticaria	histamine	Mishandled fish (i.e., tuna)	**Food:** Histamine levels
Ciguatera poisoning	1–6 hours	D, N, V, paresthesias, reversal of temperature sensation	ciguatoxin	Large ocean fish (i.e., barracuda, snapper)	**Food:** Stick test for ciguatoxin (not widely available)
D. Other poisonous food sources	Variable	Variable	Variable		

*B = bloody stools, C = cramps, D = diarrhea, F = fever, H = headache, N = nausea, V = vomiting, EM = electron microscopy, ELISA = enzyme-linked immunosorbent assay

Appendix E

Investigation of a Foodborne Outbreak Form

DEPARTMENT OF HEALTH AND HUMAN SERVICES
PUBLIC HEALTH SERVICE
CENTERS FOR DISEASE CONTROL
ATLANTA, GEORGIA 30333

CDC USE ONLY ☐☐☐☐ (1-4)

FORM APPROVED
OMB NO. 0920-0004

INVESTIGATION OF A FOODBORNE OUTBREAK

1. Where did the outbreak occur ?

State ______ (5-6) City or Town ______ County ______

2. Date of outbreak: (Date of onset 1st case)

______ MO / DA / YR (7-12)

3. Indicate actual(a) or estimated (e) numbers:

Persons exposed ______ (13-17)

Persons ill ______ (18-22)

Hospitalized ______ (23-27)

Fatal case ______ (28-31)

4. History of Exposed Persons;

No. histories obtained ______ (32-35)

No. persons with symptoms ______ (36-39)

Nausea ______ (40-43) Diarrhea ______ (44-47)

Vomiting ______ (48-51) Fever ______ (52-55)

Cramps ______ (56-59) Other, specify ______

______ (60-79)

5. Incubation period (hours):

Shortest ______ (80-83) Longest ______ (84-87)

Approx. for majority ______ (88-91)

6. Duration of illness (hours):

Shortest ______ (92-95) Longest ______ (96-99)

Approx. for majority ______ (101-104)

7. Food - specific attack rates:

Food Items Served	Number of persons who ATE specified food				Number who did NOT eat specified food			
	Ill	Not Ill	Total	Percent Ill	Ill	Not Ill	Total	Percent Ill

8. Vehicle responsible (food item incriminated by epidemiological evidence): (105-106) ______

9. Manner in which incriminated food was marketed: (Check all Applicable)

Yes 1 / No 2

(a) Food Industry
- Raw ☐☐ (107)
- Processed ☐☐ (108)

Home Produced
- Raw ☐☐ (109)
- Processed ☐☐ (110)

(b) Vending Machine ☐☐ (111)

(c) Not Wrapped ☐☐ (112)
- Ordinary Wrapping ☐☐ (113)
- Canned ☐☐ (114)
- Canned—Vacuum Sealed ☐☐ (115)
- Other (specify) ☐☐ (116)

______ (117-129)

(d) Room Temperature ☐☐ (130)
- Refrigerator ☐☐ (131)
- Frozen ☐☐ (132)
- Heated ☐☐ (133)

If a commerical product, indicate brand name and lot number

______ (134-150)

10. Place of Preparation of Contaminated Item: (151)
- Restaurant ☐ 1
- Delicatessen ☐ 2
- Cafeteria ☐ 3
- Private Home ☐ 4
- Caterer ☐ 5

Institution:
- School ☐ 6
- Church ☐ 7
- Camp ☐ 8
- Other, specify ☐ 9

______ (152-171)

11. Place where eaten: (172)
- Restaurant ☐ 1
- Delicatessen ☐ 2
- Cafeteria ☐ 3
- Private Home ☐ 4
- Picnic ☐ 5

Institution:
- School ☐ 6
- Church ☐ 7
- Camp ☐ 8
- Other, specify ☐ 9

______ (173-192)

This questionnaire is authorized by law (Public Health Service Act, 42 USC §241). Although responses to the questions asked is voluntary, cooperation of the patient is necessary for the study and control of the disease. Public reporting burden for the collection of information is estimated to average 15 minutes per response. Send comments regarding this burden estimate or any other aspect of this collection of information, including suggestions for reducing this burden to PHS Reports Clearance Officer, Rm 721-H, Humphrey Bldg, 200 Independence Ave, SW, Washington, DC 20201, ATTN: PRA, and to the Office of Information and Regulatory Affairs, Office of Management and Budget, Washington, DC 20503.

CDC 52.13 REV. 8/88

Index